D1431714

GOAL STATEMENT

The goal of the *Pediatric Clinics of North America* is to keep practicing physicians and residents up to date with current clinical practice in pediatrics by providing timely articles reviewing the state-of-the-art in patient care.

ACCREDITATION

The *Pediatric Clinics of North America* is planned and implemented in accordance with the Essential Areas and Policies of the Accreditation Council for Continuing Medical Education (ACCME) through the joint sponsorship of the University Of Virginia School Of Medicine and Elsevier. The University Of Virginia School of Medicine is accredited by the ACCME to provide continuing medical education for physicians.

The University of Virginia School of Medicine designates this enduring material activity for a maximum of 15 *AMA PRA Category 1 Credit*(s)™ for each issue, 90 credits per year. Physicians should only claim credit commensurate with the extent of their participation in the activity.

The American Medical Association has determined that physicians not licensed in the US who participate in this CME enduring material activity are eligible for a maximum of 15 *AMA PRA Category 1 Credit*(s)™ for each issue, 90 credits per year.

Credit can be earned by reading the text material, taking the CME examination online at http://www.theclinics.com/home/cme, and completing the evaluation. After taking the test, you will be required to review any and all incorrect answers. Following completion of the test and evaluation, your credit will be awarded and you may print your certificate.

FACULTY DISCLOSURE/CONFLICT OF INTEREST

The University of Virginia School of Medicine, as an ACCME accredited provider, endorses and strives to comply with the Accreditation Council for Continuing Medical Education (ACCME) Standards of Commercial Support, Commonwealth of Virginia statutes, University of Virginia policies and procedures, and associated federal and private regulations and guidelines on the need for disclosure and monitoring of proprietary and financial interests that may affect the scientific integrity and balance of content delivered in continuing medical education activities under our auspices.

The University of Virginia School of Medicine requires that all CME activities accredited through this institution be developed independently and be scientifically rigorous, balanced and objective in the presentation/discussion of its content, theories and practices.

All authors/editors participating in an accredited CME activity are expected to disclose to the readers relevant financial relationships with commercial entities occurring within the past 12 months (such as grants or research support, employee, consultant, stock holder, member of speakers bureau, etc.). The University of Virginia School of Medicine will employ appropriate mechanisms to resolve potential conflicts of interest to maintain the standards of fair and balanced education to the reader. Questions about specific strategies can be directed to the Office of Continuing Medical Education, University of Virginia School of Medicine, Charlottesville, Virginia.

The faculty and staff of the University of Virginia Office of Continuing Medical Education have no financial affiliations to disclose.

The authors/editors listed below have identified no financial or professional relationships for themselves or their spouse/partner:
Amy J. Bohlander, PhD; Diane C. Chugani, PhD; Erin Duchan, MD; Mohammad Ghaziuddin, MD; Jennifer M. Gillis, PhD, BCBA-D; Kerry Holland, (Acquisitions Editor); Marisela Huerta, PhD; Manmohan K. Kamboj, MD; Gabriel Kaplan, MD; Linda A. LeBlanc, PhD, BCBA-D; Jennifer L. McDonough, MS, CRC; Bruce Mills, PhD; Ahsan Nazeer, MD; Felice Orlich, PhD; Dilip R. Patel, MD (Guest Editor); Patricia J. Prelock, PhD, CCC-SLP; Isabelle Rapin, MD; Karen Rheuban, MD (Test Editor); Carol Schall, PhD; Wendy G. Silver, MD, MA; Neelkamal S. Soares, MD; Michelle A. Suarez, MOT, OTR/L; Ruqiya Shama Tareen, MD; Helga V. Toriello, PhD; Christopher K. Varley, MD; Paul Wehman, PhD; and Nickola Wolf Nelson, PhD, CCC-SLP.

The authors/editors listed below identified the following professional or financial affiliations for themselves or their spouse/partner:
Donald E. Greydanus, MD, FSAHM, FIAP (H), Dr HC (Athens) (Guest Editor) is on the Speakers' Bureau for GSK.
Catherine Lord, PhD receives royalties from Western Psychological Services.
James T. McCracken, MD receives research funding from Otsuka and Seaside Therapeutics, is a consultant for Novartis, and is a DSMB member for PharmaNet and BioMarin.
Luis H. Toledo-Pereyra, MD, PhD conducts research for Informa USA.

Disclosure of Discussion of Non-FDA Approved Uses for Pharmaceutical Products and/or Medical Devices:
The University of Virginia School of Medicine, as an ACCME provider, requires that all faculty presenters identify and disclose any off-label uses for pharmaceutical and medical device products. The University of Virginia School of Medicine recommends that each physician fully review all the available data on new products or procedures prior to clinical use.

TO ENROLL

To enroll in the Pediatric Clinics of North America Continuing Medical Education program, call customer service at 1-800-654-2452 or visit us online at www.theclinics.com/home/cme. The CME program is available to subscribers for an additional fee of $223.00.

Contributors

GUEST EDITORS

DILIP R. PATEL, MD
Professor, Department of Pediatrics and Human Development, Michigan State University College of Human Medicine, Pediatric Residency Program, Kalamazoo Center for Medical Studies, Kalamazoo, Michigan

DONALD E. GREYDANUS, MD
Professor, Department of Pediatrics and Human Development, Michigan State University College of Human Medicine, Program Director, Pediatric Residency Program, Kalamazoo Center for Medical Studies, Kalamazoo, Michigan

AUTHORS

AMY J. BOHLANDER, PhD
Clinical Psychologist, Department of Psychiatry, Seattle Children's Hospital, Autism Clinic, Seattle, Washington

DIANE C. CHUGANI, PhD
Professor, Carman and Ann Adams Department of Pediatrics, Division of Clinical Pharmacology and Toxicology; Department of Radiology, Children's Hospital of Michigan, Detroit Medical Center, Wayne State University School of Medicine, Detroit, Michigan

ERIN DUCHAN, MD
Instructor, Department of Pediatrics and Human Development, Michigan State University College of Human Medicine and Kalamazoo Center for Medical Studies, Kalamazoo, Michigan

MOHAMMAD GHAZIUDDIN, MD
Professor of Child Psychiatry, Department of Psychiatry, University of Michigan Medical School, Ann Arbor, Michigan

JENNIFER M. GILLIS, PhD, BCBA-D
Associate Professor of Psychology, Department of Psychology, Auburn University, Auburn, Alabama

DONALD E. GREYDANUS, MD
Professor, Department of Pediatrics and Human Development, Michigan State University College of Human Medicine, Program Director, Pediatric Residency Program, Kalamazoo Center for Medical Studies, Kalamazoo, Michigan

MARISELA HUERTA, PhD
Clinical Instructor, Department of Psychiatry, Weill Cornell Medical College, White Plains, New York

MANMOHAN K. KAMBOJ, MD
Associate Professor, Section of Endocrinology, Metabolism and Diabetes, Nationwide Children's Hospital, Columbus, Ohio

GABRIEL KAPLAN, MD
Department of Psychiatry, Hoboken University Medical Center, Hoboken, New Jersey; Department of Psychiatry, University of Medicine and Dentistry of New Jersey, Newark, New Jersey

LINDA A. LEBLANC, PhD, BCBA-D
Professor of Psychology, Department of Psychology, Auburn University, Auburn, Alabama

CATHERINE LORD, PhD
Director, Institute for Brain Development, Department of Psychiatry, Weill Cornell Medical College, White Plains, New York

JAMES T. MCCRACKEN, MD
Department of Psychiatry and Biobehavioral Sciences, David Geffen School of Medicine at UCLA, Los Angeles, California

JENNIFER L. MCDONOUGH, MS, CRC
Rehabilitation Research and Training Center, Virginia Commonwealth University, Richmond, Virginia

JOAV MERRICK, MD, MMedSci, DMSc
Medical Director, Health Services and National Institute of Child Health and Human Development, Division for Intellectual and Developmental Disabilities Ministry of Social Affairs; Division of Pediatrics, Hadassah Hebrew University Medical Centers, Jerusalem, Israel; Professor of Pediatrics, Kentucky Children's Hospital, University of Kentucky, Lexington, Kentucky

BRUCE MILLS, PhD
Professor, Department of English, Kalamazoo College, Kalamazoo, Michigan

AHSAN NAZEER, MD
Associate Professor, Child and Adolescent Psychiatry, Michigan State University, Kalamazoo Center for Medical Studies, Kalamazoo, Michigan

NICKOLA WOLF NELSON, PhD, CCC-SLP
Director, PhD Program in Interdisciplinary Health Sciences, Professor, Department of Speech Pathology and Audiology, Western Michigan University, Kalamazoo, Michigan

FELICE ORLICH, PhD
Clinical Associate Professor, Autism Psychology Services, Department of Psychiatry, Seattle Children's Hospital, Autism Clinic, Seattle, Washington

DILIP R. PATEL, MD
Professor, Department of Pediatrics and Human Development, Michigan State University College of Human Medicine, Pediatric Residency Program, Kalamazoo Center for Medical Studies, Kalamazoo, Michigan

PATRICIA J. PRELOCK, PhD, CCC-SLP
Dean, Professor, Department of Communication Sciences and Disorders, College of Nursing and Health Sciences, University of Vermont, Burlington, Vermont

ISABELLE RAPIN, MD
Professor, Neurology Saul R. Korey Department of Neurology, Department of Pediatrics (Neurology), Rose F. Kennedy Center for Research on Intellectual and Developmental Disabilities, Albert Einstein College of Medicine, Bronx, New York

CAROL SCHALL, PhD
Director of Technical Assistance, Assistant Professor, Special Education and Disability Policy, Virginia Autism Resource Center, VCU Autism Center for Excellence, Medical College of Virginia, Rehabilitation Research and Training Center, Virginia Commonwealth University, Richmond, Virginia

WENDY G. SILVER, MD, MA
Instructor, Neurology and Pediatrics, Albert Einstein College of Medicine/Montefiore Medical Center, Bronx; Assistant Professor, Neurology and Pediatrics, New York Medical College/Maria Fareri Children's Hospital, Valhalla, New York

NEELKAMAL S. SOARES, MD
Assistant Professor of Pediatrics and Family and Community Medicine, University of Kentucky, Lexington, Kentucky; Assistant Professor of Pediatrics, West Virginia University, Morgantown, West Virginia

MICHELLE A. SUAREZ, MOT, OTR/L
Assistant Professor, Occupational Therapy Department, College of Health and Human Services, Western Michigan University, Kalamazoo, Michigan

RUQIYA SHAMA TAREEN, MD
Associate Professor, Department of Psychiatry, Michigan State University College of Human Medicine, East Lansing; Psychiatry Residency Program, Kalamazoo Center for Medical Studies, Kalamazoo, Michigan

LUIS H. TOLEDO-PEREYRA, MD, PhD
Departments of Research and Surgery, Michigan State University/Kalamazoo Center for Medical Studies; Department of History, Western Michigan University, Kalamazoo, Michigan

HELGA V. TORIELLO, PhD
Professor, Department of Pediatrics and Human Development (MSU), College of Human Medicine, Secchia Center, Michigan State University; Director of Medical Genetics, Spectrum Health Hospitals, Grand Rapids, Michigan

CHRISTOPHER K. VARLEY, MD
Professor, Division of Child and Adolescent Psychiatry, Department of Psychiatry and Behavioral Sciences, University of Washington School of Medicine, Seattle, Washington

PAUL WEHMAN, PhD
Rehabilitation Research and Training Center, Virginia Commonwealth University, Richmond, Virginia

Contents

Foreword: Autism Spectrum Disorders: Practical Overview for Pediatricians   xv

Joav Merrick

Preface: Autism Spectrum Disorders: Practical Overview for Pediatricians   xix

Dilip R. Patel and Donald E. Greydanus

**Historical Perspectives on Autism: Its Past Record of Discovery and Its Present State
of Solipsism, Skepticism, and Sorrowful Suspicion**   1

Donald E. Greydanus and Luis H. Toledo-Pereyra

> Concepts of autism have evolved over the twentieth century after Bleuler coined the term to refer to symptoms of self-absorption in those with schizophrenia. Autism nosology changed to the current sesquipedalian constellation of autism spectrum disorders with a confusing archipelago of 5 conditions that often serve as islands of confusion to both the general public and professionals. This article reviews historical links that have led to the current confusing and controversial situation that is encouraging some people to return to magic, mysticism, and mantics for health care, despite the amazing accumulation of progress in vaccinology over the past 2 centuries.

In the Doctor's Office: A Parent Perspective   13

Bruce Mills

> This article explores emblematic examples of autistic ways of processing the world and effective practices for pediatrician interactions with children on the spectrum. It offers a parent perspective in relation to this dynamic, considering personal anecdotes that reflect on the communication, social, and sensory challenges for those with autism.

Autism Spectrum Disorders: Clinical Features and Diagnosis   19

Ahsan Nazeer and Mohammad Ghaziuddin

> The last decade has seen an increase of interest in autism spectrum disorders (ASD). With the prevalence now approaching 1%, children with ASD are usually first evaluated by clinicians working in primary care, such as pediatricians and family practitioners. Although classic autism is easy to recognize, differentiating autism from other spectrum disorders and comorbid conditions is not always simple.

Epidemiology of Autism Spectrum Disorders   27

Erin Duchan and Dilip R. Patel

> Epidemiologic data gathered over the last 40 years report that the conservative estimate of autistic spectrum disorder prevalence is 27.5 per 10,000 individuals; however, the prevalence estimate based on newer surveys is 60 per 10,000 individuals. Several factors are considered in various

epidemiologic surveys of autism, especially the evolution of the concept of autism and changing criteria for diagnosis. This article reviews the incidence, prevalence, and risk factors for autism.

Neurobiological Basis of Autism   45

Wendy G. Silver and Isabelle Rapin

Autism (autism spectrum disorders) is a complex, strongly genetically influenced, behaviorally defined disorder of the immature brain associated with very uneven intellectual abilities. Among its most salient and potentially treatable neurologic features that this article focuses on are epilepsy, disorganized sleep patterns, and sensory and motor deficits. Its many causes and wide range of severity means that there is no symptom, no pathology, imaging, electroencephalography, or other biologic feature, and no biologic treatment that is universal or diagnostic of this developmental syndrome.

Neuroimaging and Neurochemistry of Autism   63

Diane C. Chugani

Positron emission tomography, single-photon emission tomography, and magnetic resonance spectroscopy (MRS) are powerful tools for the monitoring of diverse neurochemical functions. Neuroimaging studies targeting neurotransmitter systems in autism have provided clues about how differences in development of these systems might lead to new intervention approaches. Direct measurement of diverse neurochemicals with MRS provides unique probes of neuronal integrity in vivo. Future directions include the combination of imaging modalities made possible by advances in software and hardware. Many tracers have not been applied in autism, and new molecules and signaling pathways might be targeted as genes associated with autism are identified.

Role of Endocrine Factors in Autistic Spectrum Disorders   75

Ruqiya Shama Tareen and Manmohan K. Kamboj

It is possible that autism spectrum disorders (ASDs) have a multifactorial cause along with more than one predisposing and perpetuating factor, all of which culminate in expression of these disorders. Endocrine and neuropeptide factors are among the list of possible etiologic or predisposing contenders. The search for an endocrine model to explain the etiopathogenesis of ASD is a new endeavor. In this article, the authors look at some of the emerging literature that is available regarding any possible relationship between the endocrine hormones and factors and whether it can possibly be etiologic or merely coincidental with autism and ASDs.

Office Screening and Early Identification of Children with Autism   89

Neelkamal S. Soares and Dilip R. Patel

Autism spectrum disorders (ASDs), also called pervasive developmental disorders in the *Diagnostic and Statistical Manual of Mental Disorders* (Fourth Edition, Text Revised), constitute a group of neurodevelopmental disorders that coalesce around a common theme of impairments in social functioning, communication abilities, and repetitive or rigid behaviors. The

ASDs considered here include autism/autistic disorder, Asperger disorder/ Asperger syndrome (AS), and pervasive developmental disorder not otherwise specified. This article focuses on autism/autistic disorder screening and its early identification, with a brief mention for AS screening, as there are limited tools and no recommendation for universal screening for AS.

Diagnostic Evaluation of Autism Spectrum Disorders   103

Marisela Huerta and Catherine Lord

Research on the identification and evaluation of autism spectrum disorders is reviewed, and best practices for clinical work are discussed. The latest research on diagnostic tools, and their recommended use, is also reviewed. Recommendations include the use of instruments designed to assess multiple domains of functioning and behavior, the inclusion of parents and caregivers as active partners, and the consideration of developmental factors throughout the diagnostic process.

Approach to the Genetic Evaluation of the Child with Autism   113

Helga V. Toriello

Autism is a heterogeneous entity that clearly has a substantial genetic component to its cause. There is likely enough evidence to suggest that there are common genetic mechanisms that predispose to various psychiatric disorders. More recent studies have attempted to identify the specific genes involved in predisposition to autism. In general, such conditions can be subdivided into metabolic, mitochondrial, chromosomal, and monogenic (ie, caused by mutation in a single gene). This article examines what conditions should be considered in the child who does not appear to have a syndromic cause as the reason for the autistic phenotype.

Language and Communication in Autism: An Integrated View   129

Patricia J. Prelock and Nickola Wolf Nelson

Children with autism spectrum disorders can have varying degrees of difficulty acquiring spoken and written language, but symptoms of communication impairment associated with social impairment are uniformly present, distinguishing autism spectrum disorders from other neurodevelopmental disabilities. Early diagnosis and early intervention involving parents can improve prognosis. Red flags for social communication problems can be observed early. This article summarizes findings from the National Standards Project of the National Autism Center, which identified 11 types of treatment, 8 of which address communication. Both contemporary behavioral approaches and naturalistic developmental approaches are included in this set.

Behavioral Interventions for Children with Autism Spectrum Disorders   147

Linda A. LeBlanc and Jennifer M. Gillis

Early intensive behavioral intervention is the only well-established treatment for young children with autism spectrum disorders (ASDs). Less intensive behavioral interventions are also effective for targeted concerns with older children and adolescents. This article describes the core features of behavioral treatments, summarizes the evidence base for

effectiveness, and provides recommendations to facilitate family understanding of these interventions and identification of qualified providers.
Recommendations are also provided for collaboration between pediatric
providers and behavior analysts who are serving families of individuals
with ASDs.

Social Skills Training for Children with Autism   165

Amy J. Bohlander, Felice Orlich, and Christopher K. Varley

This article summarizes the current literature on social skills training for
children and adolescents with autism spectrum disorders. The article describes several different methods of social skills training, along with a summary of research findings on effectiveness. Interventions described
include social skills groups, peer mentoring/training, social stories, and
video modeling. The article also describes information about accessing
social skills training services, and concludes with future directions and recommendations for pediatricians.

Psychopharmacology of Autism Spectrum Disorders   175

Gabriel Kaplan and James T. McCracken

At present, no evidence-based effective pharmacologic options are available for treating the core deficits of autism spectrum disorders (ASDs),
which are best addressed by behavioral and educational interventions.
However, such evidence exists for several of the frequently associated/co-
morbid symptoms such as aggression and severe irritability, hyperactivity,
and repetitive behaviors, which can become a major source of additional
distress and interference in functioning. This article offers information on
the psychopharmacology of ASD that is current, relevant, and organized
in a user-friendly manner, to form a concise but informative reference
guide for primary pediatric clinicians.

Transition from School to Work for Students with Autism Spectrum Disorders: Understanding the Process and Achieving Better Outcomes   189

Carol Schall, Paul Wehman and Jennifer L. McDonough

Individuals and their parents frequently turn to pediatricians, adolescent
medicine specialists, and psychologists to answer questions about the
course and outcomes of their disorder. This article provides a description
of the characteristics of autism spectrum disorders (ASD) in adolescence
and early adulthood. It also describes essential elements of high school
programs designed to increase positive outcomes for youth with ASD
and provides detailed information about various employment support
models. Finally, the implications of transition programming for medical
specialists and psychologists are discussed.

Sensory Processing in Children with Autism Spectrum Disorders and Impact on Functioning   203

Michelle A. Suarez

Children with autism experience many challenges that affect their ability to
function. Sensory processing disorder and, specifically, sensory modulation disorder can compound dysfunction and further inhibit participation

in productive activities. Through detection of and referral for sensory modulation disorders, treatment can be accessed. Emerging treatment evidence points to functional gains for autism and sensory modulation disorder that can ease the burden that this combination of symptoms has on the everyday life of children with autism.

Index   **215**

FORTHCOMING ISSUES

April 2012
Pediatric Rheumatology
Ronald M. Laxer, MDCM, FRCPC,
Guest Editor

June 2012
Pediatric Urology
Pasquale Casale, MD, and
Walid Farhat, MD,
Guest Editors

August 2012
Children, Adolescents, and the Media
Victor Strasburger, MD, *Guest Editor*

RECENT ISSUES

December 2011
Update in Childhood and Adolescent Obesity
Miriam Vos, MD, MSPH, and
Sarah Barlow, MD, MPH, *Guest Editors*

October 2011
Pediatric Endocrinology
Robert Rapaport, MD, *Guest Editor*

August 2011
Interface Between Pediatrics and Children's Mental Health
Sandra L. Fritsch, MD, and
Harsh K. Trivedi, MD,
Guest Editors

THE CLINICS ARE NOW AVAILABLE ONLINE!

Access your subscription at:
www.theclinics.com

Foreword

Autism Spectrum Disorders: Practical Overview for Pediatricians

Autism spectrum disorders (ASD) have a history and it started with the Jewish physician Leo Kanner (1894–1981), born in a small village in Galicia, which at that time was part of Austria-Hungary. He studied medicine in Berlin and graduated in 1921, but emigrated to the United States in 1924 to take a position at the State Hospital in Yankton County, South Dakota. In 1930, he was selected to develop the first child psychiatry service at Johns Hopkins Hospital, Baltimore, Maryland, where he in 1933 became associate professor of psychiatry. He was in reality the first physician in the world identified as a child psychiatrist, the founder of the first academic child psychiatry department at Johns Hopkins University Hospital, and his first textbook "Child Psychiatry"[1] from 1935 was the first English language textbook in this field. In his 1943 article[2] on autistic disturbances of affective contact, he described the specific syndrome of autism. He applied the Greek word *autos* or self to what he termed early infantile autism (Kanner's syndrome) characterized by the inability to relate to and interact with people from the beginning of life; the inability to communicate with others through language; an obsession with maintaining sameness and resisting change; a preoccupation with objects rather than people; and the occasional evidence of good potential for intelligence.

In Austria, the pediatrician Hans Asperger (1906–1980) in 1944 described a neurobiological disorder with a pattern of behavior in several young boys who had normal intelligence and language development, but exhibited autistic-like behaviors and marked deficiencies in social and communication skills. Despite the publication of his article in 1944,[3] it was not until 1994 that Asperger's syndrome was added to the Diagnostic and Statistical Manual of Mental Disorders (DSM) IV, and only in the past few years has Asperger's syndrome been recognized by professionals and parents.

The term pervasive developmental disorders (PDD) was first used in the 1980s to describe a class of disorders. This class of disorders has in common the following characteristics: impairments in social interaction, imaginative activity, verbal and nonverbal communication skills, and a limited number of interests and activities that tend to be repetitive. In the manual DSM used by physicians and mental health professionals as a guide to diagnose disorders, five disorders are identified under the category of pervasive developmental disorders: (i) autistic disorder, (ii) Rett disorder or syndrome, (iii) childhood disintegrative disorder, (iv) Asperger's disorder or syndrome, and (v) pervasive developmental disorder not otherwise specified, or PDD-NOS.

Autism and PDD-NOS are developmental disabilities that share many of the same characteristics. Usually evident by age three, autism and PDD-NOS are neurological disorders that affect a child's ability to communicate, understand language, play, and relate to others. Due to the similarity of behaviors associated with autism and

Pediatr Clin N Am 59 (2012) xv–xvii
doi:10.1016/j.pcl.2011.10.017
0031-3955/12/$ – see front matter
pediatric.theclinics.com

PDD, use of the term pervasive developmental disorder has caused some confusion among parents and professionals. However, the treatment and educational needs are similar for both diagnoses. The causes of autism and PDD are unknown. Although the prognosis for children with ASD is variable, the disorder generally has lifelong effects on the ability to socialize, to care for him/herself, and to participate meaningfully in the community. The disorder may adversely impact not just the affected child, but also his/her family members. Currently there is no effective means for prevention, no biomarkers for early diagnosis, and no specific treatment approach or a drug that can "cure" the disorder.

Interest in ASD has exploded in the past decade following the vast increase in the prevalence of ASD to 1:100-1:150 in the most recent reports. The dramatic increase in ASD cases has been accompanied by an increase in public and professional awareness and an abundance of new research and treatment strategies. What was once thought to be a rare, severe disorder is now recognized to be a common neurobehavioral disorder, which occurs along a broad continuum. Autism is probably not a single disorder, but rather reflects many different disorders with broad behavioral phenotypes causing atypical development.

Evidence from twin and family studies indicates that autism is heritable. However, no single specific gene has been consistently identified to be playing a major role in most cases. Rather, autism is thought to involve a complex interaction between multiple and variable susceptibility genes and epigenetic effects. Although brain abnormalities in autism are complex and not consistently identified, an intriguing pattern of brain growth has been discovered that involves rapid growth of head circumference during the first 3-4 years of life that slows down later in development. Enlarged white matter, variation in myelination, and impaired connectivity between brain regions were discovered and are thought to be related to functional impairments and poor information processing.

Early identification of ASD and early provision of treatment can improve outcomes for many affected children. The need for early focused intervention that will result in meaningful outcomes in cognitive, language, and adaptive skills provides a fertile ground for intervention research across many disciplines. The majority of children with ASD will need intensive and regular therapy aimed at improving communication, socialization, and behavior and to improve cognition, language, and adaptive skills. Behavioral, educational, and psychosocial interventions have been the cornerstone of treatment for individuals with ASD. The complexity of the disorder frequently requires complex treatment strategies, which include the integration of many treatments that are tailored to the child's needs and may need to change throughout development.

This issue of the *Pediatric Clinics of North America* is therefore timely, because of the many changes in this field and the need for primary physicians to pay attention to early symptoms and secure early and intensive intervention for the affected children and support for their families.

Joav Merrick, MD, MMedSci, DMSc
National Institute of Child Health and Human Development
Division of Pediatrics
Hadassah Hebrew University Medical Centers
Jerusalem, Israel IL-91012
Health Services
Division for Mental Retardation

Ministry of Social Affairs
Jerusalem, Israel IL-91012
Kentucky Children's Hospital
Department of Pediatrics
University of Kentucky College of Medicine
Lexington, KY, USA

E-mail address:
jmerrick@zahav.net.il

REFERENCES

1. Kanner L. Child psychiatry. Springfield (IL): CC Thomas; 1935.
2. Kanner L. Autistic disturbances of affectice contact. Nervous Child 1943;2:217–50.
3. Asperger H. Die autistischen psychopathen im kindersalter. Arch Psychiatr Nervenkrankheit 1944;117:76–136 [in German].

Preface

Autism Spectrum Disorders: Practical Overview for Pediatricians

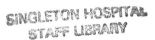

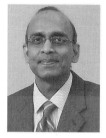 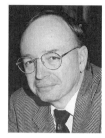

Dilip R. Patel, MD   Donald E. Greydanus, MD
Guest Editors

We are grateful and humbled to have the opportunity to edit this special issue of *Pediatric Clinics of North America* devoted to autism spectrum disorders. Because our understanding of the spectrum of autism continues to evolve, this collection of practical reviews presents the state of the knowledge at this time. We thank all the authors for sacrificing their invaluable time and sharing their passion and expertise to contribute articles for this issue. We thank the editorial and technical staff at Elsevier for their guidance, patience, and excellent work. We hope that the information presented here is of practical value for the pediatricians and other medical practitioners who take care of children and adolescents in their practice.

Dilip R. Patel, MD

Donald E. Greydanus, MD
Department of Pediatrics & Human Development
Michigan State University/Kalamazoo Center for Medical Studies
Michigan State University College of Human Medicine
1000 Oakland Drive, Kalamazoo, MI 49009-1284, USA

E-mail addresses:
patel@kcms.msu.edu (D.R. Patel)
greydanus@kcms.msu.edu (D.E. Greydanus)

Pediatr Clin N Am 59 (2012) xix
doi:10.1016/j.pcl.2011.10.016
0031-3955/12/$ – see front matter

Historical Perspectives on Autism: Its Past Record of Discovery and Its Present State of Solipsism, Skepticism, and Sorrowful Suspicion

Donald E. Greydanus, MD[a],*, Luis H. Toledo-Pereyra, MD, PhD[b,c,d]

KEYWORDS

- Autism • History • Vaccine controversy • Media effects

The boundary between biology and behavior is arbitrary and changing. It has been imposed not by the natural contours of disciplines but by lack of knowledge.
—Kandel, 1991[1]

Hominoids have had a perplexing time for millennia dealing with disability, disease, and death in their societies.[2] Placed in an often unforgiving world, hominoids have often turned to mantics, magic, religion, mysticism, and haruspex to explain or justify imperfection in fellow *Homo sapiens*. Sometimes the reaction has been positive and sometimes negative. There is evidence from 60,000 years ago that Neanderthals carefully buried their dead, even those with disabilities such as from rickets, which was very common in this group of hominoids.[3]

[a] Department of Pediatrics & Human Development, Michigan State University/Kalamazoo Center for Medical Studies, Michigan State University College of Human Medicine, 1000 Oakland Drive, Kalamazoo, MI 49009-1284, USA
[b] Department of Research, Michigan State University/Kalamazoo Center for Medical Studies, 1000 Oakland Drive, Kalamazoo, MI 49009-1284, USA
[c] Department of Surgery, Michigan State University/Kalamazoo Center for Medical Studies, 1000 Oakland Drive, Kalamazoo, MI 49009-1284, USA
[d] Department of History, Western Michigan University, Kalamazoo, MI, USA
* Corresponding author.
E-mail address: Greydanus@kcms.msu.edu

Pediatr Clin N Am 59 (2012) 1–11
doi:10.1016/j.pcl.2011.10.004
0031-3955/12/$ – see front matter © 2012 Elsevier Inc. All rights reserved.

However, prejudice and avoidance were common for countless thousands of years in many cultures toward those with defects such as mental retardation and epilepsy (the sacred disease of Hippocrates), both of which were traditionally blamed on demon possession in Western cultures.[4] One scholar in ancient China notes that mentally retarded children during the Zhou Dynasty (841 BC–221 BC) were identified as being "…stupid, a child born stupid and fearful."[5]

Babies deemed defective after careful inspection in ancient Sparta (700 BC–300 BC) were thrown into a chiasm at a cliff on the famous Mount Taygetus, which is located in Peloponnese, Greece. The ancient Athenians also allowed those with disabilities to be killed if they could not care for themselves.[6] Plato (424 BC–347 BC) concluded that disabilities interfered with a world of perfection and wrote, "The offspring of the inferior, or of the better when they chance to be deformed, will be put away in some mysterious, unknown place, as they should."[6]

The Old Testament did not allow those with blindness or lameness to "enter the house of believers," whereas the New Testament taught that those with mental illnesses were possessed by demons, a fate as noted in those with epilepsy.[6] A long-held belief in some religions was that birth defects and disabilities were the result of God's punishment due to the sins of the parents.[6]

William Shakespeare (AD 1564–1616) called those with mental retardation court fools. They could say what they wanted to the royal court because they (those with mental subnormality) were considered to have no intelligence.[7] Those with mental retardation from any cause were called village idiots in nineteenth century Western Europe and lived as beggars, church dependents, or court jesters. Because humans with mental retardation were viewed as having the same brain pathology as others who were called insane, individuals with mental retardation were often confined to asylums. Perhaps the most famous asylum in Europe was the Bethlehem Hospital in London, which came to be known as Bedlam.

Although autism was not formally recognized until the twentieth century, examples of probable autism are found earlier. For example, Martin Luther (1483–1546), through his note taker Mathesius, has a story about a 12-year-old boy with features of severe autism.[8] Perhaps the first well-documented case of autism was that of Hugh Blair of Borgue, Scotland, in a 1747 court case that involved the brother of this person seeking to gain Hugh Blair's inheritance.[9] A medical student (Jean Itard) treated a wild child with autistic features who was called by history the Wild Boy of Aveyron and was a feral child caught in 1798.[10]

The British Mental Deficiency Act was passed into law in 1913 in England and ruled in a Plato-like decision that those with mental retardation from any cause must be taken from general society and placed into custodial care.[11] The United States Supreme Court supported the sterilization of a young woman with mental retardation in 1927 during the era of twentieth century Nazi Germany, where those with mental retardation were euthanized.[12] Permitting handicapped children to be killed has been noted in twentieth century China.[5]

The birth of a girl with mental retardation who was a sister of President John F. Kennedy (1917–1963) led the United States into a new era with regard to dealing with handicapped humans. Instead of isolation, punishment, or death, science has attempted to understand the cause of various conditions with the idea of improving their lives. The US government developed disability councils starting in 1963, and US laws were passed in the 1970s at both the federal and state levels seeking to guarantee the civil rights of institutionalized individuals.[13]

In 1975, Public Law 94-142 was passed as the Education for All Handicapped Act, mandating financial support for all children with developmental disability who should receive comprehensive education no matter how severe the disability. These children were to be placed in the least-restrictive environment that was possible. The Individuals with Disabilities Education Act developed a public special education system in the United States with the extension of services down to birth while formalizing early developmental intervention systems across the nation.[13]

The Americans with Disabilities Act was passed in 1990 to further expand civil rights protection for all Americans with disabilities, including developmental disabilities. In 1997, Public Law 94-142 was updated to allow parents of those with developmental and other disabilities the right to be equal partners with school personnel in establishing an individualized education plan for this individual.[13] However, concern about the cause of disability remains intense, as now seen with autism. To understand the current milieu of thinking in this regard, historical perspectives and personalities in the arena of autism are presented.

ALFRED RUSSEL WALLACE

About 181 years after the English physician, Dr Edward Jenner, inoculated 8-year-old James Phipps with cowpox vaccine in 1796, smallpox vaccination has eliminated one of the greatest scourges of humankind, smallpox.[14] Instead of universal praise for the development of a way to prevent smallpox, controversy entered by way of a strong antivaccination movement, with such leaders as Alfred Russel Wallace (1823–1913) in England. The antivaccine movement was launched by the 1853 Vaccination Act in England, which mandated smallpox vaccination for the public in England.[15]

Wallace was a codiscoverer of natural selection and was a famous explorer, biologist, anthropologist, geographer, and naturalist. He published his own theory of evolution, which stimulated Charles Darwin to publish his own now famous theory regarding evolution. In the 1880s, Wallace was one of the leaders of a strong antivaccination movement based on claims that the smallpox vaccine was not safe and was dangerous and the idea that compulsory vaccination was unethical.[16] His first objection was that one should not be forced to take a vaccine, but then eventually he became concerned with the safety of smallpox vaccine itself. Wallace was also adamant that the vaccine would upset what he perceived was the balance of nature with potentially disastrous results for human beings. He took on the medical establishment and encouraged some to avoid the smallpox vaccination. He was joined by other prominent scientists of the Victorian age who dismantled the compulsory vaccination act and lent considerable discredit to vaccination in general. Wallace's disagreement with the well-known journal, *The Lancet*, portended controversies to come in the next century.

PAUL EUGEN BLEULER

Paul Eugen Bleuler, MD (1857–1939), a Swiss psychiatrist, introduced the term schizophrenia based on his belief that psychosis contained psychological roots and would improve with psychoanalytic therapy. His book *Lehrbuch der Psychiatrie* (*Textbook of Psychiatry*) was published in 1916 and became a standard book in this field for many years. This pioneer, heavily influenced by the work of Sigmund Freud (1856–1939), also coined the term autism based on the Greek (autos, αὐτός) or Latin (autismus) for self, which he felt was one of the symptoms of schizophrenia. Bleuler first used this term in 1912 in an article in the *American Journal of Insanity* to describe patients who seemed to lose contact with reality, live in their own world of fantasy, and were incapable of normal communication with others.[17,18]

LEO KANNER

Leo Kanner, MD (1894–1981), was a Jewish American psychiatrist whose pioneering studies led to the basis of child and adolescent psychiatry in the United States and beyond.[19] Kanner began his studies at the University of Berlin in 1913; however, his studies were interrupted by World War I when he served with the Austrian army. He was the first physician to be called a child psychiatrist as child psychiatry began to evolve from adult psychiatry. Leo Kanner founded the first academic child psychiatry department at Johns Hopkins University, and his classic 1935 textbook, *Child Psychiatry*, was the first such book in the English language.

Kanner's classic article on autism (early infantile autism), *Autistic Disturbances of Affective Contact*, was published in 1943 based on his observations of 11 children (8 boys and 3 girls) with an "…inability to relate themselves in the ordinary way to people and situations from the beginning of life."[20] The first case that was reported was that of Donald T, first seen in October, 1938, at age 5 years and 1 month, who arrived to see Dr Kanner with a 33-page typewritten report prepared by his father detailing his son's social dysfunctions. Before Donald T was 2 years old, he had an "unusual memory for faces and names, and knew the names of a great number of houses in his home town."[20]

Dr Kanner concluded: "We must, then, assume that these children have come into the world with innate inability to form the usual, biologically provided affective contact with people, just as other children come into the world with innate physical or intellectual handicaps. If this assumption is correct, a further study of our children may help to furnish concrete criteria regarding the still diffuse notions about the constitutional components of emotional reactivity. For here we seem to have pure-culture examples of inborn autistic disturbances of affective contact."[20]

Dr Kanner continued with his studies on what was then called early infantile autism or Kanner autism, which was defined as a severe behavioral or psychiatric disorder that was identified in early infancy.[21] Leon Eisenberg, MD, his coauthor in a classic summary article in 1956, went on to replace Dr Kanner as chief of child psychiatry at Johns Hopkins Hospital.[22] Leo Kanner became the editor of the *Journal of Autism and Developmental Disorders* (then called *Journal of Autism and Childhood Schizophrenia*) from 1971 to 1974.

HANS ASPERGER

Hans Asperger (1906–1980) was an Austrian pediatrician who became chair of pediatrics at the University of Vienna. During his career, he described 4 boys (out of more than 400 children) with autistic features but who were also called little professors because of their extraordinary ability to learn specific facts.[23,24] He concluded: "We are convinced, then, that autistic people have their place in the social community. They fulfill their role well, perhaps better than anyone else could, and we are talking of people who as children had the greatest difficulties and caused untold worries to their care-givers."[23]

His classic article was published in German in 1944 and was not translated into English until 9 years after his death (1980); thus, it was mostly ignored in the English-speaking community until the 1990s. Hans Aspeger started a school for children with what he called autistic psychopathy; however, the school was destroyed near the end of World War II, and much of his early work was lost in this combat-induced annihilation. During the past 2 decades, Asperger syndrome has come to represent a higher functioning person with autism. One of Hans Asperger's patients became a professor of astronomy and another became a Nobel laureate in literature.

The term Asperger syndrome was first used in 1981 by Lorna Wing, a British psychiatrist, who had a daughter with this diagnosis.[25] Hans Asperger summarized his work in an article he wrote in German in 1977.[26] Some scholars have speculated that Hans Asperger had Asperger syndrome himself.[27] The term Asperger syndrome was used in the fourth edition of the American Psychiatric Association's *Diagnostic and Statistical Manual of Mental Disorders* (*DSM*), which was published in 1994.[28]

BRUNO BETTELHEIM

Bruno Bettelheim, PhD (1903–1990), was an Austrian-born American with a doctoral degree in philosophy that included a dissertation on Immanuel Kant and art history.[29] He became a professor of psychology and education at the University of Chicago from 1944 to 1973 and was director of the University of Chicago's Sonia Shankman Orthogenic School, a home that treated children labeled as emotionally disturbed.[29,30] Bruno Bettelheim was a survivor of the Dachau concentration camp and became known for his work seeking to interpret children's fairy tales to better understand childhood development. In 1959, he published an article about 9-year-old Joey, the mechanical boy, in *Scientific America*, which helped to introduce autism to a wide audience.[31]

Bettelheim's work on autism became controversial, particularly his opinion that autism was caused by mothers who did not communicate properly with their children and withheld needed affection from them.[31,32] This refrigerator mother concept originated with Kanner and was popular in the 1960s and 1970s in the United States as experts and the lay public alike sought to understand the cause of autistic behavior. Unfortunately, Professor Bettelheim died from suicide in 1990.[33] Opinion has moved away from this concept, leaving Dr Bettelheim in a controversial status in the early twenty-first century. This began with various individuals challenging the refrigerator mother theory, such as that of Clara Park who wrote about her own autistic child in 1967.[34]

BERNARD RIMLAND

Bernard Rimland, PhD (1928–2006), was an American psychologist who became well known for his research and views on autism, attention-deficit/hyperactivity disorder, mental retardation, and learning disorders. He was the founder of the Autism Society of America in 1965 and founder (1967) as well as director of the Autism Research Institute (San Diego, CA, USA). Rimland had a son with the diagnosis of autism who eventually became an artist.

Dr Rimland[35] did not agree with Bruno Bettelheim and stressed that autism had a neurologic basis, publishing what became a well-known book in 1964 with this thesis. The foreword of this book was by Dr Leo Kanner who was labeled as the originator and early supporter of the refrigerator mother model as the cause of infantile autism. This foreword indicated that Dr Kanner was changing his views toward a neurologic basis for autism. A meeting was held in Teaneck, New Jersey, between parents of children with autism and Bernard Rimland, leading to the founding of the Autism Society of America. Parents were very pleased not to be implicated in the cause of their children's autism.

Bernard Rimland also became known for his concern with what was perceived as an increase in autism cases and his conclusion that vaccinations might be the cause of this increase. He thought that thimerosal might be the causative agent behind this epidemic. Rimland's grandfatherly status in the lay public's perception of autism has lent credence in the eyes of many that vaccines indeed may be the missing link in seeking the cause of this condition. This assertion placed him in direct conflict with organized medicine in the United States and elsewhere. Research has carefully and meticulously looked but not found any link between vaccinations (such as the measles, mumps, and rubella [MMR] vaccine) and autism.[36–38] This conflict, however, has continued to the present day partly as a result of the high status of this psychologist with the lay public and others.

OLE IVAR LØVAAS

Ole Ivar Løvaas, PhD (1927–2010), was a clinical psychologist and professor at the University of California (Los Angeles) who applied behavior analysis to those with autism, which became known as the Lovaas method or Applied Behavioral Analysis.[39] Although some studies report benefit from this popular treatment method for autism, systemic reviews do not establish its superiority over other management methods for autism.[40,41]

ANDREW WAKEFIELD

Andrew Wakefield, MD, is a surgeon and medical researcher from England who was born in 1957. He published a now discredited report in *The Lancet* in 1998 that claimed a causative connection between the MMR vaccine and what was termed autistic enterocolitis.[42] Subsequent researchers did not confirm Wakefield's research, and an investigation by the British General Medical Council revealed that Wakefield had "failed in his duties as a responsible consultant, did his work against the interests of his patients, and acted dishonestly and irresponsibly" in his published work.[43,44] The journal that published his 1998 article, *The Lancet*, has retracted the Wakefield article, and his research has been discredited in the mainstream scientific literature.[45,46] However, the controversy continues with some continuing to believe such a link despite many scientific articles demonstrating no causative underpinning.[36–38,47]

PAUL OFFIT

Paul Offit, MD, has emerged as a scientific spokesperson for the view of mainstream medicine that vaccines do not cause autism.[48,49] He is a professor of pediatrics and vaccinology at the University of Pennsylvania and chief of the Infectious Diseases Division as well as director of the Vaccine Education Center at the Children's Hospital of Philadelphia. He is an immunologist and virologist who has written often and eloquently that epidemiologic and biological studies do not reveal any association between vaccines (MMR) and autism.

Dr Offit was publically outraged with the Wakefield study that was published in *The Lancet* in 1998. Dr Offit correctly predicted that the article, although not valid, would influence some to withhold the MMR vaccine from their children, leading to a resurgence of measles and even death.[50] Dr Offit also traces the current American antivaccine movement to a 1-hour documentary on April 19, 1982, that appeared on a Washington, DC, television show called "DTP: Vaccine Roulette," linking the pertussis vaccine with severe reactions in children.[51] Several antivaccine groups have emerged since then in the spirit of Wallace and Wakefield. However, the intensity of this Galileo Galilean debate, even with clear scientific evidence revealing no connection, has led to much controversy for Dr Offit, negative mails, and even death threats.[52]

AUTISM IN THE INTERNET AGE

The general public and parents of children with autism have much to say about autism advocacy. Much information is provided to the general public via the Internet and the general media in the early part of the twenty-first century. The opinion of Kanner, Bettelheim, and others that negative parenting induced autism in their children angered and incensed parents from the beginning. This division between professionals and parents has persisted today and has even widened.[53] The opinions of Rimland and Wakefield postulating a link between vaccines and autism has driven this controversy into the twenty-first century with considerable intensity and to an extent that Wallace of the nineteenth century would appreciate and applaud. Public education from the press, television, and the Internet feeds this flowing flame of misinformation.[54,55]

Parents, including movie stars, who saw their children vanish into the depth of autism around the same time as receiving vaccines became convinced that the cause was vaccines, and are very influential spokespersons for this cause.[51,54] Sometimes physicians, including media physicians or physicians caring for media stars' children with autism, join the antivaccine movement, which seems to lend more credibility to those agreeing with this opinion. This occurs despite clear evidence from many studies noting no connection, including epidemiologic research that the epidemiology of childhood autism is the same as that found in adults.[43,45–51,56] The concern that some physicians and pharmaceutical companies value money over patients only adds to this antivaccine flame, one that has been burning across 2 centuries. Opportunistic individuals only worsen this tragic and deplorable situation.[54] Compounding this situation is the concern that some parents have that their physicians still have negative views of autism and autistic patients as well as their parents.[57]

Also contributing to the continuous state of confusion has been the frequent changes in terminology, starting with Bleuler's term autism in reference to a symptom of schizophrenia to Kanner's early infantile autism to Asperger's autistic psychopathy. The first (1952) and second (1968) editions of the American Psychiatric Association's *DSM* used the term childhood schizophrenia. Autism was included as a separate condition in the third (1980) edition of the *DSM*, whereas the fourth edition (1994) provided 5 types of the current nosology of autistic spectrum disorders or pervasive developmental disorder: autistic disorder, pervasive developmental disorder not otherwise specified, Rett syndrome, Asperger syndrome, and childhood disintegrative disorder.[28] The 1992 *International Classification of Diseases, Tenth Edition*, provides a similar list.[58]

SUMMARY

The diagnosis of autism developed in the twentieth century after society struggled for millennia to deal with disability in children and adults. Parents were often blamed for having children with defects, and perhaps this began with the Genesis 3:6 account of the fall of Adam and Eve who represent the first *Homo sapiens* parents. Concepts of various religious interpretations of disease and deformity have long centered on evil, sin, and demon possession. Children with defects were left to die in ancient Sparta and even Athens. Those with mental retardation from any cause were called village idiots in nineteenth century Western Europe and lived as beggars, church dependents, or court jesters.

The twentieth century began with high hopes for advances in science, a product of the Renaissance coming out of the Dark Ages in Europe. Eugene Bleuler coined the terms schizophrenia and autism in the early twentieth century. Leo Kanner used the term early infantile autism in 1943 based on 11 case reports but eventually identified unloving and uncaring mothers as the cause for this complex disorder. Hans Asperger reported in 1944 on a variant of autism but the report was published in German and did not receive attention in the English-speaking community until the 1990s.

Bruno Bettelheim continued the concept of the refrigerator mother through much of the late twentieth century. Parents and scholars objected to this concept, but the damage was done, with parents becoming disenfranchised from professionals dealing with their autistic children. Bernard Rimland was a well-known professor of psychology who helped to remove the cold mother concept as a cause of autism. However, in a tragic conclusion similar to that of Wallace in the nineteenth century, Rimland identified vaccines as a cause of what he perceived as a major increase in cases of autism in children.

Anxious parents, solipsistic movie stars, other entertainment-driven media persona, and additional exploitive experts joined in the view that vaccines (thimerosal, MMR vaccines) were behind the autism issue, despite clear scientific evidence that this is not the case.[59,60] A major mistrust of physicians has arisen in a society fed impressions by nonprofessionals and a few professionals. The result is a decrease in vaccinations and an increase in antivaccinationists in the United States, Europe, and other areas, leading to an increase in vaccine-preventable diseases.[15]

This antivaccination movement actually began in the nineteenth century in response to concern about the smallpox vaccination led by Alfred Russel Wallace in England. After millennia of ignorance about biological causes of disease, scientific progress in the past 2 centuries is being seriously attacked by a return to belief in mantics, magic, mysticism, and haruspex.[61,62] The revenge of the refrigerator-labeled mothers has occurred because of refrigerator professionals.

A state of solipsism and suspicion by the general public has arisen, with the health of children at risk. There is also a rush to use the American justice system to correct the perceived damage alleged from vaccines even with scientific evidence to the contrary.[63,64] There is also a threat to the vaccine industry, which remains vulnerable to a skeptical public that may shun vaccines, leading to increased damage to the public as well as potential severe financial impact to the companies that produce current vaccines and engage in research for future vaccines.[65] As more and more research focuses on genetic concepts as the cause of autism,[66] physicians face a Sisyphean task in not falling into ancient traps of blaming parents for their children's imperfections.

If I had a world of my own, everything would be nonsense.
Nothing would be what it is because everything would be what it isn't.
And contrary-wise; what it is it wouldn't be,
And what it wouldn't be, it would. You see?
            —By Alice in Alice in Wonderland; Lewis Carroll
                    (Charles Lutwidge Dodgson), 1865

REFERENCES

1. King A. Adolescence. In: Lewis M, editor. Child and adolescent psychiatry. A comprehensive textbook. 3rd edition. Philadelphia: Lippincott Williams & Wilkins, Chapter 24; 2002. p. 332–42.
2. Greydanus DE, Pratt HD. Syndromes and disorders associated with mental retardation: selected comments. Indian J Pediatr 2005;72(10):27–32.
3. Beck S. Prehistoric cultures. In: Beck S, editor. Mideast and Africa to 1700. Santa Barbara (CA): World Peace Communications; 2000. p. 648.
4. Greydanus DE, Van Dyke D. Epilepsy in the adolescent: the sacred disease and the clinician's sacred duty. Int Pediatr 2005;20(2):6–8.
5. Su H, Van Dyke DC. Breaking the silence and overcoming the invisibility: Down syndrome in China. Int Pediatr 2005;20(1):25–33.

6. Mackelprang RW, Salsgiver RO. Disability: a diversity model approach in human service practice. Florence (KY): Cengage Learning; 1998. p. 270.
7. Sulkes SB. MR in children and adolescent. In: Greydanus DE, Pratt HD, Patel DR, editors. Behavioral Pediatrics. New York (NY): Universe, Inc; 2006. p. 66–83. [Chapter: 3].
8. Wing L. The history of ideas on autism: legends, myths, and reality. Autism 1997; 1:13–27.
9. Houston R, Frith U. Autism in history: the case of Hugh Blair of Borgue. London (England): Blackwell; 2000.
10. Wolff S. The history of autism. Eur Child Adolesc Psychiatry 2004;13:201–8.
11. Wolrich M. Mental retardation. In: Greydanus DE, Wolrich ML, editors. Behavioral pediatrics. New York: Springer-Verlag; 1992. p. 314–23. [Chapter: 22].
12. Wolfensberger W. The extermination of handicapped people in World War II Germany. Ment Retard 1981;19:1–7.
13. Greydanus DE, Bhave S. Adolescents with mental retardation. Recent Adv Pediatr 2006;17:174–92.
14. Huygelen C. Jenner's cowpox vaccine in light of current vaccinology [in Dutch]. Verh K Acad Geneeskd Belg 1996;58:479–536.
15. Tafuri S, Martinelli D, Prato R, et al. From the struggle for freedom to the denial of scientific evidence: history of antivaccinationists in Europe [in Italian]. Ann Ig 2011;23:93–9.
16. Fichman M, Keelan JE. Register's logic: the anti-vaccination arguments of Alfred Russel Wallace and their role in the debates over compulsory vaccination in England, 1870-1907. Stud Hist Philos Biol Biomed Sci 2007;38:585–607.
17. Bleuler Eugen P. Lehrbuch der psychiatrie [textbook of psychiatry]. Berlin (Germany): Springer; 1983 (original 1916). ISBN 3540118330.
18. Hell D, Scharfetter C, Möller A. Eugen Bleuler, Leben und Werk. Bern (Switzerland): Huber; 2001. ISBN 3456836465.
19. Bender L. In memoriam. Leo Kanner MD June 13, 1894–April 4, 1981. J Am Acad Child Psychiatry 1982;21:88–9.
20. Kanner L. Autistic disturbances of affective contact. Nerv Child 1943;2:217–50.
21. Kanner L. Irrelevant and metaphorical language in early infantile autism. Am J Psychiatry 1946;103:242–6, 13.
22. Kanner L, Eisenberg L. Early infantile autism 1943-1955. Am J Orthopsychiatry 1956;26:55–66.
23. Asperger H. 1944 "Autistic psychopathy" in childhood. (Translated and annotated by Frith U (1991). In: Frith U, editor. Autism and Asperger syndrome. Cambridge (United Kingdom): Cambridge University Press; 1991. p. 37–92.
24. Asperger H. Early infantile autism [in German]. Med Klin 1974;69:2024–7.
25. Wing L. Asperger's syndrome: a clinical account. Psychol Med 1981;11:115–29.
26. Asperger H. The lived life. 50 years of pediatrics [in German]. Pediatr Padol 1977; 12:214–33.
27. Lyons V, Fitzgerald M. Did Hans Asperger (1906–1980) have Asperger syndrome? J Autism Dev Disord 2007;37:2020–1.
28. American Psychiatric Association. Diagnostic and statistical manual of mental disorders (DSM-IV). 4th edition. Washington, DC: American Psychiatric Association; 1994.
29. Severson KD, Aune JA, Jodlowski D. Bruno Bettleheim, autism, and the rhetoric of scientific authority. In: Osteen M, editor. Autism and representation. Routledge research in cultural and media studies. London (England): Routledge; 2007. p. 65–77.

30. Pollack R. The creation of Dr. B: a biography of Bruno Bettelheim. New York: Simon & Schuster; 1997. p. 478.
31. Bettelheim B. Joey: a "mechanical boy." Sci Am 1959;200:116–20.
32. Bettelheim B. The empty fortress: infantile autism and the birth of the self. New York: The Free Press: Simon & Schuster; 1967. p. 484.
33. Osgood NJ. Suicide in later life. New York (NY): Lexington Books; 1992. p. 4.
34. Park CC. The siege: the first eight years of an autistic child. Boston: Little, Brown and Company; 1967.
35. Rimland B. Infantile autism: the syndrome and its implications for a neural theory of behavior. New York: Appleton-Century-Crofts; 1964.
36. DeStefano F, Chen RT. Autism and measles, mumps, and rubella vaccine: no epidemiological evidence for a causal association. J Pediatr 2000;136:125–6.
37. Mrozek-Budzyn D, Kieltyka A, Majewska R. Lack of association between measles-mumps-rubella vaccination and autism in children: a case-control study. Pediatr Infect Dis J 2010;29:397–400.
38. Institute of Medicine. Adverse effects of vaccines: evidence and causality. Released August 25, 2011. Available at: http://www.iom.edu/vaccineadverseeffects. Accessed September 1, 2011.
39. Lovaas OI. Behavioral treatment and normal educational and intellectual functioning in young autistic children. J Consult Clin Psychol 1987;55:3–9.
40. Sallows GO, Graupner TD. Intensive behavioral treatment for children with autism: four-year outcome and predictors. Am J Ment Retard 2005;110:417–38.
41. Ospina MB, Krebs SJ, Clark B, et al. Behavioural and developmental interventions for autism spectrum disorder: a clinical systematic review. PLoS One 2008;3:e3755.
42. Wakefield AJ, Murch SH, Anthony A, et al. Ileal-lymphoid-nodular hyperplasia, non-specific colitis, and pervasive developmental disorder in children. Lancet 1998;351:637–41.
43. Black C, Kaye JA, Jick H. Relation of childhood gastrointestinal disorders to autism: nested case-control study using data from the UK General Practice Research Database. BMJ 2002;325:419–21.
44. Andrew Wakefield. Wikipedia, the free encyclopedia. Available at: http://en.wikipedia.org/wiki/Andrew_Wakefield. Accessed September 1, 2011.
45. Godlee F, Smith J, Marcovitch H. Wakefield's article linking MMR vaccine and autism was fraudulent. BMJ 2011;342:c7452.
46. Eggertson L. Lancet retracts 12-year-old article linking autism to MMR vaccines. CMAJ 2010;182:E199–200.
47. Institute of Medicine, Immunizaition Safety Review Committee. Immunization safety review: vaccines and autism. Washington, DC: National Academies Press; 2004.
48. Gerber JS, Offit PA. Vaccines and autism: a tale of shifting hypotheses. Clin Infect Dis 2009;48:456–61.
49. Offit PA. Autism's false prophets: bad science, risky medicine, and the search for a cure. Columbia (NY): Columbia University Press; 2008. p. 296.
50. Rapin I. High hopes, shoddy research, and elusive therapies for autism examined and exposed. Neurology Today 2009;9:23.
51. Adashi EY, Offit PA. Paul Offit on the dangers of the anti-vaccine movement. Available at: http://www.medscape.com/viewarticle/741343?src=mp&spon=24. Accessed October 24, 2011.
52. Paul Offit. Wikipedia. Available at: http://en.wikipedia.org/wiki/Paul_Offit. Accessed September 1, 2011.
53. Baker JP. Autism in 1959: Joey the mechanical boy. Pediatrics 2010;125:1101–3.

54. Rapin IE. Autism: where we have been, where are we going? Assessment, interventions, and policy. In: Volkmar FR, Paul R, Klin A, et al, editors. Handbook of autism and pervasive developmental disorders. 3rd edition, vol. 2. New York: John Wiley, Chapter 53; 2005. p. 1304–17.
55. Speers T, Lewis J. Journalists and jabs: media coverage of the MMR vaccine. Commun Med 2004;1:171–81.
56. Brugha TS, McManus S, Bankart J, et al. Epidemiology of autism spectrum disorders in adults in the community in England. Arch Gen Psychiatry 2011;68:459–66.
57. Heidgerken AD, Geffken G, Modi A, et al. A survey of autism knowledge in a health care setting. J Autism Dev Disord 2005;35:323–30.
58. World Health Organization. International classification of diseases: diagnostic criteria for research. 10th edition. Geneva (Switzerland): World Health Organization; 1992.
59. Freed GL, Clark SJ, Butchart AT, et al. Parental vaccine safety concerns in 2009. Pediatrics 2010;125:654–9.
60. Goodman NW. MMR scare stories: some things are just too attractive to the media. BMJ 2007;335:222.
61. Greydanus DE, Patel DR, Feucht C. Preface: pediatric and adolescent psychopharmacology: the past, the present, and the future. Pediatr Clin N Am 2011; 58:xv–xxiv.
62. Chatterjee A, O'Keefe C. Current controversies in the USA regarding vaccine safety. Expert Rev Vaccines 2010;9:497–502.
63. Sugarman SD. Cases in vaccine court—legal battles over vaccines and autism. N Engl J Med 2007;357:1275–7.
64. Artigas-Pallarés J. Autism and vaccinations: the end? [in Spanish]. Rev Neurol 2010;3(50 Suppl 3):S91–9.
65. Bragesiö F, Haliberg M. Dilemmas of a vitalizing vaccine market: lesions from the MMR vaccine/autism debate. Sci Context 2011;24:107–25.
66. Ratajczak HV. Theoretical aspects of autism—a review. J Immunotoxicol 2011;8: 68–79.

In the Doctor's Office: A Parent Perspective

Bruce Mills, PhD

KEYWORDS

- Autism • Communication • Social interaction
- Parent perspective • Pediatrician • Social Stories

A former student calls me. Her nearly 3-year-old son has been dealing with several medical issues. Though eating a healthy diet, he has intestinal problems, going days without a bowel movement. And there is more. She hesitates slightly: "He has been flapping his hands near his face … and he often gets overstimulated at parties." I listen as she describes his occasional meltdowns, how she and her husband have made a habit of leaving gatherings early. She list the signs of her son's sensory overload.

She called because she knows that I have a son with autism, and she has done enough of her own research to understand that some of her son's behaviors seem to fall on the autism spectrum. Unlike when my son was diagnosed in 1995, there is now a surplus of information (and misinformation) about autism and an accompanying sense of crisis. Having scheduled an appointment with her pediatrician, she worries about how her doctor will respond to concerns regarding her son's physical condition and seemingly odd behaviors. In advance of an appointment with her pediatrician, she wants to think aloud about how to relate what she has observed. She wants to be heard, not patronized or dismissed.

After I hang up, I cannot help but think ahead to this essay, to the opportunity to speak to physicians who occupy that intimate space of a doctor's visit. What can I say as a parent of a 19-year-old son with autism? What experiences might I relate to help foster a constructive "bedside" manner concerning a developmental disorder that has no blood test, that, in fact, must rely on parents' reporting of behaviors and observations during office visits? And, beyond this especially difficult early period, what stories might suggest best practices through adolescence? Given the specific difficulties those on the autism spectrum experience in relation to communication and social interaction, I reflect here on some emblematic stories, ones that point to practices that benefit children, parents, and physicians.

"RED UDDER"

One Saturday afternoon, my wife Mary and I were on our back deck, talking with friends. Jacob, my son, came out with a pair of children's safety scissors, a long,

---

Department of English, Kalamazoo College, 1200 Academy Street, Kalamazoo, MI 49006, USA
E-mail address: bmills@kzoo.edu

Pediatr Clin N Am 59 (2012) 13–18
doi:10.1016/j.pcl.2011.10.015
0031-3955/12/$ – see front matter © 2012 Elsevier Inc. All rights reserved.

hotdog-shaped balloon that we had blown up earlier in the day, and a red scrap of construction paper.

"Red udder," he said, urgently handing me the items.

He was around 6, had been diagnosed with autism 3 years earlier, and so we had learned a disciplined patience in the face of his sometimes mysterious requests.

"Red udder! Red udder!"

The balloon skidded atop the table. Puzzled by his request, I picked it up and rhythmically thumped it against my forearm to buy time. We all looked at each other, perplexed. Jacob took the red construction paper and held it against an end of the balloon. Knowing that my son thought in pictures more than language, that he felt more comfortable drawing than speaking, I remembered not to think in words. I remained patient, wishing to meet my son's anxiety with a practiced calm; I did not want to contribute to an escalation of his own frustration. I closed my eyes and tried to imagine the image that "red udder" might be trying to "sketch" for us.

Ruminating on the long tube of the balloon and red slap of paper hanging at its bottom, I glimpsed a picture. It came to me as I imagined the shape of a red cow's udder hanging beneath the balloon. I saw the tube as a metal cylinder rising toward the sky atop a fiery burst. A rocket. He wanted us to make a rocket ship.

"Rocket ship," I said, pleased to have the translation to give to my son and relieved to have avoided an afternoon of his fretful, roving efforts to be understood. Jacob took in a deep breath and let his arms rest on Mary's lap. His leaning was now relaxed, though his eyes still intently watched my cutting.

"'Rocket,' say 'rocket,' Jacob." He was not paying attention, of course. "Red udder" had communicated his want.

As I cut and taped, I wondered what chance combination of memories enabled me to translate his words, this image evoked with sparse vowels and consonants. And then my thoughts wandered back to the associations that had flashed in my mind. I realized that what he wanted came to me when I caught an image from a nursery rhyme. During the past week, we had been reading from a book of Mother Goose rhymes, including the one about the cow jumping over the moon. I went down to the basement to get the book. Against the backdrop of a night sky, I saw the illustration of a white cow, udder hanging over the curve of the sliver moon as the blocky body seemed to lift off toward outer space. While it was a seemingly simple connection, though, I despaired over the apparent randomness of this epiphany. Who else could have decoded his want? On any other day, would the right connections have formed in my mind? Would someone else have trusted that it had meaning, that it was a gesture toward connection?

Given the profound impairment in communication that marks autism, the interactions with those on the spectrum can seem a series of mysteries, and thus can escalate into frequent frustrations. In relation to my story, then, I urge consideration of a take-away message that may seem unexpected, for it invites a focus on the mode of interaction rather than any drive to solve a particular message. The aim is not to generate epiphanies, to spend office time seeking for the secret code, or to marvel at the striking way of "knowing" embodied in such visual thinking. Rather, it is to enter into such interactions prepared to listen, to convey patience, to limit verbal input, to reduce sensory distractions, and thus to manage conduct in ways that produce less frequent meltdowns or conflicts.

For those on the spectrum, after all, the world can be an ever-shifting place of unexpected demands, intrusive sensory input, and fraught efforts to communicate. It can be a place where imposing adult figures burden interactions with a rush of words, a series of comments or questions, and, in a doctor's office, a sequence of pokes, pricks, and probings. Certainly this reality can be true for many children. Yet, given their impaired ability to pick up the comforting eye contact of parents or to understand verbal assurances of strangers, children with autism will experience a doctor's visit as a worrisome break from the security of recognizable routines and sensory familiarity of the home environment.

As a parent, I valued and came to see the effectiveness of physicians who sought my input into how to interact with my son, accepted with patience the delays that may come with a child who needs more time to process verbal and/or sensory input, and understood that the interaction was not solely a problem to be solved (or a series of procedures to be performed) but an interpersonal dynamic that can build short-term and long-term trust. In reflecting on my son's words, "Red Udder," and my response, I realize that a telling moral was that I met him in a way that fostered his willingness to come to me again and again. For parents and pediatricians, the endgame is this truth: that the child will be open to a return, that he or she will seek continued connection across different ways of processing the world.

"NICK'S STORY"

It can be useful to reframe how we come to see interactions with doctors. Though we may be inclined to view a visit to a pediatrician (or other specialists) as related to yearly checkups, vaccinations, or specific medical procedures and needs, it can also be seen as a social interaction, a relationship that ideally embodies effective interpersonal communication skills as well as knowledge of social expectations and rules. In other words, the office visit is not simply a set of discrete "tests" or tasks enacted on a more or less willing child.

In their play, children remind adults of this very social dimension of a trip to the doctor's office. That is, they frame the experience through narrative, thus seeking to give some coherent shape to the event. If disinclined to think of an appointment in this way, we might recall the typical children's activity of "playing doctor" and of the various toys that invite a recreating of listening to the heart, taking a temperature, and more. For children, this activity serves several purposes, but it can be especially important to consider how the performance of the patient-doctor dynamic transforms the unease of a visit into a familiar story. For those on the spectrum, however, this kind of imaginative play is impaired. (In diagnostic manuals, autism is often characterized as behaviors that reflect the absence of symbolic or imaginative play.) In other words, the comforting knowledge of this seemingly universal children's story—and the broader social understanding of the cues and codes involving parents, receptionists, nurses, and doctor—is not easily absorbed or learned. Again, individuals on the autism spectrum have an impairment in social interactions, an inability to build or to build from the scaffolding of such stories, and, as some evidence suggests, a brain less able to construct meaning through narrative.

To be able to provide simple stories of a routine checkup or more extensive procedures, then, can be a very useful strategy. During his tonsillectomy at age 5, Mary and I came to understand the effectiveness of building Jacob's story repertoire, of providing what he could not easily construct for himself.

Starting around age 4, we began to notice that Jacob's breathing during sleep sounded congested. We began to talk about his nighttime "slurpiness" with regularity. Going to our pediatrician, he noted that his tonsils looked inflamed and that, within a year, it would be good to schedule surgery. Hearing of our concerns in terms of how to prepare Jacob for such an event, he indicated that the hospital had a brief video describing the outpatient procedure.

Entitled "Nick's Story," the video begins with a voiceover stating that "this is a story about a boy named Nick," a child around 8 years old. As the narrator continues, we see a series of Nick's drawings of events surrounding the procedure. The screen displays pictures of the young boy waking up on the morning of his tonsillectomy, standing near the breakfast table looking sad (because he is not able to eat or drink), and holding a favorite stuffed animal that he could bring to the hospital. The video then switches to the real Nick and a succession of photographs with voiceover descriptions of their meaning: Nick arriving at the hospital with his parents, his putting on a surgical gown, his getting a blood pressure check, his saying "goodbye" to his parents, and, finally, several still shots showing the surgery room and what would happen immediately before and after the procedure. In a brief and specific narrative, the actual "social" dimensions of the day are made visually explicit. For Nick, the day is not reduced to a discrete, surgical procedure. Rather, it is a tale with characters who offer support at each step; it is a story with a journey plot that involves movement through a strange and potentially threatening space as well as a conclusion that includes the stereotypical but comforting eating of a popsicle and a playful wheelchair ride to the exit door.

For my son, these visual images were especially important, for they mirrored storybooks from home as well as his own way of processing the world through personal sketches or videos. By this time, as we had seen with his use of "The Cow Jumped Over the Moon" and other Mother Goose language and images in his communications with us, Jacob had begun to mine storybooks and videos for both words and narrative structures to apply to his own life and its sometimes confusing or worrisome social interactions. For example, when a babysitter came one evening when Jacob was 4, my son said, "Something doesn't smell right!" This line comes from the movie *Homeward Bound*, a film about two lost dogs and a cat finding their way home. One dog utters these words to his companions when left at a friend of his owners. For Jacob, his use of this script signaled both his tendency to turn to a movie dialog as a story template for his own experience and to employ language—quite idiosyncratically— to convey an emotion comparable to his own. Does not the appearance of a babysitter, after all, suggest an impending abandonment?

Looking back over the video, I am struck by one moment and how it still provides my 19-year-old son with language for doctor's visits. In the video, a picture shows a nurse taking a blood sample. The narrator states, "That did hurt but *only* for a second." Years after this particular event, Jacob still prefaces a yearly flu shot with an echo of this video talk: "It will hurt," he thinks aloud, "but *only* for a moment." We later learned that this line gets expressed in another doctor story for children, *Curious George Goes to the Hospital*: "'It's going to hurt, George,' [the nurse] said, 'but only for a moment.'"

Though tailored for outpatient tonsillectomies at our local hospital, "Nick's Story" mirrored an intervention that has been helping families since the early 1990s: Social Stories. Developed by Carol Gray, Social Stories draw from the knowledge that those with autism have difficulty discerning, anticipating, and understanding the flow and basic facts of social situations. Not wired to be attentive to and easily understand such facts or rules, children on the spectrum experience various situations with significant levels of anxiety, often communicating worry and confusion through repetitive or ritualistic actions, idiosyncratic language, and, unfortunately at times, meltdowns. Problems in communication make such situations more difficult; children do not seek comfort or social knowledge in the eyes or actions of their parent or care provider. Again, without visual and/or verbal cues, the touch of a stethoscope can be sudden and even physically painful. Simple directions or requests can be lost in the sensory confusion. And, unfortunately, these responses can be quickly judged as "stubborn" or "undisciplined" (and interpreted solely as a sign of "poor parenting") rather than an attempt to express distress through the only means available.

While the term "spectrum" in "autism spectrum disorders" does underscore the uniqueness of how individuals might respond to the strange world of a doctor's visit, it might nevertheless be useful to keep in mind that Social Stories, especially those with visual supports, can help prepare for the seemingly routine aspects of an appointment as well as unusual and sometimes painful inpatient or outpatient procedures. (Information regarding this intervention can be found at http://www.thegraycenter.org/social-stories.) Parents and doctors set up the possibility for successful interactions when the experience is not a complete surprise. Even for those individuals who are highly impaired, all parties benefit from focusing on aspects of autism that can be accommodated as well as interpreting behaviors as forms of communication. Moreover, parents and doctors build a team approach that best serves the child when not suspicious of each others' assumptions and responses concerning what transpires during the visit.

"I WILL NOT BE DEAF"

During a recent trip to our doctor, I was reminded of the potential of these "best practices." My son had been complaining of ear pain on a vacation to Florida. After a morning of swimming and a mid-afternoon shower, we thought he might just have water in his ear and encouraged him to shake his head. Rather than helping, this attention to the ear only increased his laments.

"I will not be deaf," he moaned.

When we returned home, we set up an appointment. Because Jacob is 19, we have been seeking another general practitioner. The visit to our pediatrician, then, likely marked the last time in his office.

On the way to the appointment, I described the plan for the visit to Jacob. The pediatrician, I noted, would look in your ear. "Remember when you had wax in your ear," I said. "He may find wax and take it out like that time."

"It did not hurt," I reminded him.

"No shots?" Jacob asked, as he does before every visit. "No," I replied.

After checking weight, height, and blood pressure and waiting for a time in our room, his pediatrician entered.

"So how are you, Jake?"

"Fine," he said abruptly.

I described briefly and slowly, for my son's benefit, that Jacob had complained about his left ear. I indicated that his response mirrored the time when he had to have a plug of wax removed from his ear.

"Let's take a look. Jacob, I am going to look in your ears now."

He showed Jacob the instrument, moving from the right ear ("This one looks fine!") to the left ear ("Ah, I see some wax here.") He then showed my son what he would use to try to get out the wax. As years before, Jacob wanted to see what came out of his ear. Unlike the last time, not all of the wax could be "scooped" out.

"Jacob, I will need to squirt some water in your ear to get out the rest." He broke down each step. The ear needed 3 "flushings." During this time, his interaction clearly allowed for my participation. I translated the steps in ways that fit Jacob's world of video scripts and storybooks. I even found myself uttering the familiar but slightly revised line, "It will feel funny, Jacob, but only for a little bit."

At the end of the visit, just before we left the room, his pediatrician said something unexpected to me. "That went better than I anticipated." For a moment, I glimpsed more fully the work that he had been doing, the negotiating of an uncertainty that gets magnified with those on the autism spectrum.

"You know," I replied, "Jacob tends to do well with doctor's visits."

I should have said that he has learned to trust that he will be shown or told what will happen, that he will not be inundated with verbal demands and questions, that he has had videos and stories that give structure to what had initially been without a narrative frame. I should have said that he has benefited from a doctor who accepts a father and mother as a team member. Perhaps I might have said something, but Jacob had begun looking for old videos in the cabinet at the nurses' station, his five-foot-eight, 225-pound body sprawled on the floor acting out a 5-year-old yearning.

Of course, not all interactions work out so well. Parents and pediatricians have many stories to tell, and not all of them embody trust and understanding. Among parents who have children with autism, word goes out fairly quickly when a pediatrician has shown a knowledge of their child's way of processing the world, a willingness to attend closely to behaviors, and an ability to establish effective interactions with those on the spectrum—and, less positively, when a doctor shows little familiarity with autism and its impact on families.

And so, to conclude, let me return to my former student. Her outcome was not an ideal one. Her pediatrician attended well to the medical concerns, but she negotiated the description of autistic-like behaviors less confidently. According to the mother, her specific account of her son's odd behaviors and sensory difficulties did not receive the open consideration that accompanied the details of his gastrointestinal issues. The doctor heard the mother's desire to bring forward behaviors as a request for an autism diagnosis. In my years of listening to parent stories, I hear these kinds of reactions frequently: an initial dismissal of behaviors as the sign of an overanxious parent and, in recent years, as a mark of cultural hysteria concerning the burgeoning numbers of children being diagnosed. Of course, in the flow chart of possibilities these may be factors; moreover, parents can sometimes succumb to their worst fears and/or display their own interpersonal shortcomings.

Whether or not my former student's child ultimately receives an autism diagnosis, the pediatrician's response signals the profound importance of this exchange. To come to this potentially life-changing moment with the willingness to listen without being quick to judge, with a knowledge of autism and its impairments in relation to social interaction, communication, and imaginative play, with the ability to suspend assumptions about a parent's motivations, and with a referral protocol, this practice can establish deep and sustaining relationships for years.

Autism Spectrum Disorders: Clinical Features and Diagnosis

Ahsan Nazeer, MD[a],*, Mohammad Ghaziuddin, MD[b]

KEYWORDS

- Autism • Definition • Diagnosis • Clinical features • ASD
- Primary care • Comorbidity

Although cases resembling autism were probably first reported more than 2 centuries ago, the credit for describing autism as a distinct disorder goes to Leo Kanner.[1] In his seminal article, *Autistic Disturbances of Affective Contact*,[1] he described, in unusual detail, 11 children without the ability to form social relationships. According to Kanner,[1] these children showed characteristic features including aloofness, lack of imagination, and persistence of sameness; they came from "highly intelligent families" but had "very few really warm hearted fathers and mothers." These families were "strongly preoccupied with abstractions of a scientific, literary or artistic nature and limited in genuine interest in people." One year later, Vienna-born physician, Hans Asperger,[2] identified similar symptoms in 4 children who possessed similar character-istics to those studied by Kanner[1] but lacked "language delays" and were "exception-ally gifted."[2] Subsequently, Lorna Wing[3] gave the label of Asperger syndrome to these children. Around the same time, Rutter[4] proposed 4 sets of diagnostic criteria for autism: social impairment, language disturbances, insistence on sameness, and onset before 30 months of age.

DSM IV AND ICD 10 CRITERIA

Rutter's[4] and Wing's[3] definition of autism was largely responsible for the introduction of autism as a distinct disorder in the DSM (*Diagnostic and Statistical Manual of Mental Disorders, Fourth Edition*)/ICD (International Classification of Diseases) systems of

---

The authors have no conflict of interest to declare.

[a] Child and Adolescent Psychiatry, Michigan State University, Kalamazoo Center for Medical Studies, 1722 Shaffer Road, Suite # 3, Kalamazoo, MI 49048, USA
[b] Department of Psychiatry, University of Michigan Medical School, 4250 Plymouth Road, Ann Arbor, MI 48105, USA
* Corresponding author.
E-mail address: nazeer@kcms.msu.edu

classification. At present, autism is conceptualized both in the DSM IV[5] and the ICD[6] as the main category in a group of disorders, the pervasive developmental or autism spectrum disorders (ASD), all of which are characterized by similar reciprocal social and communication deficits and rigid ritualistic interests beginning in early childhood. Other disorders in this category include Asperger syndrome, pervasive developmental disorder not otherwise specified (PDDNOS), Rett syndrome, and disintegrative disorder.

Patients with Asperger syndrome, as currently defined in the DSM IV, suffer from autistic social dysfunction but without mental retardation or language delay. Rett syndrome, caused by mutations in the MECP2 gene, is characterized by autistic features in one of its phases, whereas patients with disintegrative disorder develop normally in the first 4 to 5 years of life and then go through a period of disintegration. The last category, PDDNOS, is reserved for patients who are within the autistic spectrum but do not meet the threshold for any of the named disorders. For practical purposes, the term ASD often refers to autism, Asperger syndrome, and PDD NOS, excluding Rett syndrome and disintegrative disorder. Thus, although the diagnosis of classic autism is straightforward, the identification of the subtle forms of ASD and the delineation of its various subtypes can be particularly challenging. Partly because of this difficulty in separating the subtypes of ASD, the upcoming edition of the DSM is likely to introduce a paradigm shift in its approach to the classification of autism.

PROPOSED DSM V CRITERIA

The fifth edition of the DSM (DSM V), scheduled to be published in 2013, is likely to introduce a single category of ASD and eliminate the subcategories. In brief, the draft of the DSM V has published on its Web site[7] the following changes. First, the deficits of social interaction and communication that existed in DSM IV have now been merged into a single criterion of deficits in social communication and interaction. This is because, according to the draft criteria, deficits in communication and social behaviors are inseparable and more accurately considered as a single set of symptoms. The deficits must be clinically significant and persistent. These deficits should include marked impairment of both verbal and nonverbal communication used for social interaction; lack of social reciprocity (the degree of lack of reciprocity is not specified); and a failure to develop peer relationships at the appropriate developmental level. The second criterion consists of restricted repetitive interests shown by at least 2 of the following:

1. Stereotyped motor or verbal behaviors, or unusual sensory behaviors (unusual sensory behaviors were not included in the DSM IV)
2. Excessive adherence to routines and ritualized patterns of behavior
3. Restricted, fixated interests.

The third criterion states that the symptoms of autism must be present in early childhood (in contrast with the DSM IV, which required the symptoms to be present before 3 years of age), with the caveat that the symptoms may not become fully apparent until social demands exceed the limited capacities.

Thus, from DSM III (when autism was first introduced in the classificatory system) to the proposed DSM V, the approach to the classification of ASD seems to have gone full circle, beginning with lumping to splitting and back to lumping again. The rationale for eliminating Rett disorder and disintegrative disorder is presumably that they are now conceptualized as being more neurologic than psychiatric. Regarding the proposed elimination of Asperger syndrome (or Asperger disorder), according to the

DSM V task force,[7] the disorder is difficult to separate from autism with normal intelligence and has not been shown to be a valid category. However, a diagnosis does not have to be valid to be useful.[8] Although there is no firm evidence that Asperger syndrome is distinct from autism, there is no denying that a diagnosis of Asperger syndrome can inform clinicians about the level of functioning, a pattern of behavior, and a likely outcome. Thus, the elimination of Asperger syndrome seems both unfortunate and premature.[9]

DIAGNOSTIC CRITERIA AND PREVALENCE

One result of the changes in the diagnostic criteria has been the large increase reported in recent years in the prevalence of autism.[10] When first described, autism was regarded as a rare condition affecting no more than 4 per 10,000; however, it is now much more common, occurring in at least 1 out of every 100 children. For example, a recent South Korean study reported that 2.6% of children aged 7 to 12 years meet the diagnostic criteria of ASD.[11] Autism is no longer regarded as a single entity but as a collection of disorders grouped together as ASD. The condition described by Kanner,[1] though uncommon, was not difficult to recognize. Children with autism typically show stereoptypic behaviors, perhaps repeating words or sentences, preoccupied with routines and rituals, lost in a world of their own, often withdrawn and aloof. However, children with suspected ASD, although common, are also difficult to identify because they often present with a range of deficits ranging from the most severe to the almost invisible. The distinction between autism/autistic disorders and ASD/other psychiatric disorders often seems vague and ill defined.

ASD IN PRIMARY CARE

Because most children with ASD are first seen not by the specialist but by pediatricians and family practitioners, this article synthesizes the findings of recent studies dealing with the presentation and diagnosis of ASD in primary care and its distinction from other common psychiatric disorders of childhood. However, the ability of pediatricians to make this diagnosis depends not only on their training and background but also on the time they have at their disposal. Few pediatricians have enough time to screen for this condition. For example, in a mail survey of pediatricians, only about 8% endorsed screening for ASD. Although a significant number of the responders reported that they were not familiar with the screening procedures, others reported that they did not have enough time to conduct the assessments.[12]

SYMPTOMS OF AUTISM
Core Symptoms of Autism

It is useful to categorize the symptoms of autism into 2 broad categories: core symptoms and secondary/comorbid symptoms. The core symptoms consist of reciprocal social deficits, communication impairment, and rigid ritualistic interests.[5] Recent studies suggest that the first 2 symptoms (social deficits and communication impairment) can be merged into a single category of social-communication impairment,[7] reducing the triad of autistic symptoms to a dyad of social-communication impairment and rigid restricted interests. Although each of these symptoms can occur in a variety of psychiatric disorders(hence the importance of differential diagnosis) it is the clustering of these symptoms in the same individual that makes the disorder so unique and fascinating. However, some investigators think that the correlation between social-communication impairment and rigid ritualistic interests has been exaggerated, and that their underlying neurobiological mechanisms might be different.[10] However, from a clinical standpoint, whenever a child presents with social difficulties and restricted compulsive interests, an in-depth autism-specific evaluation should be considered. In addition to the clustering of symptoms, the clinician should also take into consideration the age of presentation because different symptoms emerge at different periods during the life span.[5] Thus, during early childhood, children with autism are likely to present with language deficits and problems with hyperactivity; however, during adolescence, the symptoms might change to problems with relationships and with regulation of mood. Apart from the pattern of symptoms and the age of presentation, another factor that should be considered is whether or not the child has intellectual disability or other psychiatric disorders, as discussed later.

Secondary or Comorbid Features

Problems such as hyperactivity, aggression, and self-injurious behaviors occur in up to half of children with ASD.[11,12] More common in patients with intellectual disability, these symptoms significantly affect the quality of life of the affected individuals and their families. Depressive symptoms often emerge during adolescence.[13] At times, depressive, psychotic symptoms and suicidal behavior can also occur.[14–17] During late adolescence and early adulthood, affected persons might become increasingly slow in their body movements and may even develop catatonia, a potentially life-threatening condition that may occur in about 10% to 15% of patients with Asperger syndrome.[18]

ASSOCIATION WITH INTELLECTUAL DISABILITY

Most patients with autism suffer from intellectual disability. Along with epilepsy, the relationship between autism and intellectual disability (sometimes referred to as mental handicap or mental retardation) was the main reason that convinced researchers that autism was a biologic condition, and not a psychogenic disorder caused by social circumstances and stressful life events. However, the association between intellectual disability is neither straightforward nor fully understood, although a few generalizations can be made. First, although the level of intellectual disability can vary from mild to profound, most cases tend to be in the moderate/severe range. Second, separating autism from profound mental retardation is difficult. Third, the likelihood of seizures is increased in those who have autism and intellectual disability. Fourth, although autism and related disorders cluster in families, there is no excess of intellectual disability alone in the family members of patients of autism. Fifth, compared with those without intellectual disability, patients with autism plus intellectual disability are more likely to have ritualistic behaviors and abnormal movements. Sixth, IQ is a reliable predictor of the long-term outcome of the disorder.

ASSOCIATION WITH EPILEPSY

As stated earlier, the occurrence of epilepsy and intellectual disability were the 2 main factors that convinced skeptics about the biologic origin of autism. Epilepsy occurs in at least 30% of cases of traditional autism, usually in the preschool years or around puberty. The most common type of seizures are of the complex partial type, although other types have also been described. The occurrence of autistic features tends to be higher in the epileptic syndromes of childhood, such as Landau-Klefner syndrome.[19] Also, certain genetic syndromes association with mental retardation, such as tuberous sclerosis (TS), are particularly associated with autism. For example, the prevalence of autistic features in TS has been stated to range from 30% to 50%. In those who are affected, the likelihood of having autism increases if the tubercles are located in the temporal region.[20]

Regressive Autism

In about one-fifth of children with autism, a history of regression is present.[21,22] Typically, children start developing normally, and then, around the age of 18 months to 2 years, lose their language and adaptive skills. A history of a precipitant, such as an infection, may or may not be present. In some children, the regression seems to coincide with the emergence of seizures. However, in general, there is no history of an obvious cause. In some children, the regression may be delayed when distinction from disintegrative disorder becomes difficult.[23]

When Should Autism be Suspected

From a clinical point of view, children who present to a pediatrician should be screened for ASD if they seem excessively shy, are socially awkward, have a language impairment, or seem to be obsessed with certain topics or interests. Also, any child who has intellectual disability or epilepsy should also be screened for autism. In addition, other conditions that should alert the pediatrician to screen for autism or an autism-related condition are language delay, severe hyperactivity, and obsessive-compulsive behavior.

MENTAL STATUS EXAMINATION

Every patient with ASD seen in primary care should have a mental status examination.[24] Apart from observing and noting the core features of autism as indexed by social-communication deficits (eg, poor eye contact, absence of social smiling, problems with personal boundaries, language abnormalities) and restricted interests (eg, tendency to fixate on certain topics or activities, compulsive behaviors and rituals), the examiner should routinely evaluate for externalizing symptoms (eg, level of activity, aggressive behavior) and internalizing behaviors (eg, depressive symptoms, suicidal and self-injurious behaviors). In late adolescence and adulthood, particular attention should be paid to any signs of regression (eg, onset of psychotic symptoms, alteration of speech, emergence of catatonia).

PHYSICAL EXAMINATION

A brief medical examination should also be performed, including assessment of vision and hearing. Any dysmorphic features should be noted. Some children with autism may have an increased head circumference. A Wood lamp examination may be necessary to look for the typical skin stigmata of TS. Although a detailed neurologic examination is usually not necessary, any soft neurologic signs such as clumsiness should be noted.

SCREENING AND SCREENING INSTRUMENTS

The diagnosis of autism is based on obtaining a detailed developmental history and performing a systematic examination. Rating scales and structured interviews are commonly used to strengthen the process of clinical diagnosis, not to replace it. Although the instruments are accurate in diagnosing classic autism, they need to be interpreted with caution when autism is complicated by severe intellectual disability or when the symptoms co-occur with complex psychiatric disorders such as psychosis.[25] Therefore, the gold standard of diagnosis should consist of collecting information in a systematic manner with rating scales, structured interviews, and observation schedules, and then performing a thorough clinical examination. The type of instruments selected depends on the time and the resources available. For example, ADI (Autism Diagnostic Interview), ADOS (Autism Diagnostic Observation Schedule), and the DISCO (Diagnostic Interview for Social and Communication Disorders), take hours to administer (3–5 hours if done properly) and require special training. Newer instruments that incorporate elements of a standard mental status examination in addition to autism-specific questions might be useful.[24] In addition, diagnosis is made from the DSM/ICD criteria and not on the findings of a structured interview.[26] It is also critical to have a multidisciplinary approach to the evaluation because children with autism may behave differently with different examiners and in different settings. At the minimum, the team should include a child psychiatrist, a speech and language therapist, a psychologist, and an educational consultant.

DIFFERENTIAL DIAGNOSIS AND COMORBIDITY

When assessing a child with suspected autism, the first question that needs to be clarified is whether the child is at a normal level of cognitive functioning. If the child has an intellectual disability, then it has to be decided whether the clinical features are the result of intellectual disability or autism or both. In brief, although there is global developmental delay in intellectual disability, the pattern of deficits is neither uniform nor global in autism. If the child is of normal intelligence, other conditions should first be ruled out, such as shyness, severe attention-deficit/hyperactivity disorder, anxiety and mood disorders, and psychotic disorders. Although a detailed description of each of these conditions is outside the scope of this article, referral to a child psychiatrist should be made if necessary.[27]

SUMMARY

ASDs are more common than generally believed, occurring in as many as 1% of the population. Most patients with ASD are first referred for diagnosis to pediatricians and family practitioners. Although typical cases are easy to recognize, milder cases and those with comorbid psychiatric disorders can pose severe challenges. Despite the advances made in understanding the disorder, the diagnosis of ASD remains clinical. There is no biologic test for the diagnosis of autism. Although rating scales and structured interviews can help in clarifying the diagnosis, the eventual diagnosis remains clinical.

REFERENCES

1. Kanner L. Autistic disturbances of affective contact. Nervous Child 1943;2: 217–50.
2. Asperger H. Die "autistischen psychopathen" im Kindesalter. Arch Psychiatr Nervenkr 1944;117:76–136.
3. Wing L. Asperger's syndrome: a clinical account. Psychol Med 1981;11:115–29.
4. Rutter M. Diagnosis and definition of childhood autism. J Autism Dev Disord 1978;8(2):139–61.
5. American Psychiatric Association. Diagnostic and statistical manual of mental disorders. 4th edition. Washington: American Psychiatric Publishing; 2000.
6. International classification of diseases. Geneva (Switzerland): World Health Organization; 1993.

7. American Psychiatric Publishing. DSM-V development. Washington, DC: APA; 2010. Available at: http://www.dsm5.org/ProposedRevisions/Pages/proposedrevision.aspx?rid=94. Accessed August 14, 2011.
8. Kendell R, Jablensky A. Distinguishing between the validity and utility of psychiatric diagnosis. Am J Psychiatry 2003;160:4–12.
9. Ghaziuddin M. Should the DSM V drop Asperger syndrome? J Autism Dev Disord 2010;40(9):1146–8.
10. Frances A. The first draft of DSM-V. BMJ 2010;340:c1168.
11. Kim YS, Leventhal BL, Koh YJ, et al. Prevalence of autism spectrum disorders in a total population sample. Am J Psychiatry 2011;168(9):904–12.
12. Dosreis S, Weiner CL, Johnson L, et al. Autism spectrum disorder screening and management practices among general pediatric providers. J Dev Behav Pediatr 2006;27:88–94.
13. Mandy WP, Skuse DH. Research review: what is the association between the social-communication element of autism and repetitive interests, behaviors and activities? J Child Psychol Psychiatry 2008;49:795–808.
14. Baghdadli A, Pascal C, Grisi S, et al. Risk factors for self-injurious behaviours among 222 young children with autistic disorders. J Intellect Disabil Res 2003; 47:622–7.
15. Aman MG, Lam KSL, Van Bourgondien ME. Medication patterns in patients with autism: temporal, regional, and demographic influences. J Child Adolesc Psychopharmacol 2005;15:116–26.
16. Ghaziuddin M, Ghaziuddin N, Greden J. Depression in persons with autism: implications for research and clinical care. J Autism Dev Disord 2002;32(4):299–306.
17. Raja M, Azzoni A, Frustaci A. Autism spectrum disorders and suicidality. Clin Pract Epidemiol Ment Health 2011;7:97–105.
18. Wing L, Shah A. Catatonia in autistic spectrum disorders. Br J Psychiatry 2000; 176:357–62.
19. Tuchman R, Rapin I. Epilepsy in autism. Lancet Neurol 2002;1(6):352–8.
20. Numis AL, Major P, Montenegro MA, et al. Identification of risk factors for autism spectrum disorders in tuberous sclerosis complex. Neurology 2011;76(11):981–7.
21. Wiggins LD, Rice CE, Baio J. Developmental regression in children with an autism spectrum disorder identified by a population-based surveillance system. Autism 2009;13(4):357–74.
22. Rogers SJ. Developmental regression in autism spectrum disorders. Ment Retard Dev Disabil Res Rev 2004;10(2):139–43.
23. Kurita H, Osada H, Miyake Y. External validity of childhood disintegrative disorder in comparison with autistic disorder. J Autism Dev Disord 2004;34(3):355–62.
24. Grodberg D, Weinger PM, Kolevzon A, et al. Brief report: The Autism Mental Status Examination: development of a brief autism-focused exam. J Autism Dev Disord 2011. [Epub ahead of print].
25. Reaven JA, Hepburn SL, Ross RG. Use of the ADOS and ADI-R in children with psychosis: importance of clinical judgment. Clin Child Psychol Psychiatry 2008; 13(1):81–94.
26. Rutter M. Research review: child psychiatric diagnosis and classification: concepts, findings, challenges and potential. J Child Psychol Psychiatry 2011; 52(6):647–60.
27. Volkmar F, Cook EH Jr, Pomeroy J, et al. Practice parameters for the assessment and treatment of children, adolescents, and adults with autism and other pervasive developmental disorders. American Academy of Child and Adolescent Psychiatry, Working Group on Quality. J Am Acad Child Adolesc Psychiatry 2000;39:938.

Epidemiology of Autism Spectrum Disorders

Erin Duchan, MD[a], Dilip R. Patel, MD[b],*

KEYWORDS

- Autism spectrum disorders • Asperger disorder • Mortality
- Morbidity • Risk factors

Since Kanner's original description of autism almost 70 years ago,[1] the medical and sociocultural construct of autism has changed greatly and continues to remain in flux. The definition of autism, initially described as "autistic disturbances of affective contact," has undergone a variety of changes and currently refers to a heterogeneous group of disorders.[1] Autism spectrum disorder (ASD) is the broad term encompassing autistic disorder (AD), Asperger disorder/syndrome (AS), and pervasive developmental disorder, not otherwise specified. These disorders all share common features of impaired social relationships, impaired communication and language, and stereotypic motor mannerisms or a narrow range of interests. This article reviews the epidemiology of ASD.

The authors performed a comprehensive search of PubMed using the term *autism* combined with the following terms: *incidence*, *prevalence*, *risk factors*, *associations*, *life span*, *mortality*, or *morbidity*. The authors reviewed articles that were published within the last 5 years and printed in English. They also performed a manual search for and reviewed related articles that were referenced in the original articles. After study of these articles, the authors performed additional searches to examine specific topics not included in the initial set, such as *autism*, *genes*. They excluded case studies and case reports.

INCIDENCE

In a retrospective review of health and education records in 2006 from participating sites in the Autism and Developmental Disabilities Monitoring (ADDM) network,

[a] Department of Pediatrics and Human Development, Michigan State University College of Human Medicine and Kalamazoo Center for Medical Studies, 1000 Oakland Drive, Kalamazoo, MI 49008, USA
[b] Department of Pediatrics and Human Development, Michigan State University College of Human Medicine, Pediatric Residency Program, Kalamazoo Center for Medical Studies, 1000 Oakland Drive, Kalamazoo, MI 49008, USA
* Corresponding author.
E-mail address: patel@kcms.msu.edu

Pediatr Clin N Am 59 (2012) 27–43
doi:10.1016/j.pcl.2011.10.003
0031-3955/12/$ – see front matter © 2012 Elsevier Inc. All rights reserved.

the incidence of ASD is 1 child in every 110 children.[2] This finding is similar to the estimates that 1 in 91 children aged 3 to 17 years in the United States will be diagnosed with ASD based on data from the 2007 National Survey of Children's Health.[3] These numbers are similar to regional data whereby, in a study of birth cohorts in Massachusetts, the incidence of ASD in 2005 was 1 per 108 in children less than 3 years of age. This finding is a 66% increase in the incidence of ASD from 4 years previously, when the incidence was reported, by the same researchers using the same methodology, to be 1 in 179 children.[4]

PREVALENCE OF AUTISM IN THE UNITED STATES

Epidemiologic data gathered over the last 40 years report that the conservative estimate of ASD prevalence is 27.5 per 10,000 individuals; however, the prevalence estimate based on newer surveys is 60.0 per 10,000 individuals.[5] A review of 23 published articles reporting the prevalence of ASD found that the pooled estimate was 20.0 per 10,000 individuals, although there was a large variation among the analyzed studies as reflected by the 95% confidence interval of 4.9 to 82.1.[6] However, the prevalence of ASD in the United States from data gathered in the last 5 years (2006–2011) is 2 to 4 times greater than those estimates: 45 to 110 individuals with ASD per 10,000.[2,3,7,8] Even data gathered from surveys published in 2000 range from 57.9 to 67.5 per 10,000 individuals, which is almost twice the conservative estimate.[9–11] Among data collected from 11 US states in 2006, the prevalence of ASD within the states varied dramatically, with Florida having the lowest prevalence (42 per 10,000 individuals) and Missouri and Arizona having the highest prevalence (121 per 10,000 individuals).[2]

PREVALENCE OF AUTISM GLOBALLY

The prevalence of typical autism across the world is generally reported to be 10 per 10,000.[5] When analyzing the prevalence of typical autism, the pooled prevalence of published reports from 37 studies was 7.1 per 10,000; however, again, there were large variations with a wide 95% confidence interval of 1.6 to 30.6.[6] Another systematic review of 32 surveys that were published from 1966 to 2001 reporting the prevalence of typical autism found that the range of prevalence estimates of AD to be from 0.7 to 72.6 per 10,000 individuals, with a median prevalence, from studies published between 1992 to 2001, to be 12.7 per 10,000.[5] Interestingly, the researchers noted that all the surveys with reported prevalence rates of AD of 7.0 per 10,000 or greater were published after 1987, prompting them to recalculate the prevalence estimates using only the surveys published after 1987. From these 19 surveys, the range of AD was 2.5 to 30.8 per 10,000 individuals, with an average prevalence of 11.1 per 10,000 individuals.[5] Demonstrating a similar increase, the range of prevalence of AD in studies published after 2000 is 16.8 to 40.5 per 10,000 individuals.[9–11] A study analyzing data over an 11-year time period, from 1997 to 2008, reported the prevalence of autism in children aged 3 to 17 years to be 47 per 10,000.[12]

PREVALENCE OF AUTISM IN ASIA

The prevalence of ASD is similar in Asia. A Taiwanese 2005 national database review revealed a cumulative prevalence of ASD to be 28.72 per 10,000 individuals.[13] This finding is a dramatic increase from the Taiwanese prevalence of 1.71 per 10,000 individuals that was reported in 1996.[13] In Japan, the prevalence of ASD is reported to be 27.2 per 10,000 individuals.[14] In Chinese children younger than 15 years of age, the prevalence of ASD as estimated from a government registry from 1986 to 2005 is 16.1 per 10,000.[15] In contrast with prevalence estimates that are similar between Asia and the United States, a South Korean study estimated the prevalence of ASD to be 1.89% of the general population of 7- to 12-year-old children. This estimation, greater than estimates elsewhere in Asia and in the United States, may be an overestimation, however, based on a low participation rate of 63%.[16] In China, the prevalence of AD in children aged 2 to 6 years was 11 per 10,000.[17]

PREVALENCE OF AUTISM IN EUROPE

The prevalence of ASD in Europe tends to be similar to the reported prevalence estimates in the United States and in Asia. A stratified, multiphase, random sample survey of adults living in England determined a prevalence of ASD of 98 per 10,000 individuals.[18] A diagnosis survey distributed to children aged 5 to 9 years who were on the Special Educational Needs register in the United Kingdom determined the prevalence of ASD to be 94 per 10,000 and the prevalence of autism to be 11 per 10,000.[19] These two studies reported a higher prevalence of ASD than other reported estimations, however. In a large population sample of children in England, the prevalence of ASD was reported to be 61.9 per 10,000. Of this group, the estimated prevalence of AD was 21.6, the estimated prevalence of atypical autism was 10.8, the estimated prevalence of AS was 16.6, and the estimated prevalence of an unspecified ASD was 13.0.[20] If education records were excluded from this analysis and the data were based solely on medical records, the prevalence would have decreased by approximately 10 individuals per 10,000.[21] A screening survey in the United Kingdom followed by a multidisciplinary assessment to standardize the diagnosis reported a prevalence of all pervasive developmental disorders to be 58.7 per 10,000 and a prevalence for AD to be 22.0 per 10,000 individuals.[9] Another study based on the screening of more than 55,000 children aged 9 to 10 years in the United Kingdom reported that the prevalence of ASD was 77.2 per 10,000 and the prevalence of autism was 38.9 per 10,000.[22] These estimations are significantly greater than the estimations outside of the United Kingdom. A report from the Danish Psychiatric Central Register estimated that the prevalence of childhood autism is 11.8 per 10,000 children less than 10 years of age and the estimated prevalence of AS is 4.7 per 10,000 children less than 10 years of age.[23] In France, autism is reported to affect approximately 5 out of every 10,000 children.[24]

CHANGE IN PREVALENCE SINCE 1940

Most studies conducted between 1960 and 1980 reported the prevalence of ASD to be 2 to 5 per 10,000, whereas studies published in early 2000 reported prevalences ranging from 30 to 60 per 10,000 individuals.[3] This rate is still approximately half the rate that recent US studies have reported, as previously discussed. The US Department of Developmental Services reported that, between 1991 and 1997, there was a 556% increase in the prevalence of childhood autism.[25] From 1997 to 2008 the rate of autism increased fourfold, from a prevalence of 0.19% in 1997 to 0.74% in 2008.[12] A large retrospective review of evaluation records of American children aged 8 years in 2002 was compared with data collected by the same method 4 years later, in 2006: of the 10 states where data were collected, 9 states had an increase in the prevalence of ASD, and every state reported an increased prevalence among boys.[2] Within Massachusetts, early ASD diagnosis in boys increased more than 70% from 2001 to 2005 (88 per 10,000 children for the 2001 birth cohort compared with 151 per 10,000 for the 2005 birth cohort), whereas early diagnoses in girls increased 39% over the same time period (23 per 10,000 for the 2001 birth cohort to 32 per 10,000 for the 2005 birth cohort).[4] From 2002 to 2006, the prevalence of identified ASD among 8-year-old children increased 57% across all sex and racial/ethnic groups.[2] This trend of increasing prevalence has also been observed outside of the United States. A study using data from the UK General Practice Research Database showed an increase in incidence from around 0.3 per 10,000 individuals in 1989 to approximately 2.0 per 10,000 individuals by 1999. In addition, the increased risks of autism were observed in successive birth cohorts.[26] The prevalence of ASD in Taiwan has increased from 1.71 per 10,000 individuals to 28.72 per 10,000 individuals from 1996 to 2005, based on data from the national health insurance enrollee registry.[13] In Western Australia, the incidence of ASD increased annually with an average annual increase of 11.9% over a 17-year period, from 1985 to 2002. The overall prevalence of ASD in Western Australia among children diagnosed by 8 years of age was 8 per 10,000 births in 1983, whereas in 1999 the prevalence was 46 per 10,000 births.[27]

One possible explanation for this change in prevalence may be an underestimation of the prevalence of autism in the past. To assess this theory, a focus group of experts in the diagnosis of AD was convened to evaluate whether the prevalence of autism may have been underestimated in a 1970s British cohort study that reported a prevalence of autism of 4.5 per 10,000, which is consistent with the prevalence reported in other studies during the same time period. This cohort reviewed the original questionnaires and found that, using contemporary diagnostic features, the prevalence of autism is 37.6 per 10,000, which is consistent with current reports.[28] In another study, a stratified, multiphase, random sample of adults in England revealed a prevalence of ASD, recognized by survey, similar to the current reported prevalence in children, thus, adults with ASD living in the community tend to be unrecognized. This finding supports the possibility that the diagnosis of ASD is increasing in the pediatric population but not necessarily an increasing prevalence of ASD.[18]

Another theory that has been proposed is that the increasing prevalence of autism is a result of early diagnosis, which is later revoked. However, a prospective study evaluating diagnostic stability for autism at 2 years of age and again at 9 years of age found that diagnostic stability was very high when autism was diagnosed by 2 years of age.[29] Another study evaluating the diagnostic stability for ASD revealed that 68% of the patients diagnosed with an ASD by 2 years of age continued to meet diagnostic criteria for an ASD 2 years after the initial diagnosis. The children who no longer met diagnostic criteria for an ASD were more likely to be less than 30 months of age at the initial evaluation and, less commonly, had milder symptoms of autism or had higher cognitive scores at 2 years of age.[30] Similar data were reported in a large survey of parents of children aged 6 to 17 years. In this study, 38.2% of all children diagnosed with autism no longer had the condition.[3]

Another possible explanation for the increase in prevalence is the changing diagnostic criteria of autism and ASD as our knowledge of these conditions evolves. A study comparing 4 different diagnostic criteria for AS highlights the variability that can exist in the diagnosis of autism and ASD. The prevalence of AS per 1000 individuals was 2.5, 2.9, 2.7, and 1.6 based on the *Diagnostic and Statistical Manual of Mental Disorders* (Fourth Edition) (DSM-IV), *International Classification of Diseases, Tenth Revision*, Gillberg and Gillberg's criteria, and Mattila and colleagues[31] criteria, respectively. Another study, which compared the current criteria for diagnosis, the DSM-IV, with the proposed revised diagnostic criteria, DSM-5, demonstrated that the DSM-5 criteria are less sensitive than the prior criteria, especially for individuals with high-functioning autism or AS.[32]

In addition to diagnostic criteria, the initial diagnosis may also be influenced by other factors. The type of evaluator, such as psychiatrist, psychologist, developmental pediatrician, neurologist, or school professionals, may sway the diagnosis. For example, school professionals are almost 6 times more likely to diagnose ASD.[33] In a review of 78 evaluations of children diagnosed with ASD by their public school, a developmental disabilities eligibility determination, or a hospital-based early childhood mental health program, the rate of agreement by different evaluators was 45%. In addition, most community evaluators did not follow best practice guidelines or use autism diagnostic tools.[34] The region of the country (Midwest, South, Northeast, and West) and urbanization of the area may also influence the diagnosis of autism: autism is significantly more likely to be diagnosed in the Northeast and in metropolitan areas.[33]

Finally, the trend of increasing diagnoses of autism and ASD may reflect the success of national efforts, such as the Centers for Disease Control and Prevention's Learn the Signs, Act Early campaign and the American Academy of Pediatrics' Autism A.L.A.R.M. The current recommendations from the American Academy of Pediatrics is that physicians perform surveillance at each preventive care visit and screen for autism with a standardized developmental tool at specific intervals, such as the 9-,18-, 24-, and 30-month visits.[35] The American Academy of Pediatrics' Autism Expert Panel has further recommended that physicians use an autism-specific screening tool on all children at the 18- and 24-month visit.[36] There has also been increased public awareness about autism as a result of increased media attention, advocacy efforts, and celebrity publicity.

CONDITIONS ASSOCIATED WITH AUTISM

Although the cause of autism and ASD has not been elucidated, it is widely accepted to be a disorder of brain development. Therefore, it stands to reason that psychiatric conditions are a common comorbidity. In a large national survey, 87.3% of children aged 6 to 17 years diagnosed with ASD also had attention-deficit disorder or attention-deficit/hyperactivity disorder (ADHD), anxiety problems, behavioral or conduct problems, depression, or developmental delay. Among these conditions, the most common was attention-deficit disorder or ADHD, with an estimated prevalence of 47.2 per 100 individuals.[3] There may also be a genetic component to the neuropsychiatric disorders that are frequently comorbid with autism. In a study of Swedish twins, the probability of the nonautistic monozygotic twin being diagnosed with ADHD was 44% compared with 15% for the dizygotic twin.[37] A study comparing the families of an autistic child with families without an autistic child found that, in the families with autism, the frequency of social phobia was 10 times more common than among the control families. This study also found that 64% of first-degree relatives of a child with autism had a diagnosis of major depressive disorder, a statistically significant difference from the 19% with major depressive disorder among the control families.[38] A Danish study reported that the risk of autism is twice as high in individuals with a maternal history of a psychiatric disorder but that there was no association between paternal history of a psychiatric disorder and the risk of autism.[39] And a study evaluating obsessive-compulsive behaviors found that children with autism who displayed highly repetitive behaviors, rituals, or restricted interests were significantly more likely to have one or both parents with obsessive-compulsive traits or disorder.[40]

Developmental delay and intellectual disability are also more common among children diagnosed with autism. One survey reports that 64.8% of all children with autism aged 6 to 17 years also have a developmental delay and 74.5% of children with moderate or severe autism have a developmental delay.[3] Although intellectual disability is not a defining criterion for autism, the mean distribution of IQs in individual with autism is lower than average,[41] and approximately 40% to 60% of individuals with autism also have intellectual disability.[2,42]

Genetic conditions are also associated with autism in a small percentage of individuals with ASD. Fifteen percent of individuals identified with pervasive developmental disorder had a known genetic disorder and, of these, 9% were thought to be causative of the pervasive developmental disorder, including Rett syndrome and fragile X syndrome.[43] In a review of population-based studies of children with autism, genetic or medical conditions were found to account for less than 10% of individuals with autism.[44,45] It should be noted, however, that an association with autism is not guaranteed in any of the diagnosable medical or genetic conditions that are associated with autism.

RISK FACTORS FOR AUTISM

There are numerous risk factors for autism that have been postulated. The following discussion is meant to discuss some of the more commonly proposed risk factors with scientific evidence to support this claim but is not inclusive of all postulated risk factors.

Maternal and Paternal Age

The maternal age at the time of conception and delivery may be associated with an increased risk for the child developing an ASD. Even after controlling for maternal, paternal, and infant characteristics, mothers younger than 20 years of age had the lowest odds of their child having an early ASD diagnosis when compared with mothers greater than 20 years of age. Infants born to mothers aged 20 to 24 years had lower odds of their child having an early ASD diagnosis when compared with mothers aged 25 to 29 years. In contrast, infants of mothers older than 30 years of age had increased odds of an early ASD diagnosis. In this study, paternal age was not independently associated with ASD.[4] A Swedish study reported that a maternal age of 40 years or older was a significant risk factor for autism, with an odds ratio of 2.5. However, this study also reported that, although there was as association between advanced maternal age and a diagnosis of AS, this was not statistically significant.[42]

Advanced paternal age may also be associated with an increased risk of autism in his offspring. After controlling for maternal age, fathers more than 50 years of age were 2.2 times more likely to have a child diagnosed with autism than a father less than 29 years of age.[46] Another study found that children born to fathers more than 40 years of age have a 3.3 times increased odds of having ASD than children born of fathers less than 20 years of age.[47] An Israeli study reported that children of men older than or equal to 40 years of age were 5.75 times more likely to have ASD compared with children of men less than 30 years of age, even after controlling for year of birth, socioeconomic status, and maternal age.[48] A Danish study found that the risk of autism increased with increasing paternal age: children with fathers more than 35 years of age were almost twice as likely to have a child with autism compared with fathers aged 25 to 29 years.[39] This study, as well as 2 others, found that advanced paternal age was an independent risk factor and that advanced maternal age did not increase the risk of the child developing autism.[39,48,49]

The combination of aging mothers and fathers may pose an additional risk to the development of autism in a child. A retrospective study of all singleton children born at Kaiser Permanente in California over a 4-year period showed that the risk of a child having ASD increased significantly with each 10-year increase in maternal age and paternal age. Additionally, the adjusted relative risks for maternal and paternal age were elevated for children with AD and children with AS.[50] A cohort study of children born in 1994 and diagnosed with ASD based on DSM-IV criteria found that both maternal and paternal age were independently associated with autism, after adjusting for birth order, maternal education, and the other parent's age. This study also found that third- or later-born children from mothers aged 20 to 34 years and fathers less than 40 years of age were 3 times less likely to develop autism than firstborn children of 2 older parents.[51]

Parental Education

The education of parents may also play a role in the diagnosis of autism. Mothers with 4 or more years of college education had lower odds of their children having an early ASD compared with mothers who had only completed high school.[4] Another survey reported that children of parents with less than 12 years of education were 68% more likely to have ASD rated as moderate and 43.5% more likely to have ASD rated as severe compared with children with ASD whose parents had more than 12 years of education.[3] This increased risk may simply be an association, and more studies should be conducted to elucidate the difference.

Child's Sex

The odds of a boy being diagnosed with ASD are approximately 4 times greater than girls.[2-4,8] Of children in the United States diagnosed with ASD, 75% to 83% are boys.[2,33,52] Internationally, the gender distribution is similar. A large-scale, retrospective study using data from the Swedish Medical Birth Registry reported that boys were 4 times more likely to be diagnosed with autism and 3.5 times more likely to be diagnosed with AS.[42] Reports of boys with autism range from 79.6% in Sweden to 84.4% in Israel.[42,53]

Heritability

A genetic link to ASD seems likely, given the high recurrence rate in families. The sibling recurrence rate of pervasive developmental disorders is 7.1%,[43] whereas the sibling recurrence rate of autism is reported to be between 4.5%.[54] The relative risk of autism is 22 times greater in children who have a sibling diagnosed with autism and 13 times greater in children with a sibling who has been diagnosed with the broader autism diagnosis.[39] In families with 2 or more children with autism, the recurrence rate is 35%.[55] A study that analyzed male and female siblings separately found that the male siblings of an individual with autism have a 7% risk of having autism and an additional 7% risk for milder autistic spectrum symptoms, whereas female siblings of an individual with autism have only a 1% risk for autism.[56]

Twin studies further support the theory that ASD may have a genetic component. There is a higher concordance for autism among monozygotic than dizygotic twins.[37] Early twin studies in the United Kingdom reported that monozygotic twins had a concordance rate greater than 60% for classic autism, and when the twin without a diagnosis of classic autism was reevaluated for broader autistic phenotypes, such as communication skills and social disorders, the concordance rate increased to 92%. In contrast, dizygotic twins had no concordance, although the concordance did increase to 10% when the twin with a diagnosis of autism was evaluated for broader autistic phenotypes. This finding supports the argument that there is a genetic predisposition to idiopathic autism.[57] This data were almost duplicated in an analysis of same-sex twins less than 25 years of age in the Nordic countries (Denmark, Finland, Iceland, Norway, and Sweden) whereby the concordance for autism was 91% in monozygotic twins and 0% in dizygotic twins.[58] Similar data were reported in the largest twin study of autism to date whereby the concordance of ASD was reported to be significantly greater among monozygotic twins (88.1%) than dizygotic twins (30.5%).[59]

This data supports a heritability component of ASD; however, only 10% of ASD can be directly attributed to an underlying medical condition, such as fragile X syndrome,[59] and single-gene defects are rare within the broader autism phenotype. Thus, more likely, a unique set of genetic polymorphisms may determine an individual's susceptibility to autism; however, a review of the studies detailing the mapping of these genes is beyond the scope of this article.

Paternal Factors

Beyond parental age, there are several paternal factors that may play a role in the development of ASD. For example, fathers of an autistic child respond to social cues more slowly than fathers of typically developing children.[60] In a study of boys with AS, 15% had fathers who were also diagnosed with AS.[61]

Low Birth Weight/Gestational Age

Another risk factor that has been repeatedly identified as a risk factor for the later diagnosis of ASD is a low birth weight or low gestational age at the time of birth. The odds of a child less than 3 years of age being diagnosed with ASD are greater for infants born preterm (birth before 37 gestational weeks) or with a low birth weight (less than 2500 g) when compared with their term or normal-weight counterparts.[4,42] Other studies have shown similar associations between low birth weight and preterm delivery and the later development of autism.[62–64] One reason for this may be that some of the children born preterm or with a low birth weight have other medical conditions that also predispose them to autism. Another theory that has been proposed is that children from a nonsingleton gestation have an increased risk of autism and are also more likely to have a low birth weight or low gestation age. However, data collected from the ADDM network reviewing multiple births and a diagnosis of ASD by 8 years of age from a cohort born in 1994 found no association between the autism and multiple births.[65] In both a case-control study of Swedish children and a retrospective study of Swedish children, an association between twin gestation and autism was not identified.[42,62]

Prenatal Exposures

Despite evidence linking genetics with ASD, several studies have implicated prenatal exposures as risk factors in their development. The association between congenital rubella infection and autism was initially reported as early as 1971[66]; however, more recent data reveal that congenital rubella infection is present in only 0.75% of autistic populations, although this percentage has likely diminished with widespread usage of the measles-mumps-rubella vaccine in Western countries.[67] Multiple studies have documented that prenatal exposure to valproic acid, ethanol, thalidomide, and misoprostol are associated with an increased incidence of autism.[68,69] A 2002 study reports that maternal smoking on a daily basis in early pregnancy is associated with an increased risk of autism diagnosis of almost 1.5 times the risk of a nonsmoking mother.[62] Not all exposures increase the risk of autism, however. One retrospective study reports that use of prenatal vitamins in the periconceptual period (the 3 months before pregnancy and during the first month of pregnancy) may be associated with a reduced risk of having a child with autism, especially in genetically susceptible mothers.[70]

There are several proposed risk factors that have equivocal evidence. In 2 studies, black ethnicity was associated with an increased risk of autism[71,72]; however, in another survey that was conducted in the United States, black children had 57% lower odds of having ASD when compared with non-Hispanic white children. Multiracial children also had a decreased risk of being diagnosed with ASD: 42% lower odds than non-Hispanic white children.[3] Another proposed risk factor is season of conception. One study found that conception in the winter (December, January, February) is associated with a 6% increased risk of autism when compared with a summertime conception[73]; however, another study conducted in Sweden found no association between season of birth and the risk of developing autism.[62]

ANATOMIC TRAITS WITH AUTISM

Beginning with Kanner's original description of autism, which described an increased rate of macrocephaly, researchers continue to study anatomic traits that may be associated with autism. Dysmorphic features and minor physical anomalies are more common in individuals with autism than in the general population.[68,74] In a study using a Waldrop scale to detect the presence or absence of 41 different minor physical anomalies in children with a mean age of 7 years, 96% (n = 23) had significantly higher rates of minor physical anomalies.[75] This study also found that 17% were characterized as dysmorphic after photographs of children that had been diagnosed with syndromes associated with autism had been removed.[75]

There are 4 body areas that children with ASD had significantly higher rates of minor physical anomalies: the head, ears, mouth, and hands. In addition, there are 3 minor physical anomalies that best differentiate individuals with ASD from the control subjects: abnormal head circumference, abnormal cephalic index, and abnormal palate.[75] Of all anomalies, the most common physical anomaly is posterior rotation of the ears.[75] Other physical abnormalities include hypertelorism, deep-set eyes, wide nasal bridge, macrocephaly, micrognathia, tapering fingers, clinodactyly, pes planus, and patchy skin pigmentation.[68]

Despite Kanner's original report, a more recent study reported that only 20% of children with autism meet criteria for macrocephaly,[76] and a separate prospective study reported that the mean head circumference for all infants that were later diagnosed with ASD was in the 84th percentile.[77,78] However, most children with ASD are born with a significantly smaller head circumference and, in a study evaluating changes in head circumference over time, every subject in the ASD group experienced an increased rate of head circumference growth between 6 and 14 months of age. This increase in head circumference in the autistic subjects was related to a greater cerebral cortex volume at 2 to 5 years of age as demonstrated by magnetic resonance imaging.[77,78] Additionally, a larger head circumference at 15 to 25 months was associated with delayed onset of language and a greater number of symptoms of social impairment based on a higher autism diagnostic interview-revised social algorithm score.[78,79]

GENETIC SYNDROMES ASSOCIATED WITH AUTISM

Features of autism have been reported in several genetic syndromes, which are listed in **Table 1**.[75–91]

PROGNOSIS

The prognosis of autism reported in the literature varies with autism severity and comorbidities. However, overall, children with autism are reported to have a poorer

Table 1
Genetic syndromes associated with autism

Syndrome	Cause (if known)
Rett syndrome[80,81]	Methyl-CpG-binding protein 2 mutation
Tuberous sclerosis[82–84]	TSC1 and TSC2 mutations
Fragile X[80,82,85]	FMR1 mutation creating triplet repeats on X chromosome
Neurofibromatosis[82]	
Congenital Rubella syndrome[86]	
Moebius syndrome[82,87]	Underdevelopment of cranial nerves VI and VII
CHARGE syndrome[75,82]	CHD7 mutation
Goldenhar syndrome[75,82]	
Down syndrome[82,85,88]	Trisomy 21
Prader-Willi[82,85]	Chromosome 15 deletion inherited paternally
Angelman syndrome[82,85]	Chromosome 15 deletion inherited maternally
Cohen syndrome[82,89]	Mutations in COH1
Cowden syndrome[82,90]	PTEN tumor suppressor gene mutation
Bannayan-Riley-Ruvalcaba syndrome[82,90]	PTEN tumor suppressor gene mutation
Smith-Lemli-Opitz syndrome[82,91]	Deficiency of final enzyme in pathway that synthesizes cholesterol
De Lange syndrome[82]	
DiGeorge syndrome[82,92]	Chromosome 22q11 deletion
Wilms' tumor, Aniridia, Genito-urinary anomalies, mental Retardation Syndrome[93]	Chromosome 11p deletion
Smith Magenis syndrome[82]	

health status.[94] In very young children with autism, there is a strong association between autism severity and impaired cognitive function. Specifically, children with an IQ less than 70 have more social, play, and stereotyped behavior deficits than children with a borderline or normal IQ. In contrast, there is no significant difference in autism severity in children who have autism with borderline or normal cognitive function.[95] However, intensive intervention can improve the social-communicative behaviors of children with autism.[95] There are limited studies evaluating the life span of individuals with autism; however, one Danish study reported that the average age of death was 43 years.[96]

MORBIDITIES

There are significant morbidities associated with autism and ASD. Earlier, the prevalence of psychiatric symptoms in parents of individuals with autism was discussed; however, those with autism and ASD may also suffer from psychiatric symptoms. The mean score for the Global Assessment of Functioning (GAF) scale for a group of individuals with autism who were selected from 3 population-based studies was reported to be 21.1.[97] This GAF score is classified as serious impairment or inability to function in almost all areas. Additionally, 12% of the individuals had GAF scores between 50 and 69, which indicates moderate or mild psychiatric problems or functional impairment.[97] In a survey distributed to a large sample of university students in Virginia, the students who met diagnostic criteria for high-functioning ASD self-reported more problems with social anxiety, depression, and aggression than a matched cohort with lower autism severity scores.[98]

A second commonly encountered morbidity associated with autism is mental retardation. In a large retrospective study in the United States, mental retardation was present in 45% to 63% of children with autism.[10] Girls with autism have been found to be more likely to have severe mental deficiency (38% of girls compared with 23% of boys); however, this does not control for syndromes associated with autism.[99] A longitudinal prospective study of individuals with autism found that 30% of children diagnosed with autism tested in the mild mental retardation range (IQ 50–69) and 50% tested in the severe mental retardation range (IQ <50). In the follow-up of the same individuals 13 to 22 years later, 94% had IQs less than 70, an increase from the 80% previously.[97]

Neurologic dysfunction is another frequently encountered comorbidity of autism. In a recent study in the Netherlands, almost three-quarters of children with autism showed minor neurologic dysfunctions, a statistically significant number when compared with the control group, whereby only 6% had minor neurologic dysfunctions. The minor neurologic dysfunctions included dysfunctional posture and muscle tone, fine manipulative disability, mild abnormalities in coordination, and excessive associated movements.[100] This finding was repeated with similar results in the United States.[101] Girls with autism are more likely to have a motor deficit than boys with autism (27% vs 11%).[99]

Epilepsy is associated with neurologic dysfunction. A prospective study of individuals with autism reported that 38% of the studied population had epilepsy, most commonly experiencing partial seizures with or without secondarily generalized seizure activity.[102] The majority had onset of epilepsy before 2 years of,[102] and there is a higher risk of having epilepsy in girls with autism.[103] Another study found that 14% of autistic individuals have epilepsy; however, after eliminating individuals with perinatal or medical disorder, family history of epilepsy, severe mental deficiency, or motor deficit, only 6% of individuals with autism also have epilepsy.[99] This finding was supported by a meta-analysis of 24 studies that found that the prevalence of epilepsy among individuals with autism who also had intellectual disability (IQ <70) was 21.5% but only 8% in individuals with autism and no intellectual disability.[103]

MORTALITIES

There is excess mortality in autism, especially when comorbid with epilepsy.[104] Based on data from the California Developmental Disability System from 1998 to 2002, the mortality for individuals with autism was significantly higher than that of the general population.[105] A Swedish study of individuals with autism found the mortality rate to be 5.6 times higher than expected.[97] A Danish study reported the risk of dying in individuals with autism was nearly twice that of the general population, and this has not changed from 1993 to 2008.[96] There was an almost sixfold increase in mortality reported in a prospective study evaluating mortality in individuals with autism. Within the group of individuals with autism with early death, the rate of severe mental retardation with onset in childhood was significantly higher than in the group of living individuals with autism.[97]

There also seems to be a significant association between female gender and the risk of early death. A prospective study reported that 17% of the females with autism were dead in follow-up, after a period of 13 to 22 years, whereas only 4% of the males were deceased.[97] Other prospective studies occurring in Sweden and the United States also reported that mortality is greater in females than males.[97,106] One reason for this may be that, because autism is more common in males as previously discussed, females with autism may be more likely to have coexisting medical disorders. However, not all sources agree. Data evaluating causes of death in autism reported no significant difference in the mortality rate between males and females with autism, although the standard mortality ratio for females is greater than that of males.[105]

The increased risk of early death in individuals with autism may be associated with epilepsy.[106] There is an increased risk of death when individuals with autism are comorbid for epilepsy. Almost one-third of deaths in individuals with autism are associated with epilepsy.[96] The crude death rate (not adjusted for age) for individuals with autism increased 8.3 times when individuals also had a diagnosis of epilepsy.[104]

SUMMARY

Autism is a life-altering diagnosis for patients, their family, and the community. As autism becomes increasingly prevalent, knowledge of ASDs is crucial for health professionals. There is ongoing debate within the literature about the cause of the increased prevalence; however, regardless of cause, physicians need to be aware of the medical implications a diagnosis of autism or ASD has. This review covers incidence, prevalence, associations, comorbidities, and mortality of ASD; however, further research is necessary to clarify controversies in many of these areas. Autism has evolved over the last 70 years since the first description by Leo Kanner and, with further research, will continue to evolve over the next 70 years.

REFERENCES

1. Kanner L. Autistic disturbances of affective contact. Nerv Child 1943;2:217–50.
2. Rice C. Prevalence of autism spectrum disorders—autism and developmental disabilities monitoring network, United States, 2006. MMWR Surveill Summ 2009;58(10):1–20.
3. Kogan D, Blumberg S, Schieve L, et al. Prevalence of parent-reported diagnosis of autism spectrum disorder among children in the US, 2007. Pediatrics 2009; 124(5):1395–403.
4. Manning S, Davin C, Barfield W, et al. Early diagnosis of autism spectrum disorders in Massachusetts birth cohorts, 2001-2005. Pediatrics 2011;127(6): 1043–51.
5. Fombonne E. Epidemiological surveys of autism and other pervasive developmental disorders: an update. J Autism Dev Disord 2003;33(4):365–82.
6. Williams J, Higgins J, Brayne C. Systematic review of prevalence studies of autism spectrum disorders. Arch Dis Child 2006;91(1):8–15.
7. Schechter R, Grether J. Continuing increases in autism reported to California's developmental services system: mercury in retrograde. Arch Gen Psychiatry 2008;65(1):19–24.
8. Kogan D, Strickland B, Blumberg S, et al. A national profile of the health care experiences and family impact of autism spectrum disorder among children in the United States, 2005-2006. Pediatrics 2008;122(6):e1149–58.
9. Chakrabarti S, Fombonne E. Pervasive developmental disorders in preschool children: confirmation of high prevalence. Am J Psychiatry 2005;162(6): 1133–41.
10. Bertrand J, Mars A, Boyle C, et al. Prevalence of autism in a United States population: the brick township, New Jersey, investigation. Pediatrics 2001;108(5): 1155–61.

11. Baird G, Charman T, Baron-Cohen S, et al. A screening instrument for autism at 18 months of age: a 6 year follow-up study. J Am Acad Child Adolesc Psychiatry 2000;39(6):694–702.
12. Boyle C, Boulet S, Schieve L, et al. Trends in the prevalence of developmental disabilities in US children, 1997-2008. Pediatrics 2011;127(6):1034–42.
13. Chien I, Lin C, Chou Y, et al. Prevalence and incidence of autism spectrum disorders among national health insurance enrollees in Taiwan from 1996 to 2005. J Child Neurol 2011;26(7):830–4.
14. Honda H, Shimizu Y, Imai M, et al. Cumulative incidence of childhood autism: a total population study of better accuracy and precision. Dev Med Child Neurol 2005;47(1):10–8.
15. Wong V, Hui S. Epidemiological study of autism spectrum disorder in China. J Child Neurol 2008;23(1):67–72.
16. Kim Y, Leventhal B, Koh Y, et al. Prevalence of autism spectrum disorders in a total population sample. Am J Psychiatry 2011;168(9):904–12. [Epub ahead of print].
17. Zhang X, Ji C. Autism and mental retardation of young children in China. Biomed Environ Sci 2005;18(5):334–40.
18. Brugha T, McManus S, Bankart J, et al. Epidemiology of autism spectrum disorders in adults in the community in England. Arch Gen Psychiatry 2011;68(5):459–65.
19. Baron-Cohen S, Scott F, Allison C, et al. Prevalence of autism-spectrum conditions: UK school-based population study. Br J Psychiatry 2009;194(6):500–9.
20. Williams E, Thomas K, Sidebotham H, et al. The prevalence and characteristics of autism spectrum disorders in the ALSPAC cohort. Dev Med Child Neurol 2008;50(9):672–7.
21. Yeargin-Allsopp M. The prevalence and characteristics of autism spectrum disorders in the ALSPAC cohort. Dev Med Child Neurol 2008;50(9):646.
22. Baird G, Simonoff E, Pickles A, et al. Prevalence of disorders of the autism spectrum in a population cohort of children in South Thames: the Special Needs and Autism Project (SNAP). Lancet 2006;368(9531):210–5.
23. Lauritsen M, Pedersen C, Mortensen P. The incidence and prevalence of pervasive developmental disorders: a Danish population-based study. Psychol Med 2004;34(7):1339–46.
24. Fombonne E, Du Mazaubrun C, Cans C, et al. Autism and associated medical disorders in a French epidemiological survey. J Am Acad Child Adolesc Psychiatry 1997;36(11):1561–9.
25. Stokstad E. Development. New hints into the biological basis of autism. Science 2001;294(5540):34–7.
26. Kaye J, del Mar Malero-Montes M, Jick H. Mumps, measles, and rubella vaccine and the incidence of autism recorded by the general practitioner: a time-trend analysis. BMJ 2001;322(7284):460–3.
27. Nassar N, Dixon G, Bourke J, et al. Autism spectrum disorders in young children: effect of changes in diagnostic practices. Int J Epidemiol 2009;38(5):1245–54.
28. Heussler H, Polnay L, Marder E, et al. Prevalence of autism in early 1970s may have been underestimated. BMJ 2001;323(7313):633.
29. Lord C, Risi S, DiLavore P, et al. Autism from 2 to 9 years of age. Arch Gen Psychiatry 2006;63(6):694–701.
30. Turner L, Stone W. Variability in outcome for children with an ASD diagnosis at age 2. J Child Psychol Psychiatry 2007;48(8):793–802.

31. Mattila M, Kielinen M, Jussila K, et al. An epidemiological and diagnostic study of Asperger syndrome according to four sets of diagnostic criteria. J Am Acad Child Adolesc Psychiatry 2007;46(5):636–46.

32. Mattila M, Kielinen M, Linna S, et al. Autism spectrum disorders according to DSM-IV-TR and comparison with DSM-5 draft criteria: an epidemiological study. J Am Acad Child Adolesc Psychiatry 2011;50(6):583–592.e11.

33. Rosenberg R, Daniels A, Law J, et al. Trends in autism spectrum disorder diagnoses: 1994-2007. J Autism Dev Disord 2009;39(8):1099–111.

34. Williams M, Atkins M, Soles T. Assessment of autism in community settings: discrepancies in classification. J Autism Dev Disord 2009;39(4):660–9.

35. American Academy of Pediatrics, Council on Children With Disabilities, Section on Developmental and Behavioral Pediatrics, Bright Futures Steering Committee, Medical Home Initiatives for Children with Special Needs Project Advisory Committee. Identifying infants and young children with developmental disorders in the medical home: an algorithm for developmental surveillance and screening. Pediatrics 2006;119:1808–9.

36. Gupta V, Hyman S, Johnson C. Identifying children with autism early. Pediatrics 2007;119:152–3.

37. Lichtenstein P, Carlstrom E, Rastam M, et al. The genetics of autism spectrum disorders and related neuropsychiatric disorders in childhood. Am J Psychiatry 2010;167(11):1357–63.

38. Smalley S, McCracken J, Tanguay P. Autism, affective disorders, and social phobia. Am J Med Genet 1995;60(1):19–26.

39. Lauritsen M, Pedersen C, Mortensen P. Effects of familial risk factors and the place of birth on the risk of autism: a nationwide register-based study. J Child Psychol Psychiatry 2005;46(9):963–71.

40. Hollander E, King A, Delaney K, et al. Obsessive-compulsive behaviors in parents of multiplex autism families. Psychiatry Res 2003;117(1):11–6.

41. Yeargin-Allsopp M, Rice C, Karapurkar T, et al. Prevalence of autism in a US metropolitan area. JAMA 2003;289(1):49–55.

42. Haglund N, Kallen K. Risk factors for autism and Asperger syndrome: perinatal factors and migration. Autism 2011;15(2):163–83.

43. Chudley A, Gutierrez E, Jocelyn L, et al. Outcomes of genetic evaluation in children with pervasive developmental disorder. J Dev Behav Pediatr 1998;19(5):321–5.

44. Fombonne E. Epidemiological trends in rates of autism. Mol Psychiatry 2002; 7(Suppl 2):S4–6.

45. Chakrabarti S, Fombonne E. Pervasive developmental disorders in preschool children. JAMA 2001;285:3093–9.

46. Hultman C, Sandin S, Levine S, et al. Advancing paternal age and risk of autism: new evidence from a population-based study and a meta-analysis of epidemiological studies. Mol Psychiatry 2010. [Epub ahead of print].

47. Buizer-Voskamp J, Laan W, Staal W, et al. Paternal age and psychiatric disorders: findings from a Dutch population registry. Schizophr Res 2011;129(2–3): 128–32.

48. Reichenberg A, Gross R, Weiser M, et al. Advancing paternal age and autism. Arch Gen Psychiatry 2006;63(9):1026–32.

49. Larsson H, Eaton W, Madsen K, et al. Risk factors for autism: perinatal factors, parental psychiatric history and socioeconomic status. Am J Epidemiol 2005; 161(10):916–25.

50. Croen L, Najjar D, Fireman B, et al. Maternal and paternal age and risk of autism spectrum disorders. Arch Pediatr Adolesc Med 2007;161(4):334–40.

51. Durkin M, Maenner M, Newschaffer C, et al. Advanced parental age and the risk of autism spectrum disorder. Am J Epidemiol 2008;168(11):1268–76.
52. Giarelli E, Wiggins L, Rice C, et al. Sex differences in the evaluation and diagnosis of autism spectrum disorders among children. Disabil Health J 2010; 3(2):107–16.
53. Gal G, Abiri L, Reichenberg A, et al. Time trends in reported autism spectrum disorders in Israel, 1986-2005. J Autism Dev Disord 2011. [Epub ahead of print].
54. Jorde L, Hasstedt S, Ritvo E, et al. Complex segregation analysis of autism. Am J Hum Genet 1991;49(5):932–8.
55. Ritvo E, Jorde L, Mason-Brothers A, et al. The UCLA-University of Utah epidemiologic survey of autism: recurrence risk estimates and genetic counseling. Am J Psychiatry 1989;146(8):1032–6.
56. Miles J, Takahashi T, Bagby S, et al. Essential versus complex autism: definition of fundamental prognostic subtypes. Am J Med Genet A 2005;135(2):171–80.
57. Bailey A, Le Couteur A, Gottesman I, et al. Autism as a strongly genetic disorder: evidence from a British twin study. Psychol Med 1995;25(1):63–77.
58. Steffenburg S, Gillberg C, Hellgren L, et al. A twin study of autism in Denmark, Finland, Iceland, Norway, and Sweden. J Child Psychol Psychiatry 1989;30(3): 405–16.
59. Rosenberg R, Law J, Yenokyan G, et al. Characteristics and concordance of autism spectrum disorders among 277 twin pairs. Arch Pediatr Adolesc Med 2009;163(10):907–14.
60. Scheeren A, Stauder J. Broader autism phenotype in parents of autistic children: reality or myth? J Autism Dev Disord 2008;38(2):276–87.
61. Cederlund M, Gillberg C. One hundred males with Asperger syndrome: a clinical study of background and associated factors. Dev Med Child Neurol 2004; 46(10):652–60.
62. Hultman C, Sparen P, Cnattingius S. Perinatal risk factors for infantile autism. Epidemiology 2002;13(4):417–23.
63. Kolevzon A, Gross R, Reichenberg A. Prenatal and perinatal risk factors for autism. Arch Pediatr Adolesc Med 2007;161(4):326–33.
64. Williams K, Helmer M, Duncan G, et al. Perinatal and maternal risk factors for autism spectrum disorders in new South Wales, Australia. Child Care Health Dev 2008;34(2):249–56.
65. Van Naarden Braun K, Schieve L, Daniels J, et al. Relationships between multiple births and autism spectrum disorders, cerebral palsy, and intellectual disabilities: autism and developmental disabilities monitoring (ADDM) network-2002 surveillance year. Autism Res 2008;1(5):266–74.
66. Chess S, Korn S, Fernandez P. Psychiatric disorders of children with congenital rubella. New York: Brunner/Mazel; 1971.
67. Fombonne E. The epidemiology of autism: a review. Psychol Med 1999;29(4): 769–86.
68. Dufour-Rainfray D, Vourc'h P, Tourlet S, et al. Fetal exposure to teratogens: evidence of genes involved in autism. Neurosci Biobehav Rev 2011;35(5): 1254–65.
69. Stromland K, Nordin V, Miller M, et al. Autism in thalidomide embryopathy: a population study. Dev Med Child Neurol 1994;36(4):351–6.
70. Schmidt R, Hansen R, Hartiala J, et al. Prenatal vitamins, one-carbon metabolism gene variants, and risk for autism. Epidemiology 2011;22(4):476–85.
71. Dealberto M. Prevalence of autism according to maternal immigrant status and ethnic origin. Acta Psychiatr Scand 2011;123(5):339–48.

72. Keen D, Reid F, Arnone D. Autism, ethnicity and maternal immigration. Br J Psychiatry 2010;196(4):274–81.
73. Zerbo O, Iosif A, Delwiche L, et al. Month of conception and risk of autism. Epidemiology 2011;22(4):469–75.
74. Ozgen H, Hop J, Hox J, et al. Minor physical anomalies in autism: a meta-analysis. Mol Psychiatry 2010;15(3):300–7.
75. Tripi G, Roux S, Canziani T, et al. Minor physical anomalies in children with autism spectrum disorder. Early Hum Dev 2008;84(4):217–23.
76. Fombonne E, Roge B, Claverie J, et al. Microcephaly and macrocephaly in autism. J Autism Dev Disord 1999;29(2):113–9.
77. Courchesne E, Carper R, Akshoomoff N. Evidence of brain overgrowth in the first year of life in autism. JAMA 2003;290(3):337–44.
78. Mraz K, Green J, Dumont-Mathieu T, et al. Correlates of head circumference growth in infants later diagnosed with autism spectrum disorders. J Child Neurol 2007;22(6):700–13.
79. Lainhart J, Bigler E, Bocian M, et al. Head circumference and height in autism: a study by the Collaborative Program of Excellence in Autism. Am J Med Genet A 2006;140(21):2257–74.
80. Muhle R, Trentacoste S, Rapin S. The genetics of autism. Pediatrics 2004;113: e472–86.
81. Young D, Bebbington A, Anderson A, et al. The diagnosis of autism in a female: could it be Rett syndrome? Eur J Pediatr 2008;167(6):661–9.
82. Zafeiriou D, Ververi A, Vargiami E. Childhood autism and associated comorbidities. Brain Dev 2007;29(5):257–72.
83. Asano E, Chugani D, Muzik O, et al. Autism in tuberous sclerosis complex is related to both cortical and subcortical dysfunction. Neurology 2001;57(7):1269–77.
84. Baker P, Piven J, Sato Y. Autism and tuberous sclerosis complex: prevalence and clinical features. J Autism Dev Disord 1998;28(4):279–85.
85. Veenstra-VenderWeele J, Cook E. Molecular genetics of autism spectrum disorder. Mol Psychiatry 2004;9(9):819–32.
86. Berger B, Navar-Boggan A, Omer S. Congenital rubella syndrome and autism spectrum disorder prevented by rubella vaccination-United States, 2001-2010. BMC Public Health 2011;11(1):340.
87. Johansson M, Wentz E, Fernell E, et al. Autistic spectrum disorders in Mobius sequence: a comprehensive study of 25 individuals. Dev Med Child Neurol 2001;43(5):338–45.
88. Kent L, Evans J, Paul M, et al. Comorbidity of autistic spectrum disorders in children with down syndrome. Dev Med Child Neurol 1999;41(3):153–8.
89. Howlin P, Karpf J, Turk J. Behavioural characteristics and autistic features in individuals with Cohen syndrome. Eur Child Adolesc Psychiatry 2005;14(2):57–64.
90. Butler M, Dasouki M, Zhou X, et al. Subset of individuals with autism spectrum disorders and extreme macrocephaly associated with germline PTEN tumour suppressor gene mutations. J Med Genet 2005;42(4):318–21.
91. Manzi B, Loizzo A, Giana G, et al. Autism and metabolic diseases. J Child Neurol 2008;23(3):307–14.
92. Niklasson L, Rasmussen P, Oskarsdottir S, et al. Autism, ADHD, mental retardation and behavior problems in 100 individuals with 22q11 deletion syndrome. Res Dev Disabil 2009;30(4):763–73.
93. Xu S, Han J, Morales A, et al. Characterization of 11p14-p12 deletion in WAGR syndrome by array CGH for identifying genes contributing to mental retardation and autism. Cytogenet Genome Res 2008;122(2):181–7.

94. Boulet S, Boyle C, Schieve L. Health care use and health and functional impact of developmental disabilities among US children. Arch Pediatr Adolesc Med 2009;163(1):19–26.
95. Ben Itzchak E, Lahat E, Burgin R, et al. Cognitive, behavior and intervention outcome in young children with autism. Res Dev Disabil 2008;29(5):447–58.
96. Mouridsen S, Bronnum-Hansen H, Rich B, et al. Mortality and causes of death in autism spectrum disorders: an update. Autism 2008;12(4):403–14.
97. Gillberg C, Billstedt E, Sundh V, et al. Mortality in autism: a prospective longitudinal community-based study. J Autism Dev Disord 2010;40(3):352–7.
98. White S, Ollendick T, Bray B. College students on the autism spectrum: prevalence and associated problems. Autism 2011. [Epub ahead of print].
99. Tuchman R, Rapin I, Shinnar S. Autistic and dysphasic children. I: clinical characteristics. Pediatrics 1991;88(6):1211–8.
100. De Jong M, Punt M, De Groot E, et al. Minor neurological dysfunction in children with autism spectrum disorder. Dev Med Child Neurol 2011;53(7):641–6.
101. Jansiewicz E, Goldberg M, Newschaffer C, et al. Motor signs distinguish children with high functioning autism and Asperger's syndrome from controls. J Autism Dev Disord 2006;36(5):613–21.
102. Danielsson S, Gillberg I, Billstedt E, et al. Epilepsy in young adults with autism: a prospective population-based follow-up study of 120 individuals diagnosed in childhood. Epilsepsia 2005;46(6):918–23.
103. Amiet C, Gourfinkel-An I, Bouzamondo A, et al. Epilepsy in autism is associated with intellectual disability and gender: evidence from meta-analysis. Biol Psychiatry 2008;64(7):577–82.
104. Pickett J, Xiu E, Tuchman R, et al. Mortality in individuals with autism, with and without epilepsy. J Child Neurol 2011;26(8):932–9.
105. Pickett J, Paculdo D, Shavelle R, et al. 1998-2002 update on "causes of death in autism." J Autism Dev Disord 2006;36(2):287–8.
106. Billstedt E, Gillberg I, Gillberg C. Autism after adolescence: population-based 13- to 22-year follow-up study of 120 individuals with autism diagnosed in childhood. J Autism Dev Disord 2005;35(3):351–60.

Neurobiological Basis of Autism

Wendy G. Silver, MD, MA[a,b,c,*], Isabelle Rapin, MD[a,b,d]

KEYWORDS

- Autism • Neurology • Epilepsy • Sleep • Sensorimotor

DIAGNOSTIC ISSUES

Autism, used here as short for autism spectrum disorders (ASDs), is not a disease as it does not have a unique biologic cause. It is a behaviorally defined syndrome of early life, with varied symptoms reflecting many biologic and environmental influences that are unique to each individual's brain and that shape its unique developmental trajectory. The goal of neurologic, genetic, electrophysiologic, imaging, and other biologic tests performed on some of the children is not to diagnose autism but to attempt to define some of its many potential etiologies and understand their pathogenic effects on the brain.

Currently, the defining deficits of ASDs involve social skills, communicative language and imagination, and narrowness of focus resulting in rigidity, preoccupations, and repetitive movements (motor stereotypies) and speech. People with autism have many other symptoms besides these core characteristics, in particular uneven intellectual abilities, depending on the extent and distribution of their affected brain circuitry.

The diagnosis of autism and its subtypes is dimensional, not dichotomous (yes/no). It is based on the severity of affected individuals' symptoms, for example number of aberrant behaviors endorsed on a standardized checklist or clinical evaluation. Diagnostic cutoffs were arrived at by multidisciplinary field trials. As in obesity, diabetes, and many other multifactorial conditions, there is quasiunanimous diagnostic agreement about persons at the center of the bell-shaped severity distribution. However, this is not the case for those in its 2 tails, where diagnostic margins are inherently fuzzy. At

---

The authors have nothing to disclose.

[a] Saul R Korey Department of Neurology, Albert Einstein College of Medicine, Bronx, NY, USA
[b] Department of Pediatrics, Albert Einstein College of Medicine, Bronx, NY, USA
[c] Neurology and Pediatrics, New York Medical College/Maria Fareri Childrens Hospital, Valhalla, NY, USA
[d] Rose F. Kennedy Intellectual and Developmental Disabilities Research Center, Albert Einstein College of Medicine, Bronx, NY, USA
* Corresponding author. Division of Pediatric Neurology, Children's & Women's Physicians of Westchester, 755 North Broadway, Medical Services Building Suite 540, Sleepy Hollow, NY 10591.
E-mail address: wendy_silver@nymc.edu

Pediatr Clin N Am 59 (2012) 45–61
doi:10.1016/j.pcl.2011.10.010
0031-3955/12/$ – see front matter

the lower end, where underlying brain dysfunction and intellectual impairment are severe, there is so much overlap between the autistic and intellectual deficits that deciding whether or not autism applies as the main diagnosis is contentious. At the upper end, especially when the autism is mild and intelligence is average or greater than average, there may be so much overlap with normalcy that the diagnosis of autism is often equivocal and, in some cases, a matter of expediency. Despite their inherent lack of rigorous yes/no diagnostic criteria, well-defined and agreed upon dimensional criteria have improved the diagnostic consistency of both medical and behavioral disorders. It is essential to keep in mind that autism is behaviorally defined and has no unique biologic cause. Consequently no single sign, symptom, clinical feature, and no specific cause (biologic or environmental etiology), gene, or neuropathology invalidates its diagnosis.[1]

In the October 2008 issue of the Pediatric Clinics concerned with developmental disabilities, members of our group discussed the differential diagnosis of autism. In this contribution, we focus on clinical evidence regarding its main neurobiological basis, anatomy and imaging, epilepsy, disturbed sleep patterns, and sensorimotor symptoms.

THE BRAIN IN AUTISM

In most cases, the cause of the ASD remains unidentified and can not be found within the anatomic, radiographic, electroencephalographic (EEG), biogenetic, or pathologic evidence that neurologists routinely depend on for clinical diagnosis. Newer research evidence points to the need for more data at the brain network, cellular, and biochemical levels if the common pathophysiology that links the multiple genetic and nongenetic disorders that underlie the ASDs is going to be understood (**Table 1**).[2–4]

Brain Anatomy and Imaging

Head circumference is generally normal at birth. On average, the velocity of brain growth exceeds norms in infancy and early childhood, then plateaus early so that most older children and adults have average brain volumes,[5] with exceptions at both ends of the distribution reflecting disparate pathophysiologies. Head enlargement has been linked to mutation of the PTEN gene[6] in a subset of carriers, without its mechanism of action being fully understood. Enlargement affects white matter radial (short) corticocortical intrahemispheric connectivity selectively,[7] which magnetic resonance imaging (MRI) tractography substantiates.[8] Dysfunctional longer white matter tracts, for example between the frontal lobes and basal ganglia, or cerebellum, basal ganglia, and neocortex, may contribute to narrow repetitive behaviors.[8] Interhemispheric connections (corpus callosum and commissures) and the normal focal asymmetries in gray matter may be affected as well.

On a microscopic level, abnormalities have been detected in the Purkinje cells of the cerebellum,[9] which plays a greater role in many cognitive functions than previously appreciated, the fusiform gyrus of the ventral temporal lobe (important for facial recognition), the amygdala (involved in fear and other emotions), hippocampus (required for short-term memory and learning), and limbic system, as well as the vertical minicolumnar structure of the neocortex,[2,3] among many others.

The mirror neuron system is proposed as contributing to the dysfunctional circuitry.[10] It consists of a set of neurons that are activated by both observed and imitated actions. Brain activity consistent with that of mirror neurons has been recorded by functional MRI in the human premotor cortex, supplementary motor area, primary somatosensory cortex, and inferior parietal cortex. In humans, their

Table 1		
Some brain areas implicated in neurologic networks associated with autism		
Lobe	**Putative Areas**	**Examples of Dysfunctions**
Frontal lobes	Prefrontal cortex	Executive skills, working memory, attention
	Inferior frontal (Brocca) area	Expressive language
	Primary and supplementary motor areas	Motor skills
	Orbital frontal cortex	Repetitive, ritualistic behaviors
Temporal lobes	Superior temporal gyrus, Wernicke area	Auditory processing, language comprehension
	Fusiform gyrus	Facial recognition
	Hippocampus	Short-term memory, verbal, spatial learning
Parietal lobes	Postcentral gyrus	Somatosensory perception
	Posterior parietal lobe	Body image, complex somatosensory and spatial perceptions
Occipital lobes	Visual cortices	Visual perception
Insula	Insular cortex	Pain, smell, taste, autonomic perceptions
Limbic system	Cingulate gyrus, amygdala, septum, hypothalamus	Emotion, drive, affect, fear, aggression
Cerebellum	Vermis, hemispheres	Balance, gait, motor coordination and learning, language, cognition

Data from Refs.[2–4]

activation is not limited to motor actions but also contributes to complex activities like language, facial expression, and joint attention.[11]

To show gross anatomic findings and altered connectivity of the autistic brain requires MRI morphometry analyzed with complex statistical techniques, tractography, functional MRI, or, to illustrate neurotransmitter and other biochemical alterations, MRI spectroscopy and positron emitting tomography (PET) scanning. These techniques are for the most part research tools that have no role in the clinic, unless there is a specific clinical problem that calls for their use. In particular, an asymptomatic child with a big head does not require automatic computed tomography (CT) or MRI imaging. These spectacular new imaging technologies are research tools because they do not provide any evidence for or against an ASD clinically-defined diagnosis and rarely point to a specific cause (biologic or other etiology) for the autism. We strongly discourage routine brain imaging in the clinic without a compelling indication.

Neuropathology

There is a limited amount of brain tissue available for the neuropathologic study of ASD. However, propelled largely by parent groups, increasing numbers of samples from affected individuals who died accidentally and unaffected controls are being collected in tissue banks, notably the Autism Tissue Program (ATP; atp@brainbank.org), which assists postmortem tissue retrieval anywhere in the United States and ensures that the appropriate diagnosis and clinical data are obtained from the family. This resource is providing previously unavailable neuropathologic and genetic evidence on the pathogenesis of autism that complements information from behavioral, imaging, and electrophysiologic studies. Therefore, it behooves pediatricians and other physicians caring for affected children (and adults) to bring this resource to families' awareness. Some may want to volunteer and sign up in advance, just in case.

Thus far, no neuropathology specific to autism has been detected, which is not to say that there is none. The findings are at the cellular level and it is difficult to determine whether they arise from the particular cause(s) of the individual case or are the consequences of acquired disorders such as perinatal problems, epilepsy or its treatment, intercurrent infections, or trauma. Bauman and Kemper's[9] original findings were dropout of Purkinje cells in the cerebellum and stunted neurons in particular diencephalic pathways. The Pardo laboratory[12] attracted considerable attention when it reported increased microglial cells and inflammatory cytokines in some cases, especially because they seemed to confirm, on average, increased inflammatory cytokines in the cord blood of infants who went on to be autistic or intellectually impaired without autism.[13] Although there is extensive research on the role of potential infectious and immunologic contributors to autism, the significance of the findings remains unclear. Defining the neuropathology of autism therefore remains a high priority and research is in progress.

EPILEPSY AND AUTISM

Epilepsy is defined as at least 2 unprovoked clinical seizures. Seizures are stereotyped, brief (paroxysmal) interruptions of ongoing behavior, associated with a variety of involuntary motor and behavioral manifestations and electrographic seizure patterns.[14] Approximately 30% of children with autism have epilepsy by adolescence, and a substantial, but smaller, proportion of children with epilepsy are on the autism spectrum.[15] One disorder does not necessarily cause the other; it is more likely that both are the consequence of dysfunction in related underlying neural circuitry and, in some cases, have genes in common.[16]

There are 2 prevalence peaks of epilepsy in the ASDs population, 1 in early childhood and 1 in adolescence.[14,17] Approximately 6% to 7% of those with seizure onset in the first year of life go on to develop autism with intellectual disability.[18] Children with malignant epilepsies of infancy or seizure onset before 3 years of age are at particularly high risk for an ASD.[18] Those with infantile spasms, the most common of the infantile epileptic encephalopathies, are at especially high risk (35%) of developing autism[19,20] and intellectual disability.[21] It seems that autism is more likely in children with symptomatic epilepsy (epilepsy associated with identifiable structural or metabolic brain disorder and some genetic conditions).[22] Children with both ASD and epilepsy are at higher risk for developmental delay and intellectual disability than those with either disorder alone.[15,23] Severe intellectual disability is a proxy for the severity and extent of the underlying brain dysfunction, which itself is predictive of uncontrollable epilepsy (unless it is the expression of an untreated metabolic disorder affecting neuronal excitability).

The second peak of epilepsy, in adolescence, is poorly understood. It may encompass children with idiopathic ASD (children without a known brain disorder, or genetic or metabolic syndrome), whereas the onset of epilepsy tends to occur earlier in those with symptomatic autism.[18] The observation that the prevalence of epilepsy declines with age in individuals with static processes like cerebral palsy and intellectual disability but increases in those with an ASD raises the possibility of an ongoing degenerative process in individuals with autism and epilepsy, as is the case in Down syndrome.[17] Epilepsy generally persists into adult life, with remission reported in only 16% of adults with autism.[24]

There are several genetic disorders in which epilepsy is strongly associated with autism (see article by Toriello and Helga elsewhere this issue for further exploration of this topic). Whether epilepsy and autism are joint consequences of disorganized cortical development, or whether epilepsy is a major contributor to the autism, is debated. The most notorious of these genetic disorders is tuberous sclerosis complex (TSC), which accounts for 8% to 14% of the autism-epilepsy phenotype. Neurologists report high rates of epilepsy (60%) in TSC, half following infantile spasms, as well as a 50% risk of autism.[17,25] Three factors contribute to the risk of autism: tubers located in the temporal lobes, a history of infantile spasms, and seizures before the age of 3 years.[26,27] Infantile spasms in tuberous sclerosis are particularly ominous because at least half of the infants go on to develop autism, epilepsy with other seizure types, and variably severe intellectual compromise. How well the figures agree with population studies of TSC is uncertain because an unknown proportion of carriers of either of the 2 tuberous sclerosis genes may have minimal or no clinically significant neurologic or behavioral involvement. The partial dissociation between cognitive level, epilepsy, and autism underlines that these symptoms are not direct consequences of one another but have at least partially independent neurologic pathophysiologies.

Fragile-X and Angelman syndromes are also genetic conditions associated with intellectual impairment and a high proportion of autism, epilepsy, or both. Intellectual deficiency is almost always severe in Angelman, and more variable in fragile-X. In animals, loss of the fragile-X protein promotes excessive growth of immature-looking dendritic spines, alters the balance between excitatory and inhibitory neurotransmitters, and impairs synaptic plasticity,[28] findings that bolster the view of autism as a disorder of brain connectivity. Inhibiting the catalytic activity of a particular kinase improved spine morphogenesis and behavior in mice.[29] These experiments raise hope for future research-based novel treatment of fragile-X.[30]

Seizures in children with ASDs are treated by the well-established rules for the management of epilepsy. What to do about children with ASDs who do not have clinical seizures, even on long-term EEG monitoring, but whose EEG reveals epileptiform activity remains a dilemma. There is emerging evidence, particularly from animal models, that early-life seizures can alter the development of brain circuitry and neurotransmitter systems, contributing to cognitive and learning impairments.[31] One human study using magnetoencephalography (MEG) revealed abnormalities in almost all participants with early-onset autism despite having had no surface abnormalities on standard scalp EEG.[32] This finding raises the possibility that epileptiform EEG abnormalities in infants or toddlers is detrimental to brain development and plays a contributory role in fostering autistic symptoms, although there is still no definitive supporting evidence. There are no well-designed clinical trials that define a role for antiepileptic drug therapy to prevent or treat ASD symptoms. In particular, treating EEG epileptiform activity with antiepileptic drugs in the absence of clinical epilepsy does not reverse autistic symptoms.[24]

Seizure types depend on age and cause, and all seizure types have been reported in ASDs.[14] Seizure type or epilepsy syndrome dictates the choice of anticonvulsants in all children, including those with an ASD in whom behavioral side effects of medications have to be considered particularly carefully. Early identification and treatment of epilepsy in children who are at risk for an ASD may be the most effective approach to management. As already stressed, no empirical study shows that currently available antiepileptic drugs can prevent or improve ASDs. Early and aggressive treatment of infantile spasms and of seizures before the age of 3 years can improve outcomes, at least in infants with previously normal development.[33–35] If seizures do not come promptly under control, the children should be seen in consultation in an epilepsy center because other options such as vigabatrin, which has potentially serious retinal side effects, the ketogenic diet, or epilepsy surgery and other invasive treatments may have to be considered. These treatments must be combined with vigorous developmental interventions and therapies and with family support and counseling.

AUTISTIC/LANGUAGE REGRESSION AND EPILEPSY

Approximately one-third of parents report a developmental regression consisting of loss of whatever language had already developed, disappearance of the drive to communicate and share experiences, dwindling interest in playing with toys, and appearance of other autistic features. This regression, in some toddlers best characterized as developmental stagnation rather than regression, usually occurs insidiously between 15 and 30 months. In some children, it follows a nondescript illness, a move, or the arrival of a younger sibling. Because of much rarer but more dramatic loss of language in an epileptic context (discussed later), epilepsy seemed a plausible cause for autistic/language regression. A major problem is that children with regression rarely come to medical attention promptly, often because parents are falsely reassured. Studied at later random times, 10% to 20% of children with autistic regression without known epilepsy have an abnormal EEG, many with epileptiform discharges (spikes and spike/waves).[36] These abnormalities also occur in autistic children without regression, although less prevalently.[37] Antiepileptic treatment in the absence of clinical epilepsy is ineffective. Prognosis for language varies from extremely poor to recovery, but variably severe autistic features generally persist. Many potential mechanisms for a condition in which regression is usually followed by a prolonged plateau, then variable recovery, have been considered without real evidence thus far. Knowledge is unlikely to improve until children are referred promptly for thorough evaluation.

Other rare, perhaps overlapping syndromes in young children with regression are generally associated with dramatic EEG abnormalities that, so far, have not been shown to be causal.[38–40] The best known is acquired epileptic aphasia or Landau-Kleffner syndrome. It is always noticed when a preschooler with well-developed language stops talking or understanding language, in the context of either clinical seizures or a frankly epileptiform EEG strongly exacerbated during slow wave sleep. The children may be frustrated by their inability to communicate but are not autistic, strive to communicate nonverbally, and their nonverbal skills do not deteriorate. Treatment with anticonvulsants or steroids rarely brings about recovery, which may take months or longer and, in some cases, does not occur, leaving such children permanently aphasic for auditory, but not visual, language. Those who could read may communicate in writing, and some have acquired functional sign language or the use of an electronic sound device.

Electrical status epilepticus during slow wave sleep (ESES) describes an EEG pattern that shares features with Landau-Kleffner syndrome. ESES is occasionally found in a child without behavioral concomitant, but is more often associated with global regression. Few cases have been studied in depth so it remains poorly defined.

The most devastating of these overlapping regressive syndromes is disintegrative disorder. *Diagnostic and Statistical Manual of Mental Disorders DSM-IV-TR Fourth Edition (Text Revision)* (DSM IV-TR) defines it as language, behavioral, and cognitive regression occurring after the age of 2 years in a normally developing child who spoke in sentences.[1] It is the rarest of the pervasive developmental disorders (PDDs) and is almost never associated with a definable cause.[41] The regression is global, often involves such skills as toilet training and dressing, but is not associated with motor signs and not always with epilepsy. Prognosis for a meaningful recovery is dismal.[39] One of us evaluated a set of mute, indiscriminately hyperactive, identical twin boys said to be bright and multilingual before the regression who had made no progress between the ages of 5 and 14 years.

Progress depends on children with regression being studied vigorously at or close to the time of the regression. They need to undergo thorough medical/neurologic and neurobehavioral evaluations, searching for evidence of an immune disorder, EEG sleep monitoring, and in-depth genetic study. Regressive syndromes are biologically diverse. Progress in management will continue to stagnate unless their causes and effects on the brain are discovered.

SLEEP PROBLEMS ASSOCIATED WITH AUTISM

Sleep is a major issue in autism because between 44% and 83% of parents report problems.[37,42–44] These problems include failure to establish a regular 24-hour sleep cycle, resistance to going to sleep at bedtime, and difficulty maintaining sleep once it is initiated. In contrast, only 20% to 30% of typically developing infants and preschool children, and 11% of school-aged children, present with sleep problems.[45]

Besides insomnia and difficulty with sleep initiation and sleep maintenance, other sleep disturbances include parasomnias such as rapid eye movement (REM) and non-REM arousal disorders, rhythmical movement disorders, and periodic limb movements of sleep.[46–48] Wiggs and Stores[49] used sleep diaries from 69 parents, together with actigraphy (a device to record movement), to monitor sleep pattern; they confirmed the multiplicity of sleep problems in children with ASDs. Sleep disturbances were recorded even when parents had not identified them. Timing of sleep onset was late and final waking early; time to fall asleep and duration of nighttime awakenings abnormally long; the number of nighttime awakenings was high; sleep efficiency (time spent asleep/time in bed) was abnormally low; and the overall pattern of activity was unusual, either uniformly or episodically increased throughout the night.[49] These findings have been confirmed by EEG polysomnography and other actigraphy studies.[44,50,51]

Investigators divide sleep issues into 2 broad categories: behavioral (ie, poor sleep hygiene) versus circadian (biologic). Problems with sleep onset and limit-setting are the main contributors to poor sleep hygiene. The limit-setting type is exemplified by difficulty falling asleep and stalling/refusing to go to bed, followed by normal sleep quality and quantity once asleep. The sleep-onset type is characterized by sleeplessness unless certain conditions are met (eg, television on, parent present), followed by normal sleep quantity and quality.[49] Decreased awareness of social cues that tell typical children it is time for bed, together with hypersensitivity and hyposensitivity to visual, auditory, and sensory stimuli, may contribute to these problems in children with ASDs.[45]

The circadian system is controlled by genes that regulate the sleep-wake cycle. The suprachiasmatic nucleus of the anterior hypothalamus serves as the brain's master clock. It receives information about the 24-hour light/dark cycle of the environment through the eyes and melatonin secreted in the pineal gland.[52] Melatonin secretion is high during the night, low during the day, and unaffected by most external factors except for light. Mutations in clock genes in people with ASDs support abnormal circadian rhythmicity related to melatonin. Several studies report abnormally high daytime and low nocturnal melatonin in those with ASDs.[42,53] A 2010 review implicates abnormal melatonin secretion to explain an inverted circadian rhythm before puberty, and a trend in the opposite direction in older subjects with ASDs.[45] Delay in phasic melatonin secretion may underlie difficulties with sleep onset and reduced amounts secreted for problems with sleep maintenance.[53]

Cortisol tends to increase in the early morning just after waking and to decrease during the day to its lowest levels in the evening. Cortisol profiles seem to differ in children with ASDs. For instance, the morning peak may be displaced as well as drifting over time.[45] Corbett and colleagues[54,55] measured cortisol levels over several days and found that children with autism had a more variable circadian rhythm than age-matched typical children, and higher cortisol increases following exposure to a novel nonsocial stimulus.[54] In a 6-day study period, they recorded gradual flattening of morning cortisol peaks and evening decreases, as well as more variability in levels within and among people with ASDs.[55]

Asking about sleep in children with autism should be routine because multiple reports indicate that poor sleep is associated with poorer daytime behavior, which improves when the quality of sleep improves.[42,44,46,47,56] Parents and teachers of high-functioning children with autism and insomnia reported more autistic behaviors such as compulsive and ritualistic behaviors and hyperactivity than in good sleepers.[57] Waking after sleep onset correlated with hyperactivity and sleep fragmentation correlated with restricted/repetitive behaviors.[44] Good sleepers had fewer affective problems and better social interactions than poor sleepers.[46] Reed and colleagues[58] reported significant improvement in hyperactivity, stereotypies, and restricted and compulsive behavior in children with ASDs after behavioral intervention helped decrease sleep-onset delay and number of night awakenings. The link between poor sleep and difficult daytime behavior is well known in typically developing children; its implication for learning in children with autism is even more important given their inherent learning difficulties.

Treatment of sleep issues must be directed to the child's specific problem, whether behavioral, circadian, a medication side effect, sleep apnea, or it is comorbid with epilepsy. Parents' attendance at a sleep education workshop has fostered improvements in sleep-onset delay, sleep habits, and daytime behavior, but not nighttime awakening.[58] This type of intervention may be appropriate for well-structured families that wish to avoid medication for their children, as well as for children with inadequate sleep hygiene. It is inappropriate for children with difficulty maintaining sleep.

Great success with few adverse side effects is reported for the use of melatonin. Decrease in sleep-onset time with significant reduction in nighttime awakenings was reported in an open-label trial of controlled-release melatonin over 24-month follow-up.[56] Parents reported improvement in mood and daytime behavior as their children began to sleep more normally. A randomized, double-blind, placebo-controlled study of melatonin showed an increase in mean night sleep duration, a shorter mean sleep-onset latency, and an earlier mean sleep-onset time.[59]

In summary, difficulties with sleep are among the most common and burdensome complaints of parents of children with ASDs. The National Sleep Foundation has made treating them a priority. In a 2006 consensus statement, they agreed that pediatric insomnia needed to be addressed, potentially including pharmacologic means. Priority was given to both children with attention deficit hyperactivity disorder (ADHD) and to those with PDDs or ASDs.[60] Each child needs individual assessment of the sleep problem to tailor its rational management. A parental sleep diary and list of the child's medications for concurrent problems is a cheap and efficient way to start. Improvement in behavior with improved sleep should make treating sleep issues in children with ASDs a priority in general pediatric practice.

SENSORY ISSUES ASSOCIATED WITH AUTISM

Kanner in his original description drew attention to sensory abnormalities in autism. Today, many parents report sensory peculiarities early in their children's development.

Temple Grandin, PhD,[61] a woman with high-functioning autism, describes her unusual sensory experiences, including her delight as a child watching the movement of automatic doors and observing the shapes and reflections of tiny grains of sand, as well as her displeasure at experiencing light touch. A meta-analysis indicates that at least 50% of each included study's population reported sensory issues.[62]

Atypical sensory processing involves any or all modalities including vision, smell, taste, hearing, vestibular and somatosensory perception, proprioception, and kinesthesis (Table 2).[61,63–65] These sensory processing abnormalities may be overresponsivity or underresponsivity, the latter leading to sensory seeking like rubbing or licking the hands. A child may present with both blunting and oversensitivity in the same modality, notably to sound, for instance selectively responding to different pitches or kinds of sounds.[62,66–68] Atypical sensory behavior may contribute to stereotypic preoccupation with nonfunctional elements of materials; for example, sniffing or mouthing people or furniture, or chewing on inedible items such as clothing, a particular toy, or paper.

Although descriptions of sensory peculiarities in persons with ASDs abound, most studies suffer from small sample size and lack of controls. Oversensitivity, for example to clothes made of certain fabrics, is widely attributed to lowering of the threshold for

Table 2
Frequently described sensory processing abnormalities seen in autism

Sensory Input	Hyperresponsiveness	Hyporesponsiveness
Visual	Sensitivity to bright or flickering lights Gaze aversion Response to certain colors, eg, eating only certain colored foods	Staring at moving objects, eg, spinning tops, wheels, or sliding doors Impaired facial recognition
Olfactory	Avoidance of certain foods, people, or places because of odor	Unaware of unpleasant odor
Taste/sensory oral	Extreme food selectivity Refusal to brush teeth Avoidance of certain textures of food Avoidance of certain foods because of taste (difficult to separate from olfaction)	Overstuffing of the mouth Mouthing or licking inappropriate objects
Auditory	Intolerance to sounds, particularly loud or unfamiliar sounds (hyperacusis), eg, covering the ears	Ignoring sounds or voices (ie, acting deaf) Listening to the same sound (eg, music) repetitively
Vestibular	Motion or car sickness	Prolonged spinning or rocking Poor balance
Somatosensory	Intolerance of light touch Avoidance of certain textures of clothing Dislike of mushy textures	Remarkable tolerance to pain or cold Self-injurious behavior Need for deep touch
Proprioceptive/kinesthetic	Rigid, dystonic posture	Clumsiness or ataxic gait, poor balance

Data from Refs.[61,63–65]

touch despite almost complete lack of physiologic evidence. Frustration is probably appropriately blamed for self-injurious behaviors like biting of the hand or wrist and head banging, but without consideration that blunted pain sensation might be a contributing factor, especially if associated with seeming unawareness of cold.[67] There is no convincing explanation for children who peer at objects or wriggling fingers out of the corner of the eyes, a behavior that may be a marker for autism.[69] Gaze avoidance, also considered a key symptom of autism, consists of reluctance to look directly at another individual's face or eyes, and contributes to or may be a symptom of the social deficit of autism.[70] Hyperacusis is exemplified by the case of a teenage boy who stated that he needed sound-deadening headphones to be able to concentrate and tolerate his classes at school. This example contrasts with auditory under-responsiveness, exemplified by children who may appear deaf and unaware of their surroundings despite normal auditory function.[71,72]

Food selectivity is frequent, troublesome, and involves taste, smell, color, or texture. A review of the empirical literature of the last 25 years highlights that severe diet restriction may contribute to gastrointestinal (GI) problems and lead to nutritional deficiencies. For example, one of us examined a severely affected young man who spent his days sitting in a Jacuzzi tub and whose diet was so restricted that he was hospitalized with complications of severe vitamin deficiencies including corneal ulcerations and scurvy as well as appalling oral hygiene because of refusal to brush his teeth.

Sensory abnormalities persist lifelong, although hyporesponsiveness is stated to characterize toddlers and younger children and hyperresponsiveness and sensory-seeking older children and adults.[67,73,74] Atypical sensory responses are seen across the age and intelligence quotient (IQ) range but seem more clearly related to the severity of the autism in young than in older children.[67,71] Preliminary data suggest that restricted and repetitive behaviors are more likely in children who show sensory hyperresponsiveness than those with hyporesponsiveness even when controlling for mental age.[75,76] This suggests that sensory threshold may contribute to the pathophysiology of stereotypies.

Deficits in intersensory integration have long been reported by occupational therapists. Russo and colleagues[77] used event-related potentials (ERP) to find that the automatic integration of simultaneous auditory and somatosensory inputs is less extensive in children with ASDs than in typically developing children. The impact of this difference on the pathogenesis of ASDs remains to be determined.

Much work needs to be done before the neural basis of the many sensory peculiarities of autism is understood. It is unlikely that peripheral receptors or sensory nerves are dysfunctional. Deviant synaptic neurotransmitters or modulators of attention seem plausible but are unproven. There is no empirically proven treatment of the sensory issues associated with autism. However, parents can be a rich source of creative and thoughtful ideas on how to cope with them, as well as ways to shorten or decrease overreactions to stimuli.

MOTOR ISSUES ASSOCIATED WITH AUTISM

Motor abnormalities are prominent in autism, but are even more sparsely studied neurologically than sensory symptoms. The main motor findings include stereotypies, toe walking, low muscle tone/increased joint laxity, and clumsiness/dyspraxia. The neurologic basis of the motor findings in autism remain undefined (**Table 3**).[65,78–80]

Motor stereotypies are apparently purposeless rhythmical repetitive movements that are strongly enhanced by anxiety, boredom, excitement, sensory deprivation like blindness, or other environmental circumstances, characteristics they share

Table 3 Examples of motor findings associated with autism		
Deficit		**Examples**
Stereotypies	Arms	Hand flapping
		Finger tapping, twisting
		Shoulder shrugging
	Legs	Stamping feet
	Axial	Rocking or crunching
	Head/face	Head tilting or shaking
		Grimacing or lip pursing
	Sensory	Peering at object or fingers
		Mouthing or smelling objects
		Covering the ears
		Object manipulation
Gait		Toe walking
		Poor balance
		Decreased arm swing
		Poor bilateral coordination
		Walking over or into objects
Fine motor control	Dyspraxia	Difficulties with utensils
		Poor handwriting
		Difficulty tying shoes
		Difficulty buttoning
Hypotonia	Increased joint mobility	W-sitting

Data from Refs.[65,78–80]

with all movement disorders, including tics.[76] For many years, stereotypies were viewed as deliberately produced sensory-seeking or pleasurable self-stimulating behaviors, or as avoidance tactics. Recent studies view stereotypies as genetically influenced movement disorders modulated by environmental and endogenous circumstances. Support for an organic basis includes correlation of stereotypies with severity of the autism and cognitive impairment. We stress that they are not universal, but they do tend to persist lifelong, albeit sometimes in miniature form. They are assumed to involve basal ganglia, cerebellum, and cortical motor circuitry, although definite evidence is still lacking.

Most of the available evidence on stereotypies is indirect and garnered through parent interviews or questionnaires.[81,82] A recent study of videos of a large sample of school age children with stereotypies recorded during standardized play and scored blind as to diagnosis linked number and variety of stereotypies to young age, severity of the autism (gait and finger stereotypies), and low nonverbal IQ (head/trunk stereotypies). Atypical gazing at fingers and objects was rare but limited to those with autism.[79] Neurologic examination of the same children confirmed that stereotypies and motor impersistence distinguish high-functioning and low-functioning children with autism from nonautistic developmentally-disordered peers. The neurologists found that the inability/unwillingness to perform motor tasks in imitation or to verbal command in children with low IQ strongly suggested a diagnosis of autism.[78]

Many parents of children with ASDs cite motor delay, toe walking, and clumsiness as part of their initial concerns. Studies of gait[83,84] and postural stability,[85,86] as well as gross or fine motor skills, confirm what these parents have known for many years.[87–89] Although some children are agile, others have difficulty walking a straight line (ataxia) or have stride-length variability and postural abnormalities of the head and trunk. Stance on a tilting platform can bring out significantly larger sway, consistent with deficient integration of the visual, vestibular, proprioceptive, and other sensory inputs required for postural control.[85,86]

Dyspraxia refers to difficulty mastering intricate motor tasks. Many children with ASDs are very late learning to tie shoelaces, do up buttons, and put on clothing: clinicians should look at the child dressing after the physical examination. Having children write or copy their names or draw simple figures is a quick and easy way to test fine motor skills. A formal handwriting study showed that motor skills predicted children with ASDs' ability to form letters, which was worse than that of age-matched and intelligence-matched controls.[90] Handwriting difficulty persisted into adolescence but was then attributed to perceptual reasoning rather than poor motor skill.[91]

It is not clear whether the frequent hypotonia of autism, responsible for increased joint mobility in both large and small joints, is a function of cerebellar or other brain dysmaturation or to an associated genetic disorder of collagen. Involvement of large joints is indexed by sitting on the floor with the legs behind (W position), and of small joints by extremely flexible fingers. These findings may be independent of gross motor findings, are not a sign of motor weakness, and, in some cases, are familial (examine the parents!).

Children with motor difficulties are routinely prescribed occupational and physical therapy, which should be reserved for children in whom deficits are troublesome, provided they are likely to cooperate. Hypotonia typically does not respond to physical therapy, whereas children with dyspraxia and clumsiness in gross or fine motor skills, including gait and postural control, are likely to benefit from practice directed at the deficient skill, not to nonspecific sensory therapies like rocking or brushing. Teaching children with compromised penmanship to use a keyboard may raise their motivation and morale. Stereotypies are difficult to suppress, but parents who hate them because they are stigmatizing demand intervention. We recommend starting with behavioral approaches, which, in older children, may take the form of substituting smaller finger movements made in a pocket rather than arm flapping, for example. Parents have to be counseled to ignore stereotypies as much as possible, because asking the child to stop draws attention to them and reinforces them. Medications like small doses of risperidone or other psychotropic drugs are not effective and are best avoided unless stereotypies are very severe and interfere with the child's activities of daily living.

SUMMARY

The varied and complex symptoms of autism reflect atypical development of the immature brain affecting multiple widespread neural networks. ASDs and other developmental disorders, like psychiatric disorders of later life, are the behavioral phenotypes of this underlying brain dysfunction. All developmental disorders are strongly, but not exclusively, genetically influenced. Most cases arise from the interaction of genetics and environmental influences expressed as deviations from expected behavioral trajectories. The goal of genetic, electrophysiologic, imaging, and other biologic tests is not to diagnose autism but to attempt to define some of autism's many potential causes and to understand their pathogenic effects on the brain. The frequent neurologic comorbidities associated with ASDs, in particular epilepsy and sleep problems, should be treated early and as effectively as possible. Each child's work-up should be unique to that child: no protocol fits all.

REFERENCES

1. (DSM-IV-TR™, 2000). In: First MB, editor. Diagnostic and statistical manual of mental disorders. 4th edition. Washington, DC: American Psychiatric Association; 2000.

2. Abrahams BS, Geschwind DH. Connecting genes to brain in the autism spectrum disorders. Arch Neurol 2010;67(4):395–9.
3. Amaral DG, Schumann CM, Nordahl CW. Neuroanatomy of autism. Trends Neurosci 2008;31(3):137–45.
4. van Kooten IAJ, Palmen SJMC, von Cappeln P, et al. Neurons in the fusiform gyrus are fewer and smaller in autism. Brain 2008;131(4):987–99.
5. Courchesne E, Campbell K, Solso S. Brain growth across the life span in autism: age-specific changes in anatomical pathology. Brain Res 2011;1380:138–45.
6. Varga EA, Pastore M, Prior T, et al. The prevalence of PTEN mutations in a clinical pediatric cohort with autism spectrum disorders, developmental delay, and macrocephaly. Genet Med 2009;11(2):111–7.
7. Herbert MR, Ziegler DA, Makris N, et al. Localization of white matter volume increase in autism and developmental language disorder. Ann Neurol 2004; 55(4):530–40.
8. Verhoeven JS, De Cock P, Lagae L, et al. Neuroimaging of autism. Neuroradiology 2010;52(1):3–14.
9. Bauman M, Kemper TL. Histoanatomic observations of the brain in early infantile autism. Neurology 1985;35(6):866–74.
10. Rizzolatti G, Fabbri-Destro M. Mirror neurons: from discovery to autism. Exp Brain Res 2010;200(3–4):223–37.
11. Wan CY, Demaine K, Zipse L, et al. From music making to speaking: engaging the mirror neuron system in autism. Brain Res Bull 2010;82(3–4):161–8.
12. Vargas DL, Nascimbene C, Krishnan C, et al. Neuroglial activation and neuroinflammation in the brain of patients with autism. Ann Neurol 2005;57(1):67–81.
13. Nelson KB, Grether JK, Croen LA, et al. Neuropeptides and neurotrophins in neonatal blood of children with autism or mental retardation. Ann Neurol 2001; 49(5):597–606.
14. Kelly KR, Moshe' SL. Electrophysiology and epilepsy in autism. In: Tuchman R, Rapin I, editors. Autism: A neurological disorder of early brain development. 1st edition. London: Mac Keith Press for the International Child Neurology Association; 2006. p. 160–73.
15. Tuchman R, Moshe SL, Rapin I. Convulsing toward the pathophysiology of autism. Brain Dev 2009;31(2):95–103.
16. Sicca F, Imbrici P, D'Adamo MC, et al. Autism with seizures and intellectual disability: possible causative role of gain-of-function of the inwardly-rectifying K(+) channel Kir4.1. Neurobiol Dis 2011;43(1):239–47.
17. Tuchman R, Cuccaro M, Alessandri M. Autism and epilepsy: historical perspective. Brain Dev 2010;32(9):709–18.
18. Saemundsen E, Ludvigsson P, Hilmarsdottir I, et al. Autism spectrum disorders in children with seizures in the first year of life - a population-based study. Epilepsia 2007;48(9):1724–30.
19. Riikonen R, Amnell G. Psychiatric disorders in children with earlier infantile spasms. Dev Med Child Neurol 1981;23(6):747–60.
20. Taft LT, Cohen HJ. Hypsarrhythmia and infantile autism: a clinical report. J Autism Child Schizophr 1971;1(3):327–36.
21. Saemundsen E, Ludvigsson P, Rafnsson V. Autism spectrum disorders in children with a history of infantile spasms: a population-based study. J Child Neurol 2007; 22(9):1102–7.
22. Saemundsen E, Ludvigsson P, Rafnsson V. Risk of autism spectrum disorders after infantile spasms: a population-based study nested in a cohort with seizures in the first year of life. Epilepsia 2008;49(11):1865–70.

23. Amiet C, Gourfinkel-An I, Bouzamondo A, et al. Epilepsy in autism is associated with intellectual disability and gender: evidence from a meta-analysis. Biol Psychiatry 2008;64(7):577–82.
24. Levisohn PM. The autism-epilepsy connection. Epilepsia 2007;48:33–5.
25. De Vries PJ. What can we learn from tuberous sclerosis complex (TSC) about autism? J Intellect Disabil Res 2008;52(10):818.
26. Asano E, Chugani DC, Muzik O, et al. Autism in tuberous sclerosis complex is related to both cortical and subcortical dysfunction. Neurology 2001;57(7):1269–77.
27. Besag FM. The relationship between epilepsy and autism: a continuing debate. Acta Paediatr 2009;98(4):618–20.
28. Grossman AW, Aldridge GM, Lee KJ, et al. Developmental characteristics of dendritic spines in the dentate gyrus of Fmr1 knockout mice. Brain Res 2010; 1355:221–7.
29. Hayashi ML, Shankaranarayana Rao BS, Seo J-S, et al. Inhibition of p21-activated kinase rescues symptoms of fragile X syndrome in mice. Proc Natl Acad Sci U S A 2007;104(27):11489–94.
30. Hagerman RJ, Berry-Kravis E, Kaufmann WE, et al. Advances in the treatment of fragile X syndrome. Pediatrics 2009;123(1):378–90.
31. Brooks-Kayal A. Epilepsy and autism spectrum disorders: are there common developmental mechanisms? Brain Dev 2010;32(9):731–8.
32. Munoz-Yunta JA, Ortiz T, Palau-Baduell M, et al. Magnetoencephalographic pattern of epileptiform activity in children with early-onset autism spectrum disorders. Clin Neurophysiol 2008;119(3):626–34.
33. Riikonen R. Long-term outcome of West syndrome: a study of adults with a history of infantile spasms. Epilepsia 1996;37(4):367–72.
34. Jambaque I, Chiron C, Dumas C, et al. Mental and behavioural outcome of infantile epilepsy treated by vigabatrin in tuberous sclerosis patients. Epilepsy Res 2000;38(2–3):151–60.
35. Shields WD. Catastrophic epilepsy in childhood. Epilepsia 2000;41(Suppl 2): S2–6.
36. Tuchman RF, Rapin I. Regression in pervasive developmental disorders: seizures and epileptiform electroencephalogram correlates. Pediatrics 1997;99(4):560–6.
37. Giannotti F, Cortesi F, Cerquiglini A, et al. An investigation of sleep characteristics, EEG abnormalities and epilepsy in developmentally regressed and nonregressed children with autism. J Autism Dev Disord 2008;38(10):1888–97.
38. Trevathan E. Seizures and epilepsy among children with language regression and autistic spectrum disorders. J Child Neurol 2004;19(Suppl 1):S49–57.
39. Tuchman R. CSWS-related autistic regression versus autistic regression without CSWS. Epilepsia 2009;50(Suppl 7):18–20.
40. Ballaban-Gil K, Tuchman R. Epilepsy and epileptiform EEG: association with autism and language disorders. Ment Retard Dev Disabil Res Rev 2000;6(4): 300–8.
41. Rapin I. Autistic regression and disintegrative disorder: how important the role of epilepsy? Semin Pediatr Neurol 1995;2(4):278–85.
42. Johnson KP, Malow BA. Sleep in children with autism spectrum disorders. Curr Treat Options Neurol 2008;10(5):350–9.
43. Goodlin-Jones BL, Tang K, Liu J, et al. Sleep patterns in preschool-age children with autism, developmental delay, and typical development. J Am Acad Child Adolesc Psychiatry 2008;47(8):930–8.
44. Goldman SE, Surdyka K, Cuevas R, et al. Defining the sleep phenotype in children with autism. Dev Neuropsychol 2009;34(5):560–73.

45. Glickman G. Circadian rhythms and sleep in children with autism. Neurosci Biobehav Rev 2010;34(5):755–68.
46. Malow BA, Marzec ML, McGrew SG, et al. Characterizing sleep in children with autism spectrum disorders: a multidimensional approach. Sleep 2006;29(12):1563–71.
47. Liu X, Hubbard JA, Fabes RA, et al. Sleep disturbances and correlates of children with autism spectrum disorders. Child Psychiatry Hum Dev 2006;37(2):179–91.
48. Krakowiak P, Goodlin-Jones B, Hertz-Picciotto I, et al. Sleep problems in children with autism spectrum disorders, developmental delays, and typical development: a population-based study. J Sleep Res 2008;17(2):197–206.
49. Wiggs L, Stores G. Sleep patterns and sleep disorders in children with autistic spectrum disorders: insights using parent report and actigraphy. Dev Med Child Neurol 2004;46(6):372–80.
50. Allik H, Larsson JO, Smedje H. Sleep patterns of school-age children with Asperger syndrome or high-functioning autism. J Autism Dev Disord 2006;36(5):585–95.
51. Souders MC, Mason TB, Valladares O, et al. Sleep behaviors and sleep quality in children with autism spectrum disorders. Sleep 2009;32(12):1566–78.
52. Saper CB, Scammell TE, Lu J. Hypothalamic regulation of sleep and circadian rhythms. Nature 2005;437(7063):1257–63.
53. Richdale AL, Schreck KA. Sleep problems in autism spectrum disorders: prevalence, nature, possible biopsychosocial aetiologies. Sleep Med Rev 2009;13(6):403–11.
54. Corbett BA, Mendoza S, Abdullah M, et al. Cortisol circadian rhythms and response to stress in children with autism. Psychoneuroendocrinology 2006;31(1):59–68.
55. Corbett BA, Mendoza S, Wegelin JA, et al. Variable cortisol circadian rhythms in children with autism and anticipatory stress. J Psychiatry Neurosci 2008;33(3):227–34.
56. Giannotti F, Cortesi F, Cerquiglini A, et al. An open-label study of controlled-release melatonin in treatment of sleep disorders in children with autism. J Autism Dev Disord 2006;36(6):741–52.
57. Allik H, Larsson JO, Smedje H. Insomnia in school-age children with Asperger syndrome or high-functioning autism. BMC Psychiatry 2006;6:18.
58. Reed HE, McGrew SG, Artibee K, et al. Parent-based sleep education workshops in autism. J Child Neurol 2009;24(8):936–45.
59. Wirojanan J, Jacquemont S, Diaz R, et al. The efficacy of melatonin for sleep problems in children with autism, fragile X syndrome, or autism and fragile X syndrome. J Clin Sleep Med 2009;5(2):145–50.
60. Mindell JA, Emslie G, Blumer J, et al. Pharmacologic management of insomnia in children and adolescents: consensus statement. Pediatrics 2006;117(6):e1223–32.
61. Grandin T. Visual abilities and sensory differences in a person with autism. Biol Psychiatry 2009;65(1):15–6.
62. Ben-Sasson A, Hen L, Fluss R, et al. A meta-analysis of sensory modulation symptoms in individuals with autism spectrum disorders. J Autism Dev Disord 2009;39(1):1–11.
63. Kern JK, Trivedi MH, Grannemann BD, et al. Sensory correlations in autism. Autism 2007;11(2):123–34.
64. Rapin I. Atypical sensory/perceptual responsiveness. In: Tuchman R, Rapin I, editors. Autism: a neurological disorder of early brain development. 1st edition. London: Mac Keith Press; 2006. p. 202–30.

65. Rapin I, Tuchman RF. Autism: definition, neurobiology, screening, diagnosis. Pediatr Clin North Am 2008;55(5):1129–46, viii.
66. Baranek GT, David FJ, Poe MD, et al. Sensory Experiences Questionnaire: discriminating sensory features in young children with autism, developmental delays, and typical development. J Child Psychol Psychiatry 2006;47(6):591–601.
67. Leekam SR, Nieto C, Libby SJ, et al. Describing the sensory abnormalities of children and adults with autism. J Autism Dev Disord 2007;37(5):894–910.
68. Lane AE, Dennis SJ, Geraghty ME. Brief report: further evidence of sensory subtypes in autism. J Autism Dev Disord 2011;41(6):826–31.
69. Mottron L, Mineau S, Martel G, et al. Lateral glances toward moving stimuli among young children with autism: early regulation of locally oriented perception? Dev Psychopathol 2007;19(1):23–36.
70. Jones W, Carr K, Klin A. Absence of preferential looking to the eyes of approaching adults predicts level of social disability in 2-year-old toddlers with autism spectrum disorder. Arch Gen Psychiatry 2008;65(8):946–54.
71. Kern JK, Trivedi MH, Garver CR, et al. The pattern of sensory processing abnormalities in autism. Autism 2006;10(5):480–94.
72. Jones CR, Happe F, Baird G, et al. Auditory discrimination and auditory sensory behaviours in autism spectrum disorders. Neuropsychologia 2009;47(13):2850–8.
73. Lane AE, Young RL, Baker AE, et al. Sensory processing subtypes in autism: association with adaptive behavior. J Autism Dev Disord 2010;40(1):112–22.
74. Cermak SA, Curtin C, Bandini LG. Food selectivity and sensory sensitivity in children with autism spectrum disorders. J Am Diet Assoc 2010;110(2):238–46.
75. Chen YH, Rodgers J, McConachie H. Restricted and repetitive behaviours, sensory processing and cognitive style in children with autism spectrum disorders. J Autism Dev Disord 2009;39(4):635–42.
76. Boyd BA, Baranek GT, Sideris J, et al. Sensory features and repetitive behaviors in children with autism and developmental delays. Autism Res 2010;3(2):78–87.
77. Russo N, Foxe JJ, Brandwein AB, et al. Multisensory processing in children with autism: high-density electrical mapping of auditory-somatosensory integration. Autism Res 2010;3(5):253–67.
78. Mandelbaum DE, Stevens M, Rosenberg E, et al. Sensorimotor performance in school-age children with autism, developmental language disorder, or low IQ. Dev Med Child Neurol 2006;48(1):33–9.
79. Goldman S, Wang C, Salgado MW, et al. Motor stereotypies in children with autism and other developmental disorders. Dev Med Child Neurol 2009;51(1):30–8.
80. Gidley Larson JC, Mostofsky SH. Evidence that the pattern of visuomotor sequence learning is altered in children with autism. Autism Res 2008;1(6):341–53.
81. Lewis MH, Bodfish JW. Repetitive behavior disorders in autism. Ment Retard Dev Disabil Res Rev 1998;4(2):80–9.
82. MacDonald R, Green G, Mansfield R, et al. Stereotypy in young children with autism and typically developing children. Res Dev Disabil 2007;28(3):266–77.
83. Rinehart NJ, Tonge BJ, Iansek R, et al. Gait function in newly diagnosed children with autism: cerebellar and basal ganglia related motor disorder. Dev Med Child Neurol 2006;48(10):819–24.
84. Rinehart NJ, Tonge BJ, Bradshaw JL, et al. Gait function in high-functioning autism and Asperger's disorder: evidence for basal-ganglia and cerebellar involvement? Eur Child Adolesc Psychiatry 2006;15(5):256–64.

85. Fournier KA, Kimberg CI, Radonovich KJ, et al. Decreased static and dynamic postural control in children with autism spectrum disorders. Gait Posture 2010; 32(1):6–9.

86. Molloy CA, Dietrich KN, Bhattacharya A. Postural stability in children with autism spectrum disorder. J Autism Dev Disord 2003;33(6):643–52.

87. Provost B, Lopez BR, Heimerl S. A comparison of motor delays in young children: autism spectrum disorder, developmental delay, and developmental concerns. J Autism Dev Disord 2007;37(2):321–8.

88. Jansiewicz EM, Goldberg MC, Newschaffer CJ, et al. Motor signs distinguish children with high functioning autism and Asperger's syndrome from controls. J Autism Dev Disord 2006;36(5):613–21.

89. Nayate A, Bradshaw JL, Rinehart NJ. Autism and Asperger's disorder: are they movement disorders involving the cerebellum and/or basal ganglia? Brain Res Bull 2005;67(4):327–34.

90. Fuentes CT, Mostofsky SH, Bastian AJ. Children with autism show specific handwriting impairments. Neurology 2009;73(19):1532–7.

91. Fuentes CT, Mostofsky SH, Bastian AJ. Perceptual reasoning predicts handwriting impairments in adolescents with autism. Neurology 2010;75(20):1825–9.

Neuroimaging and Neurochemistry of Autism

Diane C. Chugani, PhD[a,b,*]

KEYWORDS

- Positron emission tomography (PET)
- Single-photon emission computed tomography (SPECT)
- Magnetic resonance spectroscopy (MRS) • Serotonin
- Dopamine • GABA • Receptors • *N*-acetylaspartate

Underlying the spectrum of autistic behaviors are multiple causes, only a small fraction of which have been identified. The reliance on this behavioral definition results from the lack of biologic markers for most individuals with autistic behavior and is a source of difficulty in the design and reproducibility of imaging studies of brain neurochemistry. Although there are various causes for autistic behavior, the possibility of alteration in common signaling pathways, shared by multiple causes of autism, seems be supported by new genetic studies.[1] Neurotransmitters in autism have been examined for more than 50 years. Methods for measuring neurotransmitters in autism have spanned biochemical measures of bodily fluids and postmortem brain, molecular imaging, and genetic measures of genes involved in neurotransmitter synthesis, transporters, receptors, and signaling pathways. There is some evidence for alteration in many neurotransmitters in autism. This review focuses on evidence for a role of altered neurotransmission in autism measured through neuroimaging techniques. The role of these neurotransmitters during different periods of brain development is discussed. Understanding the roles of each neurotransmitter in the brain across the lifespan and how those functions might be altered in autism will offer new routes for pharmacologic intervention in autism.

Neuroimaging technology has 3 primary tools to study neurochemistry in vivo: positron emission tomography (PET), single-photon emission computed tomography (SPECT), and magnetic resonance spectroscopy (MRS). Three neurotransmitter

[a] Carman and Ann Adams Department of Pediatrics, Division of Clinical Pharmacology and Toxicology, Children's Hospital of Michigan, Detroit Medical Center, Wayne State University School of Medicine, 3901 Beaubien Boulevard, Detroit, MI 48201 USA
[b] Department of Radiology, Children's Hospital of Michigan, Detroit Medical Center, Wayne State University School of Medicine, Detroit, MI, USA
* Division of Clinical Pharmacology and Toxicology, Children's Hospital of Michigan, 3901 Beaubien Boulevard, Detroit, MI 48201.
E-mail address: dchugani@pet.wayne.edu

Pediatr Clin N Am 59 (2012) 63–73
doi:10.1016/j.pcl.2011.10.002
0031-3955/12/$ – see front matter © 2012 Elsevier Inc. All rights reserved.

systems have been studied in autism spectrum disorders (ASD) using PET or SPECT imaging: serotonin, dopamine, and γ-aminobutyric acid (GABA). PET and SPECT make use of radiolabeled tracers to measure neurochemical metabolism and receptor binding. MRS involves the direct measurement of a small number of neurochemicals, including N-acetylaspartate (NAA), glutamate, glutamine, and GABA. Advantages of in vivo measures of neurochemistry over postmortem biochemical measures include the ability to take neurochemical measures and behavioral measures in the same individual, there is the possibility of longitudinal measures, and the issue of postmortem degradation and other effects of perimortem changes associated with mode of death is avoided. Structural imaging beginning with computed tomography (CT) and subsequently with magnetic resonance imaging (MRI) and studies of brain function by measuring changes of blood flow in the brain under different conditions, first by using oxygen 15 (^{15}O) labeled water with PET and subsequently by measuring blood oxygenation with MRI using a method called functional MRI, are beyond the scope of this review; recent reviews are available on these topics.[2,3] This review begins with a discussion of the neuroimaging technologies used to measure neurochemistry in vivo, followed by a review of neurochemistry in ASD studies with neuroimaging, and ends with a discussion of future directions.

PET AND SPECT METHODOLOGY

PET and SPECT are techniques that can measure and image the distribution of tracers that are designed to track biochemical and molecular processes in the body after intravenous injection or inhalation. This goal is accomplished by radiolabeling compounds of interest with positron-emitting or single-photon–emitting radionuclides. PET uses short-lived isotopes (most frequently used isotopes include fluorine 18 [^{18}F] with a half-life of 110 minutes, carbon 11 [^{11}C] with a half-life of 20 minutes, ^{15}O with a half-life of 2 minutes) that emit positrons during nuclear decay, which in turn collide with surrounding electrons, resulting in annihilation of both particles and the release of 2 high-energy (511 keV) γ-rays. The 2 γ-rays generated by a single event travel in opposite directions and are recorded by multiple pairs of oppositely situated detectors that constitute the PET camera.[4,5] For SPECT, single-photon–emitting radionuclides are used, in particular technetium 99m (Tc 99m) (half-life of 6 hours) and iodine 123 (half-life of 13 hours). SPECT imaging is performed using a γ-camera to acquire multiple two-dimensional images from different angles, and the data acquired are subjected to a tomographic reconstruction algorithm yielding a three-dimensional dataset.[6] Thus, the time course of changes in the distribution of the radiolabeled tracer in the body is recorded by the scanners after the radioactive decay of the radionuclide. Using the dynamic tissue time-activity data obtained in this manner and appropriate kinetic modeling of tracer behavior, physiologic parameters of interest (eg, receptor density, neurotransmitter synthesis rate) can then be calculated. Absolute quantification and estimation of relevant parameters of a given biochemical pathway in a noninvasive manner distinguish PET from SPECT when absolute quantification is difficult.

Many PET radiopharmaceuticals have been developed over the past 30 years for the study of normal physiologic processes and for application to the study of many disorders. More than 1400 PET tracers have been produced, and the rate of development of new tracers seems to continue in the exponential growth phase.[7] Radiolabeled tracers can be divided into several categories. The first group includes normal metabolic substrates or analogues of these substrates, such as glucose, amino acids, fatty acids, nucleotides, and oxygen.[8] Another group of PET tracers includes ligands that bind to proteins such as receptors and transporters.[9,10] Newer PET probes include antibodies, oligonucleotides, and tracers to image reporter genes to monitor gene therapy.[11,12] The traditional PET tracers were predominantly small molecules and were produced using synthetic chemistry techniques. These techniques have produced many specific tracers useful for clinical purposes. However, increasingly PET radiopharmaceuticals are being produced by bioengineering techniques, paralleling similar developments in the drug industry.[13] The PET tracers produced by these techniques are typically large-molecular-weight biotechnology probes. These techniques are often flexible enough to produce designer probes with the desired specificity, affinity, and other properties. Such targeted imaging can lead to imaging precise molecular abnormalities in humans in a noninvasive manner. However, these new technologies have been predominantly applied to disorders outside the brain, because the blood-brain barrier bars entry of these larger probes. Several groups of investigators are working on strategies for facilitating brain entry of these large-molecular-weight tracers. For example, targeting tracers to endogenous brain endothelial transporters such as carrier-mediated transporters, active efflux transporters, or receptor-mediated transporters has been attempted to improve brain tracer delivery.[14]

STUDIES OF NEUROTRANSMITTER FUNCTION WITH PET AND SPECT IN AUTISM

Given the number of radiolabeled probes available for the study of neurotransmission with PET and SPECT, it is surprising that few have been used in the study of autism. Studies investigating alterations in neurotransmitters with PET in autism have focused on dopamine, serotonin, and GABA.

DOPAMINE PRECURSOR AND TRANSPORTER STUDIES

Ernst and colleagues[15] studied 14 medication-free autistic children (8 boys, 6 girls, mean age 13 years) and 10 healthy children (7 boys, 3 girls, mean age 14 years) with ^{18}F-labeled fluorodopa (FDOPA) using PET. FDOPA is a precursor of dopamine, which is taken up, metabolized, and stored by dopaminergic terminals. Ernst and colleagues' calculated ratio of activity measured between 90 and 120 minutes after tracer administration in the caudate, putamen, midbrain, and lateral and medial anterior prefrontal regions (regions rich in dopaminergic terminals) to that in occipital cortex (a region poor in dopaminergic terminals). They reported a 39% reduction of the anterior medial prefrontal cortex/occipital cortex ratio in the autistic group, but there were no significant differences in any other region measured. These investigators suggest that decreased dopaminergic function in prefrontal cortex may contribute to the cognitive impairment seen in autism. More recently, the dopamine transporter was studied in children with autism (10 boys, 3–10 years) and 10 age-matched and gender-matched healthy children with the tracer Tc 99m TRODAT-1 (a tropane derivative) imaged by SPECT.[16] This study reported a whole brain increase in dopamine transporter binding in the autism group, whereas the striatum/cerebellum ratio showed no differences between the groups. Nakamura and colleagues[17] measured dopamine transporter binding in adults with autism (20 men, 18–26 years) using [^{11}C]WIN-35,428 imaged with PET. Dopamine transporter binding was significantly higher in orbital frontal cortex in the autism group compared with 20 age-matched and IQ-matched control subjects. Makkonen and colleagues[18] reported no difference in striatal dopamine transporter binding in 15 children with autism (14 boys, 1 girl; 5–16 years) compared with 10 nonautistic children using the tracer [^{123}I]nor-β-CIT, which labels both the dopamine and serotonin transporter, imaged by SPECT. Although this tracer labels both dopamine and serotonin transporters, the investigators made the assumption that binding in the striatum was predominantly due to dopamine transporter binding caused by the relative concentration of the transporters in this brain region. Together these studies suggest altered dopaminergic function in frontal cortical regions but not in striatum in children and adults with autism.

SEROTONIN PRECURSOR, TRANSPORTER, AND RECEPTOR STUDIES

Although there is evidence for the potential involvement of several neurotransmitters in autism, the most consistent abnormal neurotransmitter findings involve serotonin. Schain and Freedman[19] first reported increased blood serotonin in approximately one-third of autistic patients in 1961. Chugani and colleagues[20] applied α[11C]methyl-L-tryptophan (AMT) as a PET tracer in autistic children. AMT, which was developed as a tracer for serotonin synthesis with PET,[21] is an analogue of tryptophan, the precursor for serotonin synthesis. Two fundamentally different types of serotonergic abnormality were found in children with autism.[20,22,23] The first is a difference in whole brain serotonin synthesis capacity in autistic children compared with age-matched nonautistic children. Serotonin synthesis capacity was greater than 200% of adult values until the age of 5 years and then declined toward adult values in nonautistic children. In contrast, serotonin synthesis capacity in autistic children increased gradually between the ages of 2 years and 15 years to values 1.5 times the adult normal values.[22] These data suggested that humans undergo a period of high brain serotonin synthesis capacity during early childhood, and that this developmental process is disrupted in autistic children. The second type of abnormality reported relates to focal abnormalities in brain serotonin synthesis. Asymmetries of AMT uptake in frontal cortex, thalamus, and cerebellum were visualized in children with autism, suggesting a role of the dentatothalamocortical pathway in autism.[20] Subsequently, the same group measured brain serotonin synthesis in a large group of autistic children (n = 117) with AMT PET and related these data to handedness and language function.[23] Cortical AMT uptake abnormalities were objectively derived from small homotopic cortical regions using a predefined cutoff asymmetry threshold (>2 standard deviations of normal asymmetry). Autistic children showed several patterns of abnormal cortical involvement, including right cortical, left cortical, and absence of abnormal asymmetry. Groups of autistic children defined by presence or absence and side of cortical asymmetry differed on a measure of language as well as handedness. Autistic children with left cortical AMT decreases showed a higher prevalence of severe language impairment, whereas those with right cortical decreases showed a higher prevalence of left-handedness and mixed-handedness. These results suggest that global as well as focal abnormally asymmetric development in the serotonergic system could lead to miswiring of the neural circuits specifying hemispheric specialization.

Decreased serotonin transporter binding has been reported in both children and adults with autism. Makkonen and colleagues[18] using the SPECT tracer [123I]nor-β-CIT labeling both the dopamine and serotonin transporter described earlier, reported reduced serotonin transporter binding capacity in medial frontal cortex, midbrain, and temporal lobes. Similarly, Nakamura and colleagues[17] reported decreased serotonin transporter binding throughout the brain in adults with autism (20 men, 18–26 years) using [11C]McN-5652 imaged with PET. Furthermore, the reduction in binding in anterior and posterior cingulate cortices was correlated with impairment in social cognition, whereas the reduction in serotonin transporter binding in the thalamus was correlated with repetitive or obsessive behavior.

Serotonergic neurotransmission was also studied using tracers for receptor binding. Murphy and colleagues[24] measured 5HT2A receptors in 8 men with Asperger syndrome (mean age 26 years) using the SPECT tracer [^{123}I]5-I-R91150, compared with 10 healthy age-matched men. The group with Asperger syndrome had significantly reduced serotonin receptor binding in total, anterior, and posterior cingulate cortex, bilateral in frontal and superior temporal lobes and in the left parietal lobe. There were significant correlations with qualitative abnormalities in social interaction with binding reductions in anterior and posterior cortices, as well as right frontal cortex. Goldberg and colleagues[25] compared the parents of children with autism (19 parents from 11 families, 8 women, 11 men) with adults who do not have children with autism (9 women, 8 men). The cortical 5HT2 binding potential, using [^{18}F]setoperone, to measure cortical serotonin type-2 receptor (5-HT2) using PET, was significantly lower in the autism parent group compared with the control group. Furthermore, the 5HT2 binding potential was inversely correlated with platelet serotonin levels in the parent group. These results are interesting in light of family members having what has been described as the broader phenotype of autism.

Neuroimaging studies provide convincing evidence of altered serotonergic neurotransmission in both children and adults with autism. Altered serotonin synthesis, serotonin transporter, and serotonin receptors have been measured using PET and SPECT and different tracers in small groups of children and adults with autism compared with age-matched controls.

GABA$_A$ RECEPTOR BINDING STUDIES

Cytogenetic studies reported the abnormalities in chromosome 15 in autism, specifically 15q11 to 15q13, the region encoding several GABA$_A$ receptor subunit genes (GABRB3, GABRA5, and GABRG3).[26–28] Menold and colleagues[27] reported 2 single nucleotide polymorphisms located with in the GABRB3 gene in autism. Moreover, symptoms of autism can be associated with both Prader-Willi and Angelman syndromes, both of which involve alterations in the chromosome 15q11 to 15q13 region (for review see Ref.[29]). Deletion of the maternal chromosome in this region results in Angelman syndrome, which is characterized by severe mental retardation, epilepsy, a puppetlike gait, and lack of speech. Deletion of the paternal chromosome 15q11 to 15q13 results in Prader-Willi syndrome, which is characterized by mild or moderate mental retardation, hypotonia, obesity, and genital abnormalities. This region of chromosome 15 encodes GABA$_A$ receptor subunit genes GABRB3, GABRA5, and GABRG3.[27,28,30] [^{11}C]Flumazenil PET has been used to examine whether there are GABA$_A$ receptor binding abnormalities in patients with Angelman syndrome and Prader-Willi syndrome. Patients with Angelman syndrome with a maternal deletion of 15q11 to 15q13 leading to the loss of β3 subunits of the GABA receptor showed significantly decreased binding of [^{11}C]flumazenil in frontal, parietal, hippocampal, and cerebellar regions compared with a patient whose deletion did not include the GABRB3 gene.[31] Lucignani and colleagues[32] studied 6 adults with Prader-Willi syndrome and found decreased [^{11}C]flumazenil binding in insula and cingulate, frontal, and temporal neocortices compared with normal control subjects. Pearl and colleagues[33] studied 7 patients with succinic semialdehyde dehydrogenase deficiency with [^{11}C]flumazenil, compared with 10 unaffected parents and 8 healthy controls. Succinic semialdehyde deficiency is characterized by autistic behaviors, seizures, intellectual impairment, hypotonia, and hyporeflexia. Decreased GABA$_A$ receptor binding was lower in amygdala, cerebellar vermis, frontal, parietal, and occipital cortices in patients compared with both control groups. Thus, these imaging studies show decreased GABA$_A$ receptor binding in all of these genetic disorders in which autistic behavior is present. These studies show the usefulness of PET in elucidating the functional consequence of specific genetic abnormalities.

MRS METHODOLOGY

Unlike PET and SPECT, MRS does not require the administration of radiolabeled tracers. Instead, this neuroimaging technique exploits the magnetic properties of certain stable atomic nuclei within the brain tissue itself, such as hydrogen (^{1}H), phosphorous (^{31}P) and carbon (^{13}C). These nuclei, when placed in a magnetic field, align to the axis of magnetic field. The aligned nuclei are then perturbed by using a radiofrequency pulse that is absorbed by the nuclei and re-emitted, forming the MRS signal. This strategy allows the measurement of concentration of low-molecular-weight compounds within a volume of brain tissue. Dager and colleagues[34] have provided a more detailed review of this process. Because of the small signal, early studies used a single-voxel technique sampling a large volume of tissue. With improved methods and stronger magnets, most studies sample many, smaller voxels concurrently, a technique referred to as magnetic resonance spectroscopic imaging (MRSI). Few neurochemicals are present in high enough concentrations to be detected by this technique. These neurochemicals include NAA, creatine, choline, myoinositol, glutamate, glutamine, and GABA. The largest peak visible on the MRS spectrum in brain and the compound most frequently studied in autism is NAA. The role of NAA in brain function remains poorly understood, although it is generally regarded as a marker of neuronal integrity. NAA levels, like the neurotransmitters described earlier, change with brain development. There are large increases in NAA in the first 3 years of life, with smaller increases until adulthood.[35-37]

NAA STUDIES IN AUTISM

There have been a large number of studies of NAA in groups of children and adults with autism over the past 10 years, which are discussed in chronologic order. Most of those studies have reported decreased NAA throughout the brain. In an early, single-voxel MRS study sampling frontal lobe, temporal lobe, and cerebellum in 9 children with autism compared with 5 siblings, Chugani and colleagues[38] reported decreased NAA in the cerebellum in the group with autism. Furthermore, increased lactate level was reported in 1 boy with autism in the frontal lobe. In the same year, Otsuka and colleagues[39] measured NAA in voxels in the hippocampal-amygdala region and cerebellum in 27 children with autism (2–18 years) compared with 10 normal control children (6–14 years). These investigators reported significantly lower NAA levels in both regions in the group of children with autism. In a larger group of subjects (55 individuals with autism aged 2–21 years, 51 controls aged 3 months–15 years), Hisaoka and colleagues[40] reported lower NAA in temporal lobe regions, but not in frontal, parietal, cingulated, or brain stem regions. However, the control group included infants as young as 3 months of age. Because there are large increases in NAA in the first year of life, this study may not have detected real differences in these regions to inadequate age matching of the groups. In contrast to early studies of autism, a study of Asperger syndrome showed higher NAA in the medial prefrontal lobe of the Asperger group (14 adults) compared with 18 age-matched, gender-matched, and IQ-matched adults.[41] The increase in NAA was significantly correlated with obsessional behavior in the Asperger group. In the first report of multivoxel spectroscopic imaging in autism (45 3-year-old to 4-year-old children with ASD compared with 13 children with typical development and 15 children with delayed development), Friedman and colleagues[42] reported widespread reduction in NAA, as well as decreased creatine and myoinositol, in the group with ASD compared with both control groups. The first study directly addressing white matter in autism showed no difference in NAA in the left centrum semiovale between 21 children with autism compared with 12 healthy age-matched children.[43] Using MRSI, DeVito and colleagues[44] confirmed no difference in NAA in white matter, whereas they found widespread decreases in NAA in gray matter in 26 boys with autism (mean age 9.8 years) compared with 29 age-matched healthy boys. Also using MRSI, Friedman and colleagues[45] reported widespread decreases in gray matter NAA in 3-year-old to 4-year-old children with ASD, compared with age-matched typically developing children and a trend for decreased NAA compared with a group of children with developmental delay. In contrast to the previous studies showing no difference in white matter, Friedman and colleagues reported decreased NAA in white matter in both children with ASD and developmental delay, compared with the typically developing group. This difference may suggest a delay in the development of white matter in both groups. The most recent studies continue to confirm a decrease in gray matter NAA in groups of children and adults with autism,[46–50] although some studies have failed to find a difference in NAA brain concentration in ASD groups.[51,52] In a study combining MRS and fMRI, Kleinhans and colleagues[46] showed significant reductions in NAA in all brain regions combined, with a specific reduction in left frontal cortex. Furthermore, there was a significant positive correlation between left frontal lobe NAA concentration and frontal lobe activation measured during a letter-fluency word-generation task. In a study focusing on the thalamus, Hardan and colleagues[48] found a relationship between decreased NAA, phosphocreatine and creatine, and choline in left thalamus and sensory abnormalities in 18 boys with autism compared with 16 healthy children.

In considering the body of studies assessing NAA in ASD, there seems to be both widespread and particular decreases in the neurochemical in both children and adults with ASD. Although the function of NAA remains to be elucidated, it is clear that NAA is decreased in many neurologic disorders. Particular decreases in NAA affect brain regions showing particular decreases in serotonin synthesis, such as left frontal cortex and left thalamus.[20] Thus, changes in serotonin synthesis, NAA decreases, and fMRI activation all point to dysfunction of the corticothalamocortical pathway.

GLUTAMATE/GLUTAMINE IN AUTISM

Glutamate and glutamine are difficult to separate on the MRS spectrum, and so these compounds are often measured together in studies and reported as glutamate/glutamine or the Glx peak. In the first study of glutamate/glutamine in autism, Page and colleagues[53] found significantly higher glutamate/glutamine and creatine/phosphocreatine in the amygdala-hippocampal region, but not a parietal region, in a group of 25 adults with ASD and normal IQ, compared with 21 healthy age-matched and gender-matched adults. Whereas Page and colleagues reported increased glutamate and glutamine restricted to the amygdala-hippocampal regions, DeVito and colleagues[44] found widespread decreases in Glx gray matter, including in cerebellum, whereas there were no significant differences in white matter in 26 boys with autism (mean age 9.8 years) compared with 29 age-matched healthy boys. Most recently, Bernardi and colleagues[54] reported significantly reduced Glx in the right anterior cingulate in a group of 14 high-functioning adults with autism compared with 14 age-matched and IQ-matched healthy adults. Studies of glutamate and glutamine, as well as GABA, are still in their infancy because of the difficulty in separating the spectra of these 3 neurochemicals. Improved detection is expected as technology progresses.

SUMMARY AND FUTURE DIRECTIONS

In the 60-year history of the study of neurochemistry in autism, neuroimaging has been used for only one-fifth of that time to measure neurochemistry in vivo in children and adults with autism. These studies have only just begun to tap the surface of neurochemical measures possible. Future directions include the combination of imaging modalities made possible by advances in both software and hardware. For example, implementation of PET/MR is expected to be an important advance, particularly for pediatric applications. These modalities will allow both structural and neurochemical studies to be acquired in the same imaging session. For example, PET/MR could provide both presynaptic and postsynaptic measures of GABA function, MRS allows the measurement of GABA concentration in tissue, and [^{11}C]flumazenil allows the measurement of the GABA$_A$ receptor. Importantly for pediatrics, this neuroimaging technique will eliminate the need for 2 sedations and coregistration and will facilitate advanced image analysis procedures. Assessment of neurochemistry in vivo with neuroimaging has the potential, like no other imaging modality, to directly guide new pharmacologic interventions and provide biomarkers for predicting drug response.

REFERENCES

1. Bill BR, Geschwind DH. Genetic advances in autism: heterogeneity and convergence on shared pathways. Curr Opin Genet Dev 2009;19(3):271–8.
2. Anagnostou E, Taylor MJ. Review of neuroimaging in autism spectrum disorders: what have we learned and where we go from here. Mol Autism 2011;2(1):4–9.
3. Sivaswamy L, Chugani DC. Positron emission tomography. In: Hollander E, Kolevzon A, Coyle JT, editors. Textbook of autism spectrum disorders. Washington, DC: American Psychiatric Publishing; 2011. p. 395–408.
4. Hoffman EJ, Phelps ME. Positron emission tomography: principles and quantitation. In: Phelps ME, Mazziotta JC, Schelbert HR, editors. Positron emission tomography and autoradiography: principles and applications for the brain and heart. New York: Raven Press; 1986. p. 237–86.
5. Ter-Pogossian MM. Positron emission tomography. In: Wagner HN, Szabo Z, Buchanan JW, editors. Principles of nuclear medicine. London: WB Saunders; 1995. p. 342–6.
6. Kuhl DE, Edwards RQ, Ricci AR, et al. Quantitative section scanning using orthogonal tangent correction. J Nucl Med 1973;14:196–200.
7. Iwata R. Reference book for PET Radiopharmaceuticals. 2004. Available at: http://kakuyaku.cyric.tohoku.ac.jp/indexe.html. Accessed June, 2011.
8. Shiue CY, Welch MJ. Update on PET radiopharmaceuticals: life beyond fluorodeoxyglucose. Radiol Clin North Am 2004;42(6):1033–53.
9. Smith GS, Koppel J, Goldberg S. Applications of neuroreceptor imaging to psychiatry research. Psychopharmacol Bull 2003;37(4):26–65.
10. Gjedde A, Wong DF, Rosa-Neto P, et al. Mapping neuroreceptors at work: on the definition and interpretation of binding potentials after 20 years of progress. Int Rev Neurobiol 2005;63:1–20.
11. MacLaren DC, Toyokuni T, Cherry SR, et al. PET imaging of transgene expression. Biol Psychiatry 2000;48(5):337–48.

12. Jain M, Batra SK. Genetically engineered antibody fragments and PET imaging: a new era of radioimmunodiagnosis. J Nucl Med 2003;44(12):1970–2.
13. Weissleder R, Mahmood U. Molecular imaging. Radiology 2001;219(2):316–33.
14. Pardridge WM. Molecular biology of the blood-brain barrier. Mol Biotechnol 2005; 30(1):57–70.
15. Ernst M, Zamatkin AJ, Matochik JA, et al. Low medial prefrontal dopaminergic activity in autistic children. Lancet 1997;350(9078):638.
16. Xiao-Mian S, Jing Y, Chongxuna Z, et al. Study of 99mTc-TRODAT-1 imaging on human brain with children autism by single photon emission computed tomography. Conf Proc IEEE Eng Med Biol Soc 2005;5:5328–30.
17. Nakamura K, Sekine Y, Ouchi Y, et al. Brain serotonin and dopamine transporter bindings in adults with high-functioning autism. Arch Gen Psychiatry 2010;67(1): 59–68.
18. Makkonen I, Riikonen R, Kokki H, et al. Serotonin and dopamine transporter binding in children with autism determined by SPECT. Dev Med Child Neurol 2008;50(8):593–7.
19. Schain RJ, Freedman DX. Studies on 5-hydoxyindole metabolism in autism and other mentally retarded children. J Pediatrics 1961;59:315–20.
20. Chugani DC, Muzik O, Rothermel R, et al. Altered serotonin synthesis in the dentatothalamo-cortical pathway in autistic boys. Ann Neurol 1997;14:666–9.
21. Diksic M, Nagahiro S, Sourkes TL, et al. A new method to measure brain serotonin synthesis in vivo. I. Theory and basic data for a biological model. J Cereb Blood Flow Metab 1990;9:1–12.
22. Chugani DC, Muzik O, Behen M, et al. Developmental changes in brain serotonin synthesis capacity in autistic and nonautistic children. Ann Neurol 1999;45(3): 287–95.
23. Chandana SR, Behen ME, Juhasz C, et al. Significance of abnormalities in developmental trajectory and asymmetry of cortical serotonin synthesis in autism. Int J Dev Neurosci 2005;23:171–82.
24. Murphy DG, Daly E, Schmitz N, et al. Cortical serotonin 5-HT2A receptor binding and social communication in adults with Asperger's syndrome: an in vivo SPECT study. Am J Psychiatry 2006;163(5):934–6.
25. Goldberg J, Anderson GM, Zwaigenbaum L, et al. Cortical serotonin type-2 receptor density in parents of children with autism spectrum disorders. J Autism Dev Disord 2009;39(1):97–104.
26. Silva AE, Vayego-Lourenco SA, Fett-Conte AC, et al. Tetrasomy 15q11-q13 identified by fluorescence in situ hybridization in a patient with autistic disorder. Arq Neuropsiquiatr 2002;60(2-A):290–4.
27. Menold MM, Shao Y, Wolpert CM, et al. Association analysis of chromosome 15 gabaa receptor subunit genes in autistic disorder. J Neurogenet 2001;15(3–4): 245–59.
28. Buxbaum JD, Silverman JM, Smith CJ, et al. Association between a GABRB3 polymorphism and autism. Mol Psychiatry 2002;7(3):311–6.
29. Soejima H, Wagstaff J. Imprinting centers, chromatin structure, and disease. J Cell Biochem 2005;95:226–33.
30. Wagstaff J, Knoll JH, Fleming J, et al. Localization of the gene encoding the GA-BAA receptor beta 3 subunit to the Angelman/Prader-Willi region of human chromosome 15. Am J Hum Genet 1991;49:330–7.
31. Holopainen IE, Metsahonkala EL, Kokkonen H, et al. Decreased binding of [11C] flumazenil in Angelman syndrome patients with GABA(A) receptor beta3 subunit deletions. Ann Neurol 2001;49(1):110–3.

32. Lucignani G, Panzacchi A, Bosio L, et al. GABA A receptor abnormalities in Prader-Willi syndrome assessed with positron emission tomography and [11C]flumazenil. Neuroimage 2004;22(1):22–8.
33. Pearl PL, Gibson KM, Quezado Z, et al. Decreased GABA-A binding on FMZ-PET in succinic semialdehyde dehydrogenase deficiency. Neurology 2009;73(6): 423–9.
34. Dager SR, Corrigan NM, Richards TL, et al. Research applications of magnetic resonance spectroscopy to investigate psychiatric disorders. Top Magn Reson Imaging 2008;19(2):81–96.
35. van der Knaap MS, van der Grond J, van Rijen PJ, et al. Age-dependent changes in localized proton and phosphorus MR spectroscopy of the brain. Radiology 1990;176:509–15.
36. Huppi PS, Posse S, Lazeyras F, et al. Magnetic resonance in preterm and term newborns: 1H-spectroscopy in developing human brain. Pediatr Res 1991;30: 574–8.
37. Kreis R, Ernst T, Ross BD. Development of the human brain: in vivo quantification of metabolite and water content with proton magnetic resonance spectroscopy. Magn Reson Med 1993;30:424–37.
38. Chugani DC, Sundram BS, Behen M, et al. Evidence of altered energy metabolism in autistic children. Prog Neuropsychopharmacol Biol Psychiatry 1999; 23(4):635–41.
39. Otsuka H, Harada M, Mori K, et al. Brain metabolites in the hippocampus-amygdala region and cerebellum in autism: an 1H-MR spectroscopy study. Neuroradiology 1999;41(7):517–9.
40. Hisaoka S, Harada M, Nishitani H, et al. Regional magnetic resonance spectroscopy of the brain in autistic individuals. Neuroradiology 2001;43(6):496–8.
41. Murphy DG, Critchley HD, Schmitz N, et al. Asperger syndrome: a proton magnetic resonance spectroscopy study of brain. Arch Gen Psychiatry 2002; 59(10):885–91.
42. Friedman SD, Shaw DW, Artru AA, et al. Regional brain chemical alterations in young children with autism spectrum disorder. Neurology 2003;60(1):100–7.
43. Fayed N, Modrego PJ. Comparative study of cerebral white matter in autism and attention-deficit/hyperactivity disorder by means of magnetic resonance spectroscopy. Acad Radiol 2005;12:566–9.
44. DeVito TJ, Drost DJ, Neufeld RW, et al. Evidence for cortical dysfunction in autism: a proton magnetic resonance spectroscopic imaging study. Biol Psychiatry 2007;61(4):465–73.
45. Friedman SD, Shaw DW, Artru AA, et al. Gray and white matter brain chemistry in young children with autism. Arch Gen Psychiatry 2006;63:786–94.
46. Kleinhans NM, Schweinsburg BC, Cohen DN, et al. N-acetyl aspartate in autism spectrum disorders: regional effects and relationship to fMRI activation. Brain Res 2007;1162:85–97.
47. Endo T, Shioiri T, Kitamura H, et al. Altered chemical metabolites in the amygdala-hippocampus region contribute to autistic symptoms of autism spectrum disorders. Biol Psychiatry 2007;62(9):1030–7.
48. Hardan AY, Minshew NJ, Melhem NM, et al. An MRI and proton spectroscopy study of the thalamus in children with autism. Psychiatry Res 2008;163(2): 97–105.
49. Fujii E, Mori K, Miyazaki M, et al. Function of the frontal lobe in autistic individuals: a proton magnetic resonance spectroscopic study. J Med Invest 2010;57(1–2): 35–44.

50. Gabis L, Wei H, Azizian A, et al. 1H-magnetic resonance spectroscopy markers of cognitive and language ability in clinical subtypes of autism spectrum disorders. J Child Neurol 2008;23(7):766–74.
51. Zeegers M, van der Grond J, van Daalen E, et al. Proton magnetic resonance spectroscopy in developmentally delayed young boys with or without autism. J Neural Transm 2007;114:289–95.
52. Vasconcelos MM, Brito AR, Domingues RC, et al. Proton magnetic resonance spectroscopy in school-aged autistic children. J Neuroimaging 2008;18(3): 288–95.
53. Page LA, Daly E, Schmitz N, et al. In vivo 1H-magnetic resonance spectroscopy study of amygdala-hippocampal and parietal regions in autism. Am J Psychiatry 2006;163(12):2189–92.
54. Bernardi S, Anagnostou E, Shen J, et al. In vivo 1H-magnetic resonance spectroscopy study of the attentional networks in autism. Brain Res 2011;1380: 198–205.

Role of Endocrine Factors in Autistic Spectrum Disorders

Ruqiya Shama Tareen, MD[a,b,*], Manmohan K. Kamboj, MD[c]

KEYWORDS

- Autism • Autism spectrum disorders • Endocrine factors
- Endocrine hormones

Today the prevalence of autism spectrum disorders (ASDs) is reported to be between 3 and 6 per 1000, with a male-to-female ratio of 3:1 and a familial incidence of 2% to 8% in siblings of affected children.[1] This heightened awareness has been accompanied by a renewed interest and zeal to uncover underlying pathophysiologic mechanisms and to find possible causes of these disorders at multiple levels. However, thus far, the quest for etiologic predisposition for developing ASD remains elusive.

The bulk of the research in this area emerges from the knowledge about normal neurobiological development and its impact on normal social interactions throughout our life. Any effort to understand the neuromodulatory role of endocrine factors in the development of ASDs will be difficult without first establishing an understanding of the basic neurobiological mechanisms of social and behavioral neurodevelopment starting from early embryologic stages and continuing after birth and the important role played by various endocrine factors in it. Once the crucial role of endocrine factors and their effect on various stages and aspects of normal neurodevelopment process is understood, it will facilitate an understanding of the rationale for the search of a possible endocrine etiopathogenesis in ASDs.

A simplistic endocrine model proposes that there are chemical messengers, such as various neuropeptides, hormones, and hormonelike substances, which, along with neurotransmitters, such as serotonin, dopamine, and norepinephrine, facilitate the encoding of different social behaviors in the developing brain (**Box 1**). Therefore, any imbalance in this chemical transmission would lead to a defective encoding resulting in deficient or abnormal social behaviors that are the hallmarks of ASDs.

[a] Department of Psychiatry, Michigan State University College of Human Medicine, East Lansing, MI, USA
[b] Psychiatry Residency Program, Kalamazoo Center for Medical Studies, 1722 Shaffer Road, Suite 3, Kalamazoo, MI 49048, USA
[c] Section of Endocrinology, Metabolism and Diabetes, Nationwide Children's Hospital, 700 Children's Drive (ED425), Columbus, OH 43205, USA
* Corresponding author. Psychiatry Residency Program, Kalamazoo Center for Medical Studies, 1722 Shaffer Road, Suite 3, Kalamazoo, MI 49048.
E-mail address: tareen@kcms.msu.edu

Pediatr Clin N Am 59 (2012) 75–88
doi:10.1016/j.pcl.2011.10.013
0031-3955/12/$ – see front matter © 2012 Elsevier Inc. All rights reserved.

Box 1
Endocrine-related factors and neuropeptides investigated in autism

Hypothalamus

    Corticotropin-releasing hormone

    Thyrotropin-releasing hormone

Pineal gland

    Melatonin

Pituitary gland

    Growth hormone and related factors

    Oxytocin

    Vasopressin

    Apelin

Thyroid hormone

Intestinal neuropeptides

    Secretin

    Neurotensin

Adrenal medulla

    Cortisol

Gonadal steroids

    Testosterone

    Estrogen

Endocrine disruptors

Vitamin D

Basic facial expressions and social signals are universal and are beyond the boundaries of cultural and regional variations. Humans learn to process these signals both consciously and subconsciously by not only understanding their own feelings, intentions, and beliefs but also by realizing that the other person may have different feelings, intentions, and beliefs, thus, modulating their own social interaction in anticipation of the other person's response. This concept is a well-known psychological theory known as the theory of mind. It is a fundamental basis that one has to use for self-reflection and for coordinated social interaction.[2]

According to the theory of mind, we all have to invoke a mental state in ourselves to predict a social behavior by others. Most people with ASDs fail to understand the facial and emotional cues and real meanings associated with them and also exhibit differences in the processing of facial social cues when compared with controls matched for age, IQ level, level of education, and occupation.[3] Autistic children display qualitative impairment in reciprocal social interaction, inadequate understanding of social and emotional cues, along with a poor understanding and response to social signals.[3] A model of the endocrine contribution to social recognition and approach and avoidance behaviors is depicted in **Fig. 1**.

Neuronal activation patterns in the cerebellum and mesolimbic areas, especially in the medial temporal lobe, amygdala, hippocampus, insula, and striatum, were notably different in children with ASDs.[3] Several endocrine hormones are directly or indirectly

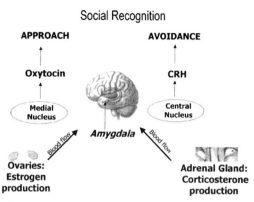

Fig. 1. One model of the endocrine contribution to social recognition and approach and avoidance behaviors. CRH, corticotropin-releasing hormone. (*From* Schulkin J. Autism and the amygdala: an endocrine hypothesis. Brain Cogn 2007;65:87–99; with permission.)

linked with the encoding of social behavior via their action at the amygdala, hippo-campus, and other related structures known to be involved in different aspects of social development.[4] Some of the hormones, which have been investigated in terms of their role in neurocognitive and neurobehavioral development, are discussed here.

GROWTH HORMONE AND RELATED FACTORS

The relationship between autism, growth hormone, and growth factors has been mentioned in the literature because of the role of neurotrophic factors, including insu-linlike growth factor (IGF)-1, in brain development. IGF-1 levels in cerebrospinal fluid of children with autism were noted to be significantly lower in children with autism versus controls indicating that there might be some pathogenic role of IGF-1 in autism.[5] IGF-1 is important in the normal development of cerebellum, and its deficiency may lead to cerebellar growth disruption. Riikonen has proposed "premature growth without guid-ance" possibly mediated by a disrupted IGF system as a possible neurobiological mechanism contributing to autism.[6] Children with autism are known to have larger brain size and brain volume. Rates of increase in head circumference of children with ASDs were compared with brain volume on magnetic resonance imaging. It was noted that the clinical onset of autism was preceded by a rapid and excessive increase in head size at 1 to 2 months and then also at 6 to 14 months of age.[7]

Mills and colleagues[8] further investigated whether children with ASDs only have a larger head circumference, whether they are also taller and heavier, and whether these growth measurements are correlated with higher levels of growth factors. Children with ASDs were found to have significantly higher levels of IGF1, IGF2, insulin-like growth factor binding protein 3, and growth hormone binding protein; significantly higher weights and body mass indices; and larger head circumferences; but no significant difference in heights was found in comparison with age-matched controls.[8] It has been suggested that accelerated head growth should be considered an early marker of ASDs.[9] Although this demonstrated a correlation, further studies need to be under-taken to explain the role of growth factors in the etiopathogenesis of ASDs, if any.

OXYTOCIN

Oxytocin hormone is known to play an important role in the regulation of social recognition, affiliation, bonding, and attachment. Because one of the main deficits in ASDs is social deficit, it is not surprising that many researchers have attempted to find if there is any causative link between oxytocin and ASDs. Animal studies have shown that oxytocin and vasopressin help regulate the social behavior of prairie voles, especially the formation of partner preference. Oxytocin receptors are more directly involved in social recognition and adaptation and are found concentrated in the olfactory bulb, lateral septum, amygdala, and piriform cortex. To further elucidate the effect of oxytocin on social adaptive behavior, researchers have developed oxytocin knockout (OTKO) mice. The OTKO mice have shown failure of social adaptation on repeated exposure, which supports the hypothesis that oxytocin is responsible for integrating the social olfactory information and facilitating the consolidation of social memory in the medial amygdala.[10]

Oxytocin has also been found to mediate feelings of trust in social interactions. This finding, in turn, promotes cooperation and interaction in social settings. Negative social emotions, such as fear and anxiety, can cause difficulties in social situations, and oxytocin is known to cause attenuation of amygdala activity, which leads to the reduction of negative feelings and anxiety associated with new or uneasy social situations, thus, promoting trustworthiness in these social situations. Oxytocin receptor gene (OXTR), located at the 3p25 region, has been researched in terms of a correlation with ASDs. A single nucleotide polymorphism of OXTR was found in children and adolescents with ASD.[11] Aberrant methylation, genomic deletion, or epigenetic inhibition of the OXTR gene may also play an etiologic role.[12,13] Peripherally circulating oxytocin may not serve as an accurate indicator of true oxytocin availability, but low levels of peripherally circulating oxytocin in children with autism were associated with poor performance on a cognitive test battery when compared with the control group. Children in the control group with a higher level of oxytocin correlated with greater social interaction and better daily living skills as compared with children with ASD.[14] When children with autism and Asperger syndrome were given an infusion of oxytocin, their autistic behavior decreased significantly.[15] The same group also showed that the social information retention also improved with oxytocin infusion in such individuals.[16] There is some evidence that the systemic administration of oxytocin improves emotion recognition and repetitive behavior.[17]

Most of the human studies, which showed a positive correlation of deficiency of oxytocin to the autistic behavior, were performed in a smaller number of subjects, and replications of results with a larger cohort are needed. Children with autism display qualitative impairment in reciprocal social interaction, inadequate understanding of social and emotional cues, along with a poor understanding and response to social signals, but whether or not deficiency in oxytocin is responsible for this presentation is still an open question.

VASOPRESSIN

Arginine vasopressin (AVP), commonly known as antidiuretic hormone, has a rich receptor distribution throughout the nervous system, especially in the nasal septum, cerebral cortex, hippocampus, and hypothalamus. AVP has been implicated in various psychiatric disorders, including depression, anxiety, schizophrenia, and autism. Two main types of vasopressin receptors have been implicated in ASDs: the V1a receptors (V1a R) and V1b receptors (V1b R). The V1aR gene has been associated with autism.[18] In animal models, V1aR and V1bR knock out (KO) mice showed impairment in social interaction when compared with normal mice; V1bR KO mice demonstrate a reduction in social motivation when challenged with olfactory discrimination tasks. The V1aR KO mice show a decrease in anxiety-related behavior and in depression.[18] Genetic studies have shown that the AVPR1a locus acts as a mediator of social behavior, but at this time the link between genes and related behavior is not well established.[19] Vasopressin in humans (males) is found to be associated with the generation of and reciprocation to social signals associated with courtship and aggression.

Intranasal vasopressin displayed sex-specific effects on corrugator electromyographic responses to same-sex faces after a single application in the group receiving AVP. The social communication facilitated by vasopressin was gender specific, and men and women under similar social stress used different social strategies. AVP facilitated agonistic responses in men and affiliative responses in women.[20] Multiple studies build up increasing evidence that both oxytocin receptors and AVP receptors may have an important role in the pathophysiology of ASDs, and some degree of polymorphism in AVPR1a receptor along with other neuropeptides receptors may be responsible to expression of autism and related disorders.[11,15,21,22]

APELIN

Apelin is a recently discovered neuropeptide, essentially an endogenous ligand for the G protein-coupled receptor, which can counteract the action of arginine vasopressin. The receptors for AVP and apelin are present together in magnocellular neurons of the hypothalamus. Boso and colleagues[23] have found significantly lower levels of apelin and high levels of AVP in patients with autism, again highlighting possible dysfunction in the AVP axis in the pathophysiology of autism.

MELATONIN

The pineal gland (or pineal body) is a small endocrine gland situated in the midline close to the third ventricle. It secretes melatonin, which is responsible for the recognition of photoperiod, adjustment of circadian and seasonal rhythm, sleep induction, and facilitating the immune response. Melatonin is studied in this context because about 44% to 83% of children with ASDs display various levels of sleep disturbances.[24] Some of the objective sleep disturbances noted in this population include longer sleep latency, more frequent awakenings, increased duration of stage 1 sleep, decreased non–rapid eye movement (REM) and slow-wave sleep (stages 3 and 4), and a lower number of rapid eye movements during REM, all of which results in an overall lower sleep efficiency.[25] Melatonin levels are found to be lower in 65% of children with ASD, which is attributed to the deficiency of the last enzyme in the melatonin pathway known as acetylserotonin O-methyltransferase (ASMT).[26]

Polymorphism in the ASMT gene located in the pseudoautosomal region of sex chromosomes lead to decreased transcription and, thus, a lower level of melatonin, about 50% of the concentration found in age-matched controls.[26,27] A genetic predisposition was proposed because unaffected parents of children with ASDs also showed abnormal melatonin levels in blood and platelets.[25] A study of about 400 patients with ASDs from Italy, the United Kingdom, and Finland showed several mutations in the ASMT gene.[28] Another study has also shown duplication of the ASMT gene in ASDs, which seems to be more common than other types of mutations. This duplication may cause a defect in the expression of the ASMT proteins in children with ASDs. Another important sleep-related observation in children with ASDs is a free-running sleep-wake cycle, which responds well to the exogenous administration of melatonin; however, large, controlled studies to consolidate this finding are not available.[29–31] It has been postulated that one of the initial events in the development of ASDs could be the disturbance of the sleep-wake cycle because of the deficient melatonin pathway. Melatonin is also known to impact synaptic plasticity, and its deficiency may cause a weaker neuronal network resulting in abnormal synaptogenesis.[26]

THYROID HORMONE

Fetal thyroid gland starts developing by third week, with thyroid hormone production starting by 10th week of fetal life. It is well known that adequate thyroid hormone levels are essential for the developing fetal brain and thyroid hormone deficiency during neurogenesis can adversely effect brain development.[32] Maternal thyroxine (T4) crosses the placenta and contributes to about 20% to 44% of the total thyroid hormone pool of the fetus. Thyroid hormones play several important functions in brain development, including granule cell proliferation in the cerebellum; granule cell apoptosis; mRNAs encoding nerve growth factor and neurotrophin, which influences neuronal migration; mRNA expression and translation of reelin, which encodes a large extracellular protein; glycogenesis; effect on astrocytes, which secrete laminin, a key guidance signal for the migration of neurons, synaptogenesis, and myelination.[33]

Rat models demonstrate that the unavailability of thyroid hormone at the time of active neurogenesis and of migrations of neurons into the cerebral cortex and hippocampus leads to irreversible damage to neurogenesis. It has been hypothesized, therefore, that disturbances in the thyroid hormone availability and metabolism during the critical periods of neural development may lead to behavioral disturbances as noted in ASDs.[33,34]

Thyroid-deficient animal models have been created to elucidate the effect of thyroid hormone in newborns by adding 0.02% propylthiouracil in the drinking water of rat pups from 0 to 9 days of age. Social and behavioral changes deviant from normal neurodevelopment were observed in the exposed rat pups, including hyperactivity, decreased habituation, hypersensitivity to auditory impulses, and impairment in spatial learning.[35] However, extensive data on the relationship of thyroid hormone and autism are not yet available.

CORTISONE

The hypothalamo-pituitary-adrenal (HPA) axis controls the secretion of cortisol from the adrenal gland by secretion of corticotropin-releasing factor from the hypothalamus and adrenocorticotropin hormone (ACTH) from the pituitary gland. The main function of cortisol is to facilitate the adaptation of the organism to environmental challenges, and secretion of cortisol is increased in times of stress. Cortisol has a well-established diurnal rhythm, with the highest peak in the early morning with another definite brisk peak of cortisol 20 to 30 minutes after awakening, which is known as the cortisol awakening response (CAR). The CAR seems to be under genetic influence in comparison with the diurnal variation of cortisol, which is under environmental influence.

The exact function of CAR is still not fully understood but several associations have been found with various psychiatric disorders. CAR is thought to be linked to the awakening process and to facilitate memory representations of the orientation of self, time, and place.[36] Impairment of CAR has been reported in children with Asperger syndrome versus a control group.[37] The impaired CAR could be the reason for children with ASDs having difficulties in coping with changes in environment and, thus, requiring a consistency in their environment and daily routines.[37] However, another study failed to replicate these findings when CAR was compared in 15 children with ASDs with 20 normally growing children.[38] However, other abnormalities noted in children with ASDs were delayed cortisol response to ACTH stimulation and an increased level of ACTH with normal or decreased level of serum cortisol. These abnormalities, along with findings of a delayed CAR response, may point toward a possible hyposensitivity of the adrenal gland to ACTH in children with ASDs.[37] Another study of 50 children with autism demonstrated elevated ACTH levels and low plasma cortisol levels in 10% of children, thus, indicating a low level of basal HPA activation. This finding was also strengthened by the fact that about 10% of this cohort also showed an inadequate cortisol response to exogenous ACTH administration.[39]

Corbett and colleagues[40] compared the response of the HPA axis in children with ASDs versus controls. They showed that children with ASDs showed decreased variability, a higher evening level of cortisol, and a decrease in morning cortisol over 6 days after exposure. Impairment of the limbic HPA (LHPA) was postulated. Children with ASDs demonstrated higher psychological measures of stress and sensory functioning.[40] A dysregulated LPHA axis was thought to predispose children with ASDs to atypical neurodevelopment resulting in typical behavioral issues seen in ASDs.[41]

TESTOSTERONE

ASDs exhibit a clear predilection for male gender; autism is 4 times more common in boys than girls. Asperger syndrome is more then 10 times more common in males. This finding caused the extreme male brain (EMB) theory. EMB built on the knowledge that the human brain has 2 important dimensions: empathizing and systemizing. Empathizing is the innate ability of a person to identify and understand another person's emotions and feeling and to reciprocate in an appropriate social manner. An average female responds to another person in a much more empathizing way, whereas in the normal male brain, systemizing is much more dominant than empathizing, although both genders can use systematizing and empathizing in appropriate social situations.[42] EMB proposed that in children with ASD, the systemizing is overdeveloped and empathizing is underdeveloped. It has been postulated that oversystemizing is the reason why children with ASDs display special abilities involving phenomenon that are predictable, structured, and mechanical; however, on the other hand, they struggle with the phenomenon, which is unpredictable and cannot be controlled or negotiated in a systemic, structured manner.[42] EMB theory has led the researchers to look for the possible role of testosterone in the cause of ASDs.

It has been shown that variance in androgen receptor gene encoding may predispose females to autistic disorders.[43] Digit span ratio (ie, second digit to fourth digit length ratio (2D/4D) is supposed to be fixed by the 14th week of gestation and serves as a proxy for the prenatal testosterone exposure to the fetus. The 2D/4D ratio is lower in males than females.[44] Boys with ASDs have been shown to have even lower ratios of 2D to 4D than boys of comparable age, indicating a higher level of prenatal testosterone exposure compared with the children without ASDs. The siblings and parents of children with ASDs also show more masculine digit span suggesting a genetic predisposition and familial tendency for elevated maternal testosterone levels during gestation.[45] The levels of free testosterone in amniotic fluid were measured in amniotic fluid of 129 participants (66 boys and 63 girls) and compared with the results of the psychological tests performed in children aged between 18 and 24 months.[46] Boys scored lower in variables, such as eye contact, preference of looking at the face, and vocabulary development. Testosterone levels were found to be associated with autistic traits in children aged 2 years or younger.[4]

Although this seems to be a robust association of testosterone with ASDs, it is difficult to prove causality unless one can manipulate the free testosterone in the womb, which is not possible. Children with autistic traits are thought to be sexually dimorphic, and high prenatal exposure to free testosterone predicts development of

ASD in children.[46] Adult women with ASDs in comparison with their normal counterparts were found to have an increased incidence of hirsutism, polycystic ovary syndrome, delayed puberty, irregular menstrual periods, and severe acne problems, all of which indicate a high androgenic state.[47] When mothers with children who had ASDs were compared with mothers of normal children, there was also evidence of a hyperandrogenic state, although it was less robust, suggesting that the children with ASDs may have a genetic predisposition to a hyperandrogenic state that may predispose them to ASDs.[47]

ESTROGEN

Estrogen facilitates the secretion of oxytocin, which has shown to play a central role in social development, including establishing trust, ability to take social risk, facilitation of bodily contact, and partner preference.[48] Any further direct role has not been implicated.

SECRETIN

Secretin is part of the secretin-glucagon peptide family and is produced by the secretory granules of S cells lining the mucosa of small intestine. Secretin has primary digestive functions but, like many other neuropeptides, also has autonomic endocrine functions in addition to having central nervous system (CNS) functions.[49] Secretin is also produced in the cerebellum, hippocampus, and the area postrema of the medulla, and its G-protein–coupled receptors are found in these areas along with other parts of the CNS, such as the cerebral cortex, brainstem, thalamus, amygdale, and striatum.

When 3 children with ASDs were given secretin in an effort to improve their gastrointestinal function, they showed improvement in language skills and behavior.[50] This finding, along with the knowledge that secretin has shown some effectiveness when used to treat behavioral problems in patients with schizophrenia, has led to a renewed interest not only in secretin but also in developing specific ligands for such neuropeptide receptors. Secretin-receptor–deficient mice have shown decreased synaptic plasticity in the CNS, especially in the hippocampus, and also demonstrate a significant reduction in long-term potentiation, akin to the process of consolidation of long-term memory, thus, suggesting an important role of secretin in cognition and memory.[51] The secretin-receptor–deficient mice also displayed impaired social recognition, rigid social phenotype, inability to retreat in the face of unfamiliar situations, and difficulty in reversal tasks, which are comparable to the difficulty in social interactions and stereotypic behaviors seen in children with ASDs.[51]

NEUROTENSIN

Neurotensin (NT), a vasoactive neuropeptide found in the brain and gastrointestinal tract, is known to play an important role in immunologic reactions and the inflammatory response in the gastrointestinal tract via its effect on mast cells, T-cell activation, lymphocyte proliferation, and the release of interleukin 1 from macrophages.[52] When vasoactive neuropeptide antagonists were given to pregnant mice during the critical embryogenesis phase, the male offspring developed a clear lack of sociability suggesting that this animal model may have some usefulness as a model of autism.[53] NT is released from the brain, dorsal root ganglia, and intestine under stress, which could be relevant to the finding of a higher incidence of prenatal stress in mothers of children with ASDs.

Serum samples were obtained from 19 children with ASDs and were compared with a control group of 16 healthy children. NT was found to be significantly elevated in children with ASDs. NT is a potent activator of mast cells, and children with ASDs are known to have significant problems associated with mast cell hyperactivation as indicated with a higher incidence of atopic and allergic disorders. In ASDs, these allergic reactions are not associated with the usual markers, such as immunoglobulin E elevation or positive skin allergy tests, implicating a nonimmune pathway of mast cell activation. A strong correlation of ASDs with mastocytosis (a rare disease of mast cell overproliferation) has been noted. Mastocytosis is 10 times more common in children with ASDs.[52] A higher concentration of NT in these children could be an indication of altered immunity and possibly brain inflammation, which may contribute to the development of ASD.[52]

VITAMIN D

It has been suggested that autism is linked with prenatal vitamin D deficiency. Dealberto and colleagues[54] looked at the prevalence of autism according to maternal immigrant status and ethnic origin regarding the vitamin D insufficiency hypothesis and found that black ethnicity was associated with an increased risk for autism. It was suggested that more work was needed to establish the effect of maternal vitamin D insufficiency during pregnancy on the fetal brain. Although the cause and effect is not established, 2 case reports of improvement in psychiatric symptoms with effective vitamin D treatment are noted.[55]

Epidemiologic evidence supporting maternal vitamin D deficiency as a risk factor for infantile autism was found by studying the birth month and prevalence with effective latitude for various countries, again suggesting vitamin D as a risk factor by possibly affecting fetal brain development and the state of maternal immunity.[56] Ferrnell and colleagues[57] analyzed and compared the effect of vitamin D in mothers of Somali and Swedish origin with and without children with autism and found low vitamin D levels in Somali mothers and even lower in the ones with children with autism.

DIABETES MELLITUS AND AUTOIMMUNE DISORDERS

There has been a recent report of increased prevalence of ASDs in a population of children with T1DM type 1 diabetes mellitus (T1DM).[58] A prevalence of autism of 0.9% in T1DM versus 0.34 to 0.67 in the control population was noted.[59,60] A common autoimmune pathogenesis is hypothesized. Mothers of autistic children were found to have higher incidence of autoimmune diseases in their families, along with findings of low helper-inducer cell number, and low helper to suppressor cell ratio, all indicating an autoimmune commonality.[61]

An increased risk of ASDs was also observed in children with a maternal history of rheumatoid arthritis and celiac disease as well as those with a family history of type 1 diabetes.[62] Forty six percent of families with autism reported having 2 or more family members with autoimmune disorders compared with only 26% of controls.[63]

The Danish National Registry also notes an association of infantile autism with a history of ulcerative colitis in the mothers and T1DM in the fathers.[64] However, contrary to these studies establishing a relationship of autoimmune diseases and autism, a study based on the Finnish Prospective Childhood Diabetes Registry found no support for the suggestion of a link between T1DM and ASDs.[65] Although the opinions are not conclusive, they bring up attention toward this possible association and indicate need for further research in this area.

ENDOCRINE DISRUPTORS

Endocrine disruptors, including polychlorinated biphenyls, perchlorates, mercury, and resorcinol, all may act as antithyroid substances.[66] Many of these agents work by inhibiting the D2 or D3 deiodinases or affect the hypothalamo-pituitary-thyroid axis. Multiple agents, including plant isoflavanoids, plant thiocyanates, tobacco smoke, and plant herbicides, can inhibit thyroid hormone biosynthesis in multiple ways. Any transient maternal hypothyroxinemia during the critical period of brain development may be caused by iodine deficiency, presence of antithyroid antibodies, or other environmental influences. The thyroid-stimulating hormone (TSH) and prolactin responses to thyrotropin-releasing hormone were measured in boys with autism and compared with boys with mental retardation and minimal brain dysfunction and controls. The TSH response was noted to be significantly lower in the boys with autism.[67] This finding led to the suggestion that there may be increased dopaminergic or decreased serotonergic activity in the brain, probably together with hypothalamic dysfunction, in children with autism.[67] However, other researchers have shown no correlation between neonatal thyroxine levels and neurobehavioral disorders.[68]

Older studies using triiodothyronine therapy in children with autism were also shown to offer no benefit.[69,70] The effect of some other environmental pollutants has also been looked at in a few studies. Windham and colleagues[71] tried to explore the possible associations between ASDs and environmental exposures in the San Francisco Bay area and found a potential association between autism and estimated metal concentrations and possibly solvents in the air. However, there was no relationship suggested in looking at the rates of attention-deficit/hyperactivity disorder and autism in Nevada counties in relation to the perchlorate content in the drinking water.[72]

SUMMARY

As evident from the previous writing, the literature regarding the etiopathogenic role of endocrine-related factors and ASDs is sparse and remains somewhat preliminary, controversial, and inconclusive. Many studies have tried to establish an etiologic connection between ASDs and the role of endocrine factors, whereas others are primarily epidemiologic studies establishing more of an association between the two entities. Most of the studies have built on the existing knowledge of the role of endocrine factors in neurodevelopment and psychology and in specific areas of concern in ASDs, such as social deficits, language facilitation, sleep pattern and circadian rhythms, behavioral maladaptations, and so forth. Most of the data are in the stages of preliminary observations, and a lot more research needs to be done in the future to clarify these complicated questions.

REFERENCES

1. Muhle R, Trentacoste SV, Rapin I. The genetics of autism. Pediatrics 2004;113(5): 72–86.
2. Leudar I, Costa A, Francis D. Theory of mind: a critical assessment. Theory Psychol 2004;14:571.
3. Critchley HD, Daly EM, Bullmore ET, et al. The functional neuroanatomy of social behavior: changes in cerebral blood flow when people with autistic disorder process facial expressions. Brain 2000;123:2203–12.
4. Schulkin J. Autism and the amygdala: an endocrine hypothesis. Brain Cogn 2007;65:87–99.

5. Riikonen R, Makkonen I, Vanhala R, et al. Cerebrospinal fluid insulin-like growth factors IGF-1 and IGF-2 in infantile autism. Dev Med Child Neurol 2006;48(9): 751–5.

6. Riikonen R. Insulin-like growth factors: neurobiological regulators of brain growth in autism. Current Clinical Neurology 2008;3:233–44.

7. Aylward EH, Minshew NJ, Field K, et al. Effects of age on brain volume and head circumference in autism. Neurology 2002;59(2):175–83.

8. Mills JL, Hediger ML, Molloy CA, et al. Elevated levels of growth-related hormones in autism and autism spectrum disorder. Clin Endocrinol (Oxf) 2007; 67(2):230–7.

9. Marz KD, Dixon J, Dumont-Mathieu T. Accelerated head and body growth in infants later diagnosed with autism spectrum disorders: a comparative study of optimal outcome children. J Child Neurol 2009;24(7):833–45.

10. Young LJ, Pitkow LJ, Feguson JN. Neuropeptides and social behavior: animal models relevant to autism. Mol Psychiatry 2002;7:S38–9.

11. Ebstein RP, Israel S, Lerer E, et al. Arginine vasopressin and oxytocin modulate social behavior. Ann N Y Acad Sci 2009;1167:87–102.

12. Gregory SG, Connelly JJ, Towers AJ, et al. Genomic and epigenetic evidence for oxytocin receptor deficiency in autism. BMC Med 2009;7:62.

13. Gurrieri F, Neri G. Defective oxytocin function: a clue to understanding the cause of autism? BMC Med 2009;7:63.

14. Modahl C, Green L, Fein D, et al. Plasma oxytocin levels in autistic children. Biol Psychiatry 1998;43(4):270–7.

15. Hollander E, Novotny S, Hanratty M, et al. Oxytocin infusion reduces repetitive behaviors in adults with autistic and Asperger's disorders. Neuropsychopharmacology 2003;28(1):193–8.

16. Hollander E, Bartz J, Chaplin W, et al. Oxytocin increases retention of social cognition in autism. Biol Psychiatry 2007;61(4):498–503.

17. Heinrichs M, von Dawans B, Domes G. Oxytocin, vasopressin, and human social behavior. Front Neuroendocrinol 2009;30(4):548–57.

18. Egashira N, Mishima K, Iwasaki K, et al. New topics in vasopressin receptors and approach to novel drugs: role of the vasopressin receptor in psychological and cognitive functions. J Pharm Sci 2009;109(1):44–9.

19. Donaldson ZR, Young LJ. Oxytocin, vasopressin, and the neurogenetics of sociality. Science 2008;322(5903):900–4.

20. Thompson RR, George K, Walton JC, et al. Sex specific influences of vasopressin on human social communication. Proc Natl Acad Sci U S A 2006;103(20): 7889–94.

21. Bartz JA, Hollander E. The neuroscience of affiliation: forging links between basic and clinical research on neuropeptides and social behavior. Horm Behav 2006; 50(4):518–28.

22. Bartz JA, Hollander E. Oxytocin and experimental therapeutics in autism spectrum disorders. Prog Brain Res 2008;170:451–62.

23. Boso M, Emanuele E, Politi P, et al. Reduced plasma apelin levels in patients with autistic spectrum disorder. Arch Med Res 2007;38(1):70–4.

24. Johnson KP, Malow BA. Sleep in children with autism spectrum disorders. Curr Neurol Neurosci Rep 2008;8(2):155–61.

25. Limoges E, Mottron L, Bolduc C, et al. Atypical sleep architecture and the autism phenotype. Brain 2005;128:1049–61.

26. Melke J, Botros HJ, Chaste P, et al. Abnormal melatonin synthesis in autism spectrum disorders. Mol Psychiatry 2008;13(1):90–8.

27. Jonsson L, Ljunggren E, Bremer A, et al. Mutation screening of melatonin-related genes in patients with autism spectrum disorders. BMC Med Genomics 2010;3:10.
28. Toma C, Rossi M, Sousa I, et al. Is ASMT a susceptibility gene for autism spectrum disorders? A replication study in European populations. Mol Psychiatry 2007;12(11):977–9.
29. Giannotti F, Cortesi F, Cerquiglini A, et al. An open-label study of controlled-release melatonin in treatment of sleep disorders in children with autism. J Autism Dev Disord 2006;36(6):741–53.
30. Sanchez-Barceló EJ, Mediavilla MD, Reiter RJ. Clinical uses of melatonin in pediatrics. Int J Pediatr 2001;2011:892624.
31. Anderson IM, Kaczmarska J, McGrew SG, et al. Melatonin for insomnia in children with autism spectrum disorders. J Child Neurol 2008;23(5):482–5.
32. Colborn T. Neurodevelopment and endocrine disruption. Environ Health Perspect 2004;112(9):944–9.
33. Howdeshell KL. A model of the development of the brain as a construct of the thyroid system. Environ Health Perspect 2002;110:337–48.
34. Morreale de Escobar G, Obregon MJ, Escobar de Rey F. Role of thyroid hormone during early brain development. Eur J Endocrinol 2004;151:U25–37.
35. Miyuki S, Kanai H, Xu X, et al. Review of animal models for autism: implication of thyroid hormone. Congenit Anom 2006;46(1):1–9.
36. Fries E, Dettenborn L, Kirschbaum C. The cortisol awakening response (CAR): facts and future directions. Int J Psychophysiol 2009;72(1):67–73.
37. Brosnan M, Turner-Cobb J, Munro-Naan Z, et al. Absence of a normal cortisol awakening response (CAR) in adolescent males with Asperger syndrome (AS). Psychoneuroendocrinology 2009;34(1):1095–100.
38. Zinke K, Fries E, Kliegel M, et al. Children with high-functioning autism show a normal awakening response (CAR). Psychoneuroendocrinology 2010;35(1): 1578–82.
39. Hamza RT, Hewedi DH, Ismail MA. Basal and adrenocorticotropic hormone stimulated plasma cortisol levels among Egyptian autistic children: relation to disease severity. Ital J Pediatr 2010;36:71.
40. Corbett BA, Mendoza S, Wegelin JA, et al. Variable cortisol circadian rhythm in children with autism and anticipatory stress. J Psych Neurosci 2008;33(3): 227–34.
41. Corbett BA, Schupp CW, Levine S, et al. Comparing cortisol, stress and sensory sensitivity in children with autism. Autism Res 2009;2(1):39–49.
42. Baron-Cohen S. The extreme male brain theory of autism. Trends Cogn Sci 2002; 6(6):248–54.
43. Henningsson S, Jonsson L, Ljunggren E, et al. Possible association between the androgen receptor gene and autism spectrum disorder. Psychoneuroendocrinology 2009;34(5):752–61.
44. Hönekopp J. Relationships between digit ratio 2D:4D and self-reported aggression and risk taking in an online study. Pers Individ Dif 2011;51:77–80.
45. Hönekopp J, Bartholdt L, Beier L, et al. Second to fourth digit length ratio (2D:4D) and adult sex hormone levels: new data and a meta-analytic review. Psychoneuroendocrinology 2007;32(4):313–21.
46. Auyeung B, Taylor K, Hackett G, et al. Foetal testosterone and autistic traits in 18 to 24-month-old children. Mol Autism 2010;1(1):11.
47. Ingudomnukul E, Baron-Cohen S, Wheelright S, et al. Elevated rates of testosterone-related disorders in women with autism spectrum conditions. Horm Behav 2007;51(5):597–604.

48. Choleris E, Gustafsson JA, Korach KS, et al. An estrogen dependent micronet mediating social recognition: a study with oxytocin- and estrogen receptor-alpha and –beta knockout mice. Proc Natl Acad Sci U S A 2003;100(10):6192–7.

49. Chapter MC, White CM, DeRidder A, et al. Chemical modification of class II G protein-coupled receptor ligands: frontiers in the development of peptide analogs as neuroendocrine pharmacological therapies. Pharmacol Ther 2010;125(1):39–54.

50. Horvath K, Papadimitriou JC, Rabsztyn A, et al. Gastrointestinal abnormalities in children with autistic disorder. J Pediatr 1999;135(5):559–63.

51. Nishijima I, Yamagata T, Spencer CM, et al. Secretin receptor-deficient mice exhibit impaired synaptic plasticity and social behavior. Hum Mol Genet 2006; 15(21):3241–50.

52. Angelidou A, Francis K, Vasiad M, et al. Neurotensin is increased in serum of young children with autistic disorder. J Neuroinflammation 2010;7:58.

53. Hill J, Cuasay K, Abebe D. Vasoactive intestinal peptide antagonist treatment during mouse embryogenesis impairs social behavior and cognitive function of adult male offspring. Exp Neurol 2007;206(1):101–13.

54. Dealberto MJ. Prevalence of autism according to maternal immigrant status and ethnic origin. Acta Psychiatr Scand 2011;123(5):339–48.

55. Humble MB. Vitamin D, light and mental health. J Photochem Photobiol B 2010; 101(2):142–9.

56. Grant WB, Soles CM. Epidemiologic evidence supporting the role of maternal vitamin D deficiency as a risk factor for the development of infantile autism. Dermatoendocrinol 2009;1(4):223–8.

57. Fernell E, Barnevik-Olsson M, Bågenholm G. Serum levels of 25-hydroxyvitamin D in mothers of Swedish and of Somali origin who have children with and without autism. Acta Paediatr 2010;99(5):743–7.

58. Freeman SJ, Roberts W, Daneman D. Diabetes and autism: is there a link? Diabetes Care 2005;28(4):925–6.

59. Devendra D, Liu E, Eisenbarth GS. Type 1 diabetes: recent developments. BMJ 2004;328(7442):750–4.

60. Bertrand J, Mars A, Boyle C, et al. Prevalence of autism in a United States population: the Brick Township, New Jersey, investigation. Pediatrics 2001;108(5):1155–61.

61. Denney DR, Frei BW, Gaffney GR. Lymphocyte subsets and interleukin-2 receptors in autistic children. J Autism Dev Disord 1996;26(1):87–97.

62. Atladóttir HO, Pedersen MG, Thorsen P, et al. Association of family history of autoimmune diseases and autism spectrum disorders. Pediatrics 2009;124(2): 687–94.

63. Comi AM, Zimmerman AW, Frye VH, et al. Familial clustering of autoimmune disorders and evaluation of medical risk factors in autism. J Child Neurol 1999; 14(6):388–94.

64. Mouridsen SE, Rich B, Isager T, et al. Autoimmune diseases in parents of children with infantile autism: a case-control study. Dev Med Child Neurol 2007;49(6): 429–32.

65. Harjutsalo V, Tuomilehto J. Type 1 diabetes and autism: is there a link? Diabetes Care 2006;29(2):484–5.

66. Román GC. Autism: transient in utero hypothyroxinemia related to maternal flavonoid ingestion during pregnancy and to other environmental antithyroid agents. J Neurol Sci 2007;262(1–2):15–26.

67. Hashimoto T, Aihara R, Tayama M, et al. Reduced thyroid-stimulating hormone response to thyrotropin-releasing hormone in autistic boys. Dev Med Child Neurol 1991;33(4):313–9.

68. Soldin OP, Lai S, Lamm SH, et al. Lack of a relation between human neonatal thyroxine and pediatric neurobehavioral disorders. Thyroid 2003;13(2):193–8.

69. Campbell M, Small AM, Hollander CS, et al. A controlled crossover study of triiodothyronine in autistic children. J Autism Child Schizophr 1978;8(4):371–81.

70. Abbassi V, Linscheid T, Coleman M. Triiodothyronine (T3) concentration and therapy in autistic children. J Autism Child Schizophr 1978;8(4):383–7.

71. Windham GC, Zhang L, Gunier R, et al. Autism spectrum disorders in relation to distribution of hazardous air pollutants in the San Francisco Bay area. Environ Health Perspect 2006;114(9):1438–44.

72. Chang S, Crothers C, Lai S, et al. Pediatric neurobehavioral diseases in Nevada counties with respect to perchlorate in drinking water: an ecological inquiry. Birth Defects Res A Clin Mol Teratol 2003;67(10):886–92.

Office Screening and Early Identification of Children with Autism

Neelkamal S. Soares, MD[a,b], Dilip R. Patel, MD[c,d],*

KEYWORDS

• Screening • Early identification • Autism • Pediatrician's role

Given the increasing media coverage of autism over the last decade and increasing awareness among professionals and lay persons, in part due to the Centers for Disease Control and Prevention (CDC) *Learn the Signs, Act Early* campaign (a collaboration of the CDC National Center on Birth Defects and Developmental Disabilities, American Academy of Pediatrics [AAP], Autism Speaks, First Signs, Autism Society of America, and Organization for Autism Research), autism has emerged into the mainstream consciousness and is no longer considered a rare disorder as it once was (5.2:10,000).[1–6] However, with the prevalence now estimated at 1 in 110, it is more than likely that every pediatrician, family practitioner, and nurse practitioner who provides care for children will encounter at least one child diagnosed with (or suspected of having) autism in the course of well-child and sick care.[7] Often, the pediatrician is the first professional the parents or caregivers approach with concerns about their child's development and suspicion of autism. Pediatricians are in an advantageous position of having multiple encounters for developmental surveillance.[8,9]

There is no lack of information when it comes to professional education about autism screening, diagnosis, and interventions. The AAP has published comprehensive practice guidelines and an autism tool kit.[4,10,11] Among grassroots organizations, Autism Speaks and First Signs provide information on autism mainly for lay persons,

---

The authors have nothing to disclose.

[a] University of Kentucky, 740 South Limestone, KY Clinic J-454, Lexington, KY 40536, USA
[b] West Virginia University, Morgantown, WV, USA
[c] Department of Pediatrics and Human Development, College of Human Medicine, Michigan State University, East Lansing, MI, USA
[d] Developmental and Behavioral Pediatrics, Neurodevelopmental Pediatrics, Pediatrics Residency Program, Michigan State University/Kalamazoo Center for Medical Studies, 1000 Oakland Drive, Kalamazoo, MI 49008-1284, USA
* Corresponding author. Developmental and Behavioral Pediatrics, Neurodevelopmental Pediatrics, Pediatrics Residency Program, Michigan State University/Kalamazoo Center for Medical Studies, 1000 Oakland Drive, Kalamazoo, MI 49008-1284.
E-mail address: patel@kcms.msu.edu

Pediatr Clin N Am 59 (2012) 89–102
doi:10.1016/j.pcl.2011.10.011
0031-3955/12/$ – see front matter © 2012 Elsevier Inc. All rights reserved.

but are valuable sources of information for professionals as well. The *Learn the Signs, Act Early* campaign aims to increase provider awareness of the importance of early intervention in diagnosing and managing developmental disorders including autism (**Table 1**).

Despite all this information, pediatrician surveys in 2004 revealed that only 8% actually screen for autism spectrum disorders (ASDs).[12] Although this increased to 42% in a survey in 2008, this is not close to the expectation that all children must be screened for ASDs.[13] One possible reason for the low screening rates may be unfamiliarity with the ASD screening tools.[14–20] There are currently practicing pediatricians who trained when autism was a rare condition, when no screening tools were universally available. Nowadays, pediatric residency programs have mandatory developmental-behavioral pediatric rotations, and there is a plethora of information regarding screening tools and identification. Ongoing training and awareness is a key for professionals to

Table 1 Resources	
Resource	**Materials for Physicians**
Autism Speaks http://www.autismspeaks.org	Nation's largest autism science and advocacy organization, dedicated to funding research; increasing awareness of ASDs; and advocating for the needs of individuals with autism and their families The Video Glossary (formerly under First Signs) demonstrates the phenotype and variations of social, communicative, and behavior symptoms in ASDs and how these vary from typical development. This is a helpful refresher not just for physicians, but also serves as a teaching tool for trainees and even parents and caregivers. It also contains video clips demonstrating different types of therapies available for children with ASDs
Centers for Disease Control & Prevention National Center on Birth Defects & Developmental Disabilities http://www.cdc.gov/ncbddd/autism/	"Learn the Signs, Act Early" campaign aims to educate parents and professionals about childhood development, including early warning signs of autism and other developmental disorders, and encourages developmental screening and intervention. The Web site has lots of free downloadable and print materials for physicians to use in the office, including informational cards, fact sheets, and brochures
First Signs http://www.firstsigns.org/	Public awareness and training program designed to educate pediatric practitioners, clinicians, early childhood educators, and parents about the importance of early detection and intervention of autism and other developmental disorders. Its Web site offers downloadable, free, and purchasable materials for clinicians to use in the office and in parent education

access and use the tools available for screening for autism. The CDC Act Early project in collaboration with the Association of University Centers on Disabilities convened regional "Act Early" summits to bring together key state stakeholders to address the increasing demand for evidence-based practices for children with ASDs to and create action plans including increasing awareness among professionals. Other initiatives include the Autism ALARM (Autism is prevalent; Listen to parents; Act early; Refer; Monitor) funded by a cooperative agreement between the AAP and the National Center on Birth Defects and Developmental Disabilities at the CDC and Medical Home Initiatives.

WHAT IS A PEDIATRICIAN TO DO?

The AAP recommends developmental surveillance at every well-child visit and developmental screening using standardized tools at 9-, 18-, and 24- or 30-month visits, or whenever parent or provider concern is expressed. In addition, autism-specific screenings are recommended at the 18- and 24-month visits (the AAP screening algorithm can be accessed at http://www.aap.org).[4] Surveillance and screening activities should be performed within the medical home and coordinated with tracking and intervention services available in the community.[4]

Screening tools are generally classified as Level 1 (administered to all children and meant to identify children at risk for an ASD in contrast to those with typical development) and Level 2 (administered to a referred population in early intervention and diagnostic clinics, and meant to differentiate between children at risk for an ASD and other developmental disorders) (**Table 2**). For a primary care pediatrician, Level 1 screening tools are most appropriate in terms of the accessible population and in the context of a medical home. Although the choice of screening tool itself will vary from clinician to clinician, based on cost, availability, and familiarity, the tenets of using a screening tool must always be adhered to:

1. Autism screening is not meant to provide a diagnosis, merely to offer guidance on next appropriate steps (referral for intervention or further diagnostic procedures)
2. One must thoroughly familiarize oneself with the screening tool, its sensitivity, its specificity, and how it is applicable in one's particular population
3. No alteration in the order or presentation of the tool must be done to maintain its validity; this includes paying attention to the age range on which the tool is validated and adhering to it
4. There has been no demonstrated advantage of one screening tool over another in a single comparative study between Early Screening of Autistic Traits Questionnaire, Social Communication Questionnaire, Communication and Symbolic Behavior Scales-Developmental Profile, Infant-Toddler Checklist, and key items of the Checklist for Autism in Toddlers[14]

Other tools that have been used for screening include the Checklist for Autism in Toddlers (CHAT) and the Screening Test for Autism in Toddlers (STAT).[21–23] These tools require the clinician to engage in observations and interaction with the child-patient. CHAT is a combined parent report and child observation tool from which the modified CHAT (M-CHAT) was derived.[24] Administered at 18 to 24 months of age, it consists of 14 questions or items and takes about 5 minutes to complete. It now has a revised version called the Quantitative CHAT (Q-CHAT), which is a 25-item parent report on a 5-point scale.[21] Both CHAT and Q-CHAT are freely available for download at http://www.autismresearchcentre.com/, and are available in English, Spanish, German, and other languages. A highlight of the Q-CHAT is the little cartoon

Table 2
Screening tools

Tool	Details	How to Obtain
Modified Checklist for Autism in Toddlers (M-CHAT)[a] (Robins et al,[15] 2001)	Used in children 16–30 mo old. Available in several different languages. 23 Yes/no response parent questionnaire, completes in 5 min	Free to download and use http://www2.gsu.edu/ ~psydlr/DianaLRobins/ Official_M-CHAT_website. html
Pervasive Developmental Disorders Screening Test-II (PDDST-II) (Siegel,[16] 2004)	Used in children 18–48 mo old. Available in English and Spanish. Stage I also called Primary Care Screener (PCS). 22-item parent report measure, completes in 10–15 min	Purchase from Pearson Assessments http://www. pearsonassessments.com/ $42.50 for the 25 PCS forms
Social Communication Questionnaire (SCQ) (Rutter et al,[17] 2003)	Previously known as Autism Screening Questionnaire (ASQ), it is used in children >4 y old. 40 yes/no questions can be completed in 10 min. Available in English and Spanish. More useful as a screener for research projects with parents who already know about ASD symptoms, less useful in young children	Purchase from Western Psychological Services http://portal.wpspublish. com/ $110.00, includes 20 current and 20 lifetime autoscore forms, and manual
Childhood Autism Spectrum Test (CAST) (Scott et al,[18] 2002)	Formerly called the Childhood Asperger Syndrome Test. Used in children aged 4–11 y old, also available in various languages. Despite original name, can be used in screening both Asperger and low-functioning children with autism	Free to download and use Autism Research Center http://www. autismresearchcentre.com/ tests/cast_test.asp
Autism Spectrum Screening Questionnaire (ASSQ) (Ehlers et al,[19] 1999)	Used in children aged 7–16 y. This 27-item checklist, for parents and teachers, takes 10 min to complete. It is designed for screening for symptoms of Asperger disorder (and high-functioning autism)	Available at link http://www. springerlink.com/content/ h26q7u2323251347/ fulltext.pdf but permission from publisher may be necessary

The M-CHAT Follow-Up Interview is recommended to be used along with the M-CHAT, particularly in low-risk community samples.[20] This subsequently reduces false positives and unnecessary referrals. It is available for download free at http://www2.gsu.edu/~psydlr/Diana_L._Robins,_Ph.D._ files/M-CHATInterview.pdf. At present, a cross-validation study of the M-CHAT is under way involving primary care sites in the Atlanta area. In addition, the investigators are exploring the utility of the M-CHAT in expanding autism screening to investigate multiple levels of screening, and a comparison of autism-specific screening and broad developmental screening.

[a] M-CHAT has been used extensively in research and clinical practice with sensitivity and specificity demonstrated in the target age range of 16 to 30 months of age. Its validity in those younger than 16 months has not been demonstrated.

images next to each question demonstrating the type of skill to aid parents in interpretation.

The STAT is a 12-item combined parent report and child observation tool that takes 20 minutes to complete.[22] It requires 2-day training at the TRIAD program at Vanderbilt University (and now through an online tutorial accessed at http://kc.vanderbilt.edu/triad/training/page.aspx?id=1555).

While there is no substitute for reading the manual of the tools you are using, there are some online tools that aim to further familiarize pediatricians with autism screening tools. Among these are the online learning modules from the Vermont Interdisciplinary Leadership Education for Health Professionals which, as part of its Autism extension grant, developed several learning modules to aid diverse groups of professionals in screening for autism at early ages. Several tools including M-CHAT, Pervasive Developmental Disorders Screening Test II, and Social Communication Questionnaire (SCQ) have these learning modules in different downloadable formats (Powerpoint, HTML, pdf). These modules, along with other helpful learning resources such as "how to speak to parents before and after screening," are accessible at their Web site http://www.uvm.edu/~vtilehp/autism/.

HOW EARLY IS EARLY SCREENING?

At present, the average reported age of diagnosis for autism is 5.7 years; however, it is recognized that parents or caregivers have suspicions of autism in their children prior to 2 years of age and often by 18 months of age.[25,26] Evidence shows that early identification leads to early intervention of ASDs and that early intervention is associated with improved outcomes.[27] However, there is a limitation on how early screening and diagnosis can be done reliably. It is difficult to reliably distinguish, before age 1 year, between typical and atypical social, communicative, and behavior characteristics, which are the core constructs of autism. About 1:4 children with ASD have regressive types of symptoms, that is, they had typical or near typical acquisition of developmental milestones, particularly language, and then seemed to lose these around age 18 to 24 months.[28,29] Therefore, too early screening may lead to a false sense of security if not followed by repeat screening or vigilance after 18 months of age.

Although there have been numerous studies exploring infancy diagnostics, including videotapes and screening questionnaires, they have yet to be proved sufficiently stable to be recommended for use in population-based screening.[30–32]

The Autism Observation Scale for Infants is a direct interaction, rather than parent report tool, which holds promise for identifying autism from as early as 6 months of age.[33] It is currently being validated in both premature and term populations, but its value in population screening in the office is not yet established.

Similarly, the Communication and Symbolic Behavior Scales (CSBS), particularly the Developmental Profile Infant-Toddler Checklist (CSBS-DP), is a screening tool that can be used with at-risk infants and toddlers older than 6 months, particularly for social and communication skills; however, it is not an ASD-specific screening tool. It can be downloaded for free at http://www.brookespublishing.com/store/books/wetherby-csbsdp/CSBSDP_Checklist.pdf.[34]

While there is no definite ASD screening tool available for infants younger than 15 months, this does not mean that pediatricians do not stay vigilant about autism red flags in this age group. Awareness of red flags (**Table 3**) and observing these skills, or asking anticipatory guidance questions during well-child visits, may alert the physician to monitor the child more closely.

Table 3
Early developmental skills and autism

Developmental Skill	Typical Age of Acquisition	Child with Autism
Social smile	Emerges at 6–8 wk old, usually seen by 3 mo	Some children with autism do have smile, but parents' history make determining typicality of such behaviors difficult (smile elicited by physical contact or anticipatory routine, as opposed to true social smile)
Response to name	By 8–10 mo of age, children can respond to their name being called	Children who have autism usually do not, or poorly, respond to name, needing multiple attempts or physical touch. Concerns about hearing loss are often the first alert to caregivers that something is amiss
Joint attention (JA)	8–10 mo following another's eye gaze; then following a point by 10–12 mo old	No JA, sometimes briefly glances in direction but no return to initiating individual
Gesture communication	Gestural pointing, often first to indicate something of need "protoimperative" seen at age 12–14 mo; then "protodeclarative" to draw attention toward an object at 15–16 mo old	No pointing; leading "hand-over-hand," some extension of hand, but no "3-way pointing" engaging JA with point
Babbling	Typical "bilabial babbling" with repetition of baba or dada seen at 6–7 mo old. By 8–10 mo, alternate babbling with silent opportunities to engage caregiver verbal responses. At age 10–12 mo, typical "jibber-jabber" or jargon sounds are heard	Usually delayed babbling until beyond age 12 mo. Also, isolated, noncommunicative repetitive sounds are heard before functional communication attempts

SOME PRACTICAL SUGGESTIONS FOR AUTISM SCREENING

In a survey of pediatricians regarding autism screening, among the main reasons reported for not screening for ASD were lack of familiarity with tools (62%), referral to a specialist (47%), and insufficient time (32%).[12] One can appreciate that in an environment of optimizing time-value and productivity of physician work, these are important perceived barriers to be addressed. Thus, screening for ASDs is best accomplished if it is incorporated into existing practices, remembering that change in behavior is often the most difficult to effect. There are several strategies by which ASD screening can be accomplished with minimal burden on the practitioner, while achieving its purpose.

1. Select the appropriate tool. Some screening tools (M-CHAT, Q-CHAT, Childhood Autism Spectrum Test, Autism Spectrum Screening Questionnaire) do not have

to be purchased, and many practices may opt for these rather than purchasing tools. However, the decision should be made based on the population to be screened, particularly the age group on which the tool is validated, ease of administration, and sensitivity and specificity of the tool. Validation and psychometrics of individual tools should be accessible at the Web sites of the publisher.

2. Use existing tools or materials collected in one place. Organization is a time-saving venture, and the AAP Autism Toolkit incorporates screening tools, templates, and other physician resources in one place.[11] It is helpful to have the electronic versions of tools used in a folder accessible to office staff, who will be primarily responsible for providing them to families at the time of visit. Always remember to have access to the scoring grid or template as well, particularly when staff is scoring the tool. One way to simplify scoring the M-CHAT, for example, is to have a transparency overlay of the scoring template to place over completed forms. The M-CHAT Web site has the overlay template and a Microsoft Excel scoring program that enable interpretation by entering responses directly from the form (http://www2. gsu.edu/~psydlr/DianaLRobins/Official_M-CHAT_website.html).

3. Integrate with developmental screening. Because more pediatricians report screening for general developmental problems (82%), ASD screening can be incorporated into general developmental screening practices.[12] Because general developmental screen is recommended at the 9-, 18-, and 30-month (or 24-month, depending on health insurance coverage) visits, and ASD screen at the 18- and 24-month visits, it is helpful to develop a protocol to use tools, as shown in **Table 4**.[9]

Some examples of general developmental (GD) screening tools are Ages & Stages Questionnaires, Child Development Inventory, and Pediatric Evaluation of Developmental Status (PEDS).[35–37] It may be tempting to use a single instrument for both general development and autism screening in the interests of time and simplicity; however, a study found that almost three-quarters of children who screened positive for an ASD using the M-CHAT did not elicit corresponding developmental concerns on a GD measure such as the PEDS.[38] This finding implies that a GD screen is not sufficiently specific to replace or be used as a first-stage screening tool for ASD.

In addition, GD screening tools, especially those with open-ended questions, may miss delays in the domains of social and communication skills that are important for the early identification of ASD.[39]

At all preventive visits, however, developmental surveillance should continue with history, observations, and review of other documentation (as necessary). Particular attention should be given to high-risk groups such as siblings of children already diagnosed with ASDs, children with genetic syndromes and other neurologic disorders, and premature children.[40–44]

Table 4
Use of screening instruments

Age of Visit (mo)	Developmental Surveillance	Developmental Screening	Autism Screening
9		☑	
12	☑		
15	☑		
18		☑	☑
24		☑	☑

4. Engage office personnel in screening. It is reasonable to engage clinical or nonclinical staff in the administration and scoring of screening instruments in providing the screening tool to families. The physician should interpret the score and counsel the family on an action plan. Some strategies to perform this stepwise approach are:

   a. A session to train office staff on the screening tools (access, orientation, guidelines to administer, and scoring) is a good start.
   b. Screening tool provided at the time of check-in can be completed in the waiting room. If there are literacy issues with parent or caregiver, assign a staff member to assist them. Many tools are available in several languages, so cultural awareness of the family's native language helps.
   c. For scheduled preventive visits and reliable families, the screening tool can be mailed out to the caregiver to complete and bring at the scheduled visit. Some practices are providing links on their Web pages to families to access screening tools, with instructions on completing and bringing it in for the visit.
   d. If there is inadequate time during the preventive visit to perform ASD and developmental screening, a separate visit only for screening can be set up. However, it is advisable to review billing and health insurance coverage procedures to ensure that the separate visit is reimbursable.
   e. Consider designating a specific individual to administer screening and provide parent counseling for developmental issues, or run parent training.
   f. Have an action plan for positive screens; this includes documentation, follow-up (eg, Using M-CHAT Follow-Up Interview), and discussion of implications with parents.

WHAT TO DO AFTER A POSITIVE SCREEN

In one study, even after child had positive screening for ASD, families waited an average of 7 months to pursue further diagnostic evaluation,[23] despite there not being a significant wait-list for the diagnostic clinic. Therefore, one must not assume that all families are eager to pursue formal diagnostics, particularly after a positive screen that has some degree of false positives. While pursuing diagnostic evaluation is important, equally important is parental support and education, access to interventions, and the reduction of financial barriers to the same.[44] Good practice in this regard starts with knowing your community and maintaining a resource list of autism service providers (speech, occupational, and behavioral therapists), specialists (including diagnosticians such as developmental pediatricians, pediatric neurologists, child psychiatrists, clinical psychologists), and other community agencies (Respite Care, Early Childhood Education), as well as state waiver programs for ASDs. Parents serve as a valuable source of information, particularly families who have children who have been diagnosed several years previously, as they have persevered and, in some instances, succeeded in pursuing these avenues. Autism Speaks has a searchable database of resources in the Family Resource Guide, including ability to map the resources.

Handouts provide families with information about ASDs including medical, educational, therapeutic, and other topics. Autism Speaks offers information for families, as does First Signs, providing the pediatrician with options to order materials that can be stocked in the clinic, or access to electronic resources that can be printed on demand.

Pediatricians should be familiar with the resources within the local educational system for children suspected of having, or diagnosed with, ASDs. An important start is recognizing which portion of the educational system bears the responsibility for evaluation and services for children, depending on age. Part C (Early Intervention) of the Individuals with Disabilities Education Act (IDEA) mandates that infants and toddlers with disabilities (birth up to third birthday) and their families receive services by assisting states in operating a comprehensive program of interventions, delivered as much as possible in natural settings according to families' needs.[45] Part B covers children aged 3 to 21 years, and for children in this age group the local education authority (school district) is the first access point for families.

Pediatricians can facilitate families' access to services by providing information about local policies, furnishing requisite medical documentation and letters to support eligibility, and directing families to Web sites such as the US Department of Education's Building the Legacy at http://www.idea.ed.gov/. The AAP Autism Toolkit for Clinicians has formats of letters that can be customized for pediatrician practices. Local and regional parent advocacy centers also are valuable resources for families.

Despite having all the information about resources and providing referrals and recommendations to families, there is a significant concern that lack of care coordination can lead to inefficiency of care, especially important for children with developmental problems.[46] Several pilot projects at State level exemplify access and care coordination.

1. Improving linkages among pediatric primary care providers and other community providers (Arkansas)
2. Identifying best practices for ensuring effective referrals and linkages (Illinois)
3. Systematically screen, refer, and track services for children at risk of delays; create communication and feedback loops between clinics and early intervention staff (Minnesota)
4. Infrastructure to ensure follow-up for referrals, linkage of subsystems and monitoring of performance, and resources and visibility in rural areas (Oklahoma)
5. Using Medicaid quality improvement processes, increasing the spread of developmental screening using standardized tools in primary care and assuring sustainable, patient-centered coordination (Oregon).

Pediatricians should familiarize themselves with what is happening in their communities at a macro level, in addition to strengthening the principles of care coordination within the context of their own pediatric Medical Home.[47] The AAP Web site on Medical Home, http://www.medicalhomeinfo.org/, has resources including a Care Coordination toolkit, job descriptions for care coordinators (both health personnel and layperson), and a training curriculum for coordinators.

SCREENING IS REIMBURSABLE

While pediatricians are concerned about the cost to their practice of screening procedures and hence report that they do not screen more frequently, parent report tools are cost-effective in comparison with physician-administered tools.[48] Developmental screening, including autism screening with standardized tools, is eligible for reimbursement.

Since 2005, the Centers for Medicare and Medicaid Services (CMS) included a modifier code 96110, which represents developmental testing, limited (including screening, with interpretation and report).[49] In a 2010 Current Procedural Terminology editorial revision, the language was amended to "developmental screening-limited, with interpretation and report, *per standardized instrument form*."[47,50] This code can be appended to a standard Evaluation/Management (E/M) service code with a modifier, either -25 or -59. It is important to understand the differences between the two: -25 modifier is used to report a separate significant identifiable service on the same day as the E/M service, whereas -59 is used to identify a procedure that is distinct/independent from the other E/M service provided.

In general, it is preferred to use the -25 modifier, though the -59 modifier is generally used for repeat procedures by same physician (eg, more than 1 version of a rating scale given to multiple raters). Whereas the -59 modifier is not appended to the E/M code, the -25 modifier is, particularly for 96110. There have been some instances of payors declining -59 modifiers, indicating that -76 is more appropriate; however, technically the -59 reporting (or easier still, multiple units as 96110 $\times$ 2 for developmental and M-CHAT screening at same visit) is appropriate. The -76 modifier is only for repeating the same test multiple times, which is not the case in most screening visits in early childhood, especially for ASDs.

There are several things to keep in mind with -25, 96110 reporting.

1. No physician work is required for this code, so even if a clinic staff member administers and scores the screening tool, only the physician's work of interpretation is expected; this is reflected in the nonphysician work relative value unit (RVU) assignment of the code by CMS (**Table 5**).
2. There has been a gradual reduction in RVU reimbursement for 96110 from CMS since 2005 to 2011.[50] However, this is still more than the "per-administration" cost of the screening tool (ranging from 0 for M-CHAT to $5.50 for SCQ).
3. Each time a screening tool is used, the -25 modifier can be applied. However, submission of claims for 96110 is only permissible when using a validated screening instrument, not when asking typical developmental history questions done in surveillance at preventive visits.
4. Not all health insurance plans cover for 96110 and not in all states. For example, some states do not permit "unbundling," whereas others recognize modifier -59 and not -25. It is always prudent to discuss the possibilities with billing personnel in the office, particularly as 96110 billing and reimbursement relates to one's major payors in one's population.

However, it is recommended that all denied claims should be appealed, as sometimes Medicaid and other private insurance plan administrators may not be familiar with what one is trying to accomplish, particularly if there has not been a strong history of 96110 submissions in one's practice area. The AAP provides help in this regard through their Coding Hotline, 1-800-433-9016, ext 4022 or at aapcodinghotline@aap.org.

AUTISM SCREENING AND ELECTRONIC HEALTH RECORDS

With the passage of the Patient Protection & Affordable Care Act (PPACA or ACA) in 2010, there is an increasing emphasis of transition to electronic health records (EHR).[51] Whereas traditional screening tools are paper based, increasingly tools are being adapted to conform to electronic systems. This change allows for increased

Table 5 Relative value unit (RVU) and allowable fee		
CMS Year	NF (Nonfacility) Practice Expense RVU	Medicare Allowable Fee ($)
2005	0.36	13.64
2011	0.24	8.15

efficiency with tracking of scores, possible linkage to referral, and care coordination. However, there are obstacles to seamlessly integrating existing GD screening tools into an EHR platform. Many of the tools are copyrighted, and most EHR platforms have not incorporated these screening tools. One exception of a GD tool is the PEDS, which has an electronic version available at http://www.pedstest.com/OnlineScreening.aspx.[37] This version allows for online fill-in forms for parents, automated scoring returned in real time, and printable summary reports. It can be used from multiple locations.

From an autism screening tool perspective, only the M-CHAT has an electronic version available at http://www.mchat.org/, which includes the latest scoring system, Best7.[15] The PEDS has an optional M-CHAT module that can be completed after the PEDS online.

At present, many practices are using paper versions of the screening tools, then scanning them into EHRs. This process means manual scoring and duplication of effort with scanning, making automated retrieval, tracking, and linkage to referral templates difficult without further manipulation of the EHR platform. Some Web portals (eg, Child Health and Development Interactive System, http://www.childhealthcare.org/chadis/) can integrate electronic versions of common screening tools, allowing the clinician to review results of the questionnaires, and link to clinical guides for many topics, as well as to handouts for families including resources that can be customized. However, the cost, particularly for smaller physician practices, will be a consideration with such programs.

Nevertheless, with the explosion in the use of handheld smart phones and other data-capture devices with wireless capability, there will be an impetus to have families enter screening tool information through online mechanisms in advance of the preventive visit, further potentially enhancing efficiency, as long as such mechanisms can be simple, intuitive, and in accordance with HIPAA (Health Insurance Portability and Accountability Act, 1996) privacy protections.[51]

SUMMARY

ASDs are being encountered more frequently by primary care pediatricians in office practice, with a reported prevalence of approximately almost 1 in 100. The pediatrician is often the first professional the parents or caregivers approach with concerns about their child's development. One of the keys to accomplishing universal screening for ASDs is for the pediatrician to familiarize himself or herself with the screening tools available. It is important to realize that screening tools are not meant to provide a diagnosis, merely to guide one toward next appropriate steps (referral for intervention or further diagnostic procedures).

There still are no highly validated tools for screening ASDs before the age of 15 months, so continuing developmental surveillance is essential, with particular scrutiny for red flags in high-risk populations (genetic disorders, siblings of children with ASDs, premature infants). It is also important to screen for ASD at 18 months and again at around 24 to 30 months, because 25% of children may not be screened as positive early, due to "regressive" ASD.

While pediatricians do report important perceived barriers to routine screening for ASDs in practice, the authors hope to have outlined several practice strategies to mitigate the burden on the practice, while highlighting the potential financial advantages of routine billing for screening practices. Integration with developmental screening, involving office staff in the screening procedures, and using available electronic and paper tools from the various resources is helpful. The most important aspect is care coordination to close the loop following positive screening, to ensure that linkages are made to interventions and diagnostic referrals for families.

REFERENCES

1. American Psychiatric Association. Diagnostic and statistical manual of mental disorders. 4th edition. Text Revision, Washington, DC: American Psychiatric Press; 2000.
2. Fombonne E. Prevalence of childhood disintegrative disorder. Autism 2002;6(2): 149–57.
3. American Psychiatric Association (APA) DSM-5 development Proposed draft revisions to DSM disorders and criteria, 2010. Available at: www.dsm5.org. Accessed October 25, 2011.
4. Johnson CP, Myers SM, American Academy of Pediatrics Council on Children with Disabilities. Identification and evaluation of children with autism spectrum disorders. Pediatrics 2007;120(5):1183–215.
5. Singh J, Hallmayer J, Illes J. Interacting and paradoxical forces in neuroscience and society. Nat Rev Neurosci 2007;8:153–60.
6. Fombonne E. The epidemiology of autism: a review. Psychol Med 1999;29: 769–86.
7. Rice C. Prevalence of autism spectrum disorders—autism and developmental disabilities monitoring network, United States, 2006. MMWR Surveill Summ 2009;58(SS10):1–20.
8. Hagan JF, Shaw JS, Duncan P, editors. Bright futures: guidelines for health supervision of infants, children, and adolescents. 3rd edition. Elk Grove Village (IL): American Academy of Pediatrics; 2008.
9. American Academy of Pediatrics. Identifying infants and young children with developmental disorders in the medical home: an algorithm for developmental surveillance and screening. Pediatrics 2006;118:405–20.
10. Myers SM, Johnson CP, American Academy of Pediatrics Council on Children with Disabilities. Management of children with autism spectrum disorders. Pediatrics 2007;120(5):1162–82.
11. AAP Autism Expert Panel. Autism: caring for children with autism spectrum disorders: a resource toolkit for clinicians. Elk Grove Village (IL): American Academy of Pediatrics; 2007.
12. Dosreis S, Weiner C, Johnson L, et al. Autism spectrum disorder screening and management practices among general pediatric providers. J Dev Behav Pediatr 2006;27:S88–94.
13. Zeiger VM. Screening for autism spectrum disorders: pediatric practices eight years after publication of practice guidelines. Doctoral Dissertation, Indiana University Indianapolis; 2008.
14. Oosterling IJ, Swinkels SH, van der Gaag RJ, et al. Comparative analysis of three screening instruments for autism spectrum disorder in toddlers at high risk. J Autism Dev Disord 2009;39:897–909.
15. Robins DL, Fein D, Barton ML, et al. The modified checklist for autism in toddlers: An initial study investigating the early detection of autism and pervasive developmental disorders. J Autism Dev Disord 2001;31:131–44.
16. Siegel B. The pervasive developmental disorders screening test II (PDDST-II). San Antonio (TX): Psychological Corporation; 2004.
17. Rutter M, Bailey A, Lord C. SCQ: The Social Communication Questionnaire. Manual. Los Angeles (CA): Western Psychological Services; 2003.

18. Scott F, Baron-Cohen S, Bolton P, et al. The CAST (Childhood Asperger Syndrome Test): preliminary development of UK screen for mainstream primary-school children. Autism 2002;6(1):9–31.
19. Ehlers S, Gillberg C, Wing L. A screening questionnaire for Asperger syndrome and other high functioning autism spectrum disorders in school age children. J Autism Dev Disord 1999;29:129–40.
20. Kleinman JM, Robins DL, Ventola PE, et al. The modified checklist for autism in toddlers: a follow-up study investigating the early detection of autism spectrum disorders. J Autism Dev Disord 2008;38:827–39.
21. Allison C, Baron-Cohen S, Wheelwright S, et al. The Q-CHAT (Quantitative Checklist for Autism in Toddlers): a normally distributed quantitative measure of autistic traits at 18-24 months of age: preliminary report. J Autism Dev Disord 2008;38(8):1414–25.
22. Stone WL, Coonrod EE, Ousley OY. Brief report: screening tool for autism in two-year-olds (STAT): development and preliminary data. J Autism Dev Disord 2000;30(6):607–12.
23. Dietz C, Swinkels S, van Daalen E, et al. Screening for autistic spectrum disorder in children aged 14-15 months. II: population screening with the Early Screening of Autistic Traits Questionnaire (ESAT). Design and general findings. J Autism Dev Disord 2006;36:713–22.
24. Baron-Cohen S, Allen J, Gillberg C. Can autism be detected at 18 months? The needle, the haystack, and the CHAT. Br J Psychiatry 1992;161:839–43.
25. Shattuck PT, Durkin M, Maenner M, et al. Timing of identification among children with an autism spectrum disorder: findings from a population-based surveillance study. J Am Acad Child Adolesc Psychiatry 2009;48(5):474–83.
26. De Giacomo A, Fombonne E. Parental recognition of developmental abnormalities in autism. Eur Child Adolesc Psychiatry 1998;7(3):131–6.
27. Rogers SJ, Vismara LA. Evidence-based comprehensive treatments for early autism. J Clin Child Adolesc Psychol 2008;37(1):8–38.
28. Rogers SJ. Developmental regression in autism spectrum disorders. Ment Retard Dev Disabil Res Rev 2004;10(2):139–43.
29. Landa RJ, Holman KC, Garrett-Mayer E. Social and communication development in toddlers with early and later diagnosis of autism spectrum disorders. Arch Gen Psychiatry 2007;64(7):853–64.
30. Werner E, Dawson G, Osterling J, et al. Brief report: recognition of autism spectrum disorder before one year of age: a retrospective study based on home videotapes. J Autism Dev Disord 2000;30(2):157–62.
31. Osterling J, Dawson G. Early recognition of children with autism: a study of first birthday home video tapes. J Autism Dev Disord 1994;24:247–57.
32. Pierce K, Carter C, Weinfeld M, et al. Detecting, studying, and treating autism early: the one-year well-baby check-up approach. online J Pediatr 2011;159(3):458–65. DOI: 10.1016/j.jpeds.2011.02.036.
33. Bryson SE, Zwaigenbaun L, McDermott C, et al. The Autism Observation Scale for Infants: scale development and reliability data. J Autism Dev Disord 2008;38(4):731–8.
34. Wetherby AM, Prizant G. Communication and symbolic behavior scales developmental profile. Baltimore (MD): Brookes Publishing; 2008.
35. Squires J, Bricker D. Ages & Stages questionnaires (ASQ-3™). 3rd edition. Baltimore (MD): Paul Brookes Publishing Co; 2009.
36. Ireton H. The Child Development Inventory (CDI). San Antonio (TX): Pearson Assessments; 1992.

37. Glascoe FP. Parents' Evaluation of Developmental Status (PEDS). Nolensville (TN): PEDSTest.com, LLC; 2010.

38. Pinto-Martin JA, Young LM, Mandell DS, et al. Screening strategies for autism spectrum disorders in pediatric primary care. J Dev Behav Pediatr 2008;29(5): 345–50.

39. Stone WL, Coonard EE, Turner LM, et al. Psychometric properties of the STAT for early autism screening. J Autism Dev Disord 2004;34(6):691–71.

40. Volkmar F, Paul R, Klin A, et al, editors. Handbook of autism and pervasive developmental disorders: assessment, interventions, and policy, vol. 2. 3rd edition. Hoboken (NJ): John Wiley & Sons, Inc 2005. p. 707–29.

41. Constantino JN, Zhang Y, Frazier T, et al. Sibling recurrence and the genetic epidemiology of autism. Am J Psychiatry 2010;167(11):1349–56.

42. Cohen D, Pichard N, Tordjman S, et al. Specific genetic disorders and autism: clinical contribution towards their identification. J Autism Dev Disord 2005; 35(1):103–16.

43. Johnson S, Hollis C, Kochhar P, et al. Autism spectrum disorders in extremely preterm children. J Pediatr 2010;156(4):525–31.

44. Webb SJ, Jones EJ. Early identification of autism: early characteristics, onset of symptoms, and diagnostic stability. Infants & Young Children 2009;22(2):100–18.

45. US Department of Education. Building the legacy. IDEA; 2004. Available at: http://www.idea.ed.gov/. Accessed October 25, 2011.

46. French JB, Hudson SS. Measuring care coordination for children at risk of developmental delay: challenges and opportunities. Washington, DC: National Committee for Quality Assurance; 2010.

47. American Academy of Pediatrics Council on Children with Disabilities. Care coordination in the medical home: integrating health and related systems of care for children with special health care needs. Pediatrics 2005;116:1238–44.

48. Dobrez A, Sasso L, Holl J, et al. Estimating the cost of developmental and behavioral screening of preschool children in general pediatric practice. Pediatrics 2001;108(4):913–22.

49. AAP Pediatric Coding Newsletter online Developmental Screening/Testing Coding Fact Sheet for Primary Care Pediatricians. Available at: http://coding.aap.org/. Accessed October 25, 2011.

50. Current procedural terminology (CPT). Chicago: American Medical Association; 2010.

51. Patient Protection and Affordable Care Act (2010). Available at: http://www.healthcare.gov/. Accessed October 25, 2011.

Diagnostic Evaluation of Autism Spectrum Disorders

Marisela Huerta, PhD*, Catherine Lord, PhD

KEYWORDS

- Autism spectrum disorder • Diagnosis • Assessment
- Diagnostic instruments

Michael is a 9-year-old male with a history of language delays. Currently, his expressive language seems to be at age level. However, he demonstrates difficulty following instructions at home and at school. Most notably, his peer interactions are poor. Though Michael is interested in his peers, he does not have friends. Recently, he has been struggling academically as well.

Olivia is a 5-year-old female who is described as "precocious." Her parents are most concerned about her increasing physical aggression. She hits and bites others. Olivia is also quite particular about how the activities in her day are conducted. Notably, Olivia does not play imaginatively with other children though she loves to watch and imitate her favorite videos.

Tony is a 2-year-old boy who is often fearful. He demonstrates anxiety in new environments and often clings to his parents. Tony's parents also expressed a concern about his lack of language. Tony uses a limited number of single words, but often, he does not speak at all. It is not clear how much speech Tony understands at this time.

—Adapted from clinical intake notes

As illustrated in the examples above, referrals to autism specialty clinics frequently span the full spectrum of the disorder and often involve diverse symptom presentations. Such heterogeneity in autism spectrum disorders (ASD) makes identification of the disorder a complex process. As a result, the diagnosis of ASD poses challenges and the definition of best practices in ASD evaluations may come into question.

This work was supported by grants R01MH089390-02 and RC1MH089721 from the National Institute of Mental Health to Dr Lord.

Conflicts of Interest Statement: Dr Lord receives royalties for the Autism Diagnostic Interview-Revised and Autism Diagnostic Observational Schedule; profits from these instruments when they are used in Dr Lord's projects or clinical work are donated to charity. Dr Huerta does not have any conflicts of interest.

Department of Psychiatry, Weill Cornell Medical College, 21 Bloomingdale Road, White Plains, NY 10605, USA

* Corresponding author.

E-mail address: mah2046@med.cornell.edu

The past decade has seen many advances in the availability of standardized ASD testing tools and increased knowledge about the variability in symptom expression. In addition, researchers have learned much about caregivers' varied experiences with the referral and diagnostic process that can inform clinical work. This article describes these insights with the goal of highlighting best practices for evaluating ASD. (Given that the current categorical classification system that makes distinctions between autism, Asperger disorder, and pervasive developmental disorder, not otherwise specified is highly unreliable [Lord and colleagues., in press],[1] the authors use the term "autism spectrum disorders" to refer to these disorders collectively. This is the term currently used in the proposed Diagnostic and Statistical Manual of Mental Disorders, Fifth Edition [see www.dsm5.org].)

CHALLENGES IN ASD DIAGNOSTIC ASSESSMENT

The American Academy of Pediatrics[2] and the American Psychological Association[3] have recommended an approach for the identification of ASD that involves stepwise, and at times, recursive surveillance. Starting at pediatric (eg, well-baby) appointments, the approach calls for a formal screening if behaviors of concern are noted during surveillance (see Patel's review of screening recommendations in this issue). If screening, including any caregiver concern, indicates cause for attention, the screening has to be followed by a formal diagnostic assessment. After the publication of these guidelines, the identification of ASD seems to have improved somewhat.[4] However, many children continue to be first identified by their educational programs,[5,6] and a significant minority of children with ASD are likely to be undiagnosed.[5,7]

A contributing factor to the problem of underidentification is the variability of symptom expression in ASD. The presentation of ASD can range from a child who is nonverbal and unlikely to make social initiations to a child who is verbally fluent but overly reliant on previously learned scripts of speech and social behavior (Ghaziuddin provides a detailed review of the clinical features of ASD in this issue). Because of this variability in symptom type and severity, diagnostic decision making is a complex process; no singular algorithm can be applied to the diagnosis of ASD. In a clinical sense, this has meant that no one behavior, such as responding to name or joint attention, excludes a diagnosis of ASD.[8] For example, although responding to his or her name and responding to joint attention are important characteristics of ASD in toddlers, most children with ASD can carry out both these actions by older preschool.[9] Even as a toddler, a very intelligent child who understands his name and follows a point may still merit a diagnosis of ASD because he or she does not seek to share enjoyment with others, smile back to people except during intense physical activity, show any interest in his or her siblings or same-age peers, and use language to answer questions or make socially directed comments.

Diagnosis of ASD can be difficult because behaviors seen in a child often depend on many non–autism-specific factors, including cognitive functioning and age.[10–12] The diagnosis of ASD is further complicated because of the interactions that occur between development and ASD symptoms. At certain ages, many characteristics, especially when defined by informants, that are common to ASD are not actually specific to the diagnosis and may occur in children with other disorders. In a study, as reported by parents and caregivers, stereotyped language was not more prevalent in children with ASD than in typically developing children and children with other nonspectrum diagnoses who were younger than 4 years and in children who did not have complex language.[13] These findings indicate that the types of behaviors which a clinician must attend to for diagnosis depend very much on the developmental factors, such as age and language level, as well as the source of information (ie, caregiver report through interview, questionnaire, or clinician observation).

To address these challenges, the National Research Council Committee on Educational Interventions for Children with Autism advised that each child suspected of having ASD have an evaluation that incorporates the following standards: the assessment of multiple areas of functioning including adaptive skills, an appreciation that variability in performance and ability is common in autism, and the use of a developmental perspective when assessing behavior and synthesizing results.[14] This type of evaluation is typically beyond the scope of usual pediatric practice, and so most cases depend on appropriate referral. Most recent studies, particularly those dedicated to the careful phenotyping of children who span the full spectrum of autism, have not only yielded data in support of these practices but also informed clinical practice with new methods and tools to implement these recommendations. These findings, and the practical implications of the guidelines, are discussed below.

BEST PRACTICES IN ASD DIAGNOSTIC EVALUATIONS
The Diagnostic Process

The inclusion of standardized cognitive and developmental testing, as well as an assessment of language, is particularly important to differentiate ASD from other developmental difficulties. These tests, if carefully selected and carried out by professionals experienced in the assessment of children with developmental disabilities, should provide information about the child's overall level of ability and functioning in both verbal and nonverbal areas, providing a crucial starting point for the clinician to make the best estimate of a clinical diagnosis. The separation of verbal and nonverbal estimates of functioning is particularly important because many children with ASD show much stronger nonverbal skills than one might expect from their language level or play. Standardized scores from a skilled examiner allow the clinician to consider questions such as the following: Can intellectual disability and/or language delay explain the difficulties in social interaction? Given this level of ability, are observed difficulties in communication and social behavior above and beyond what would be expected? Does the level of social ability fall short of what is expected given the cognitive or language ability?

The term "multidisciplinary" has often been used to describe best practice diagnostic evaluations. In some clinics, this term has meant that an autism evaluation is performed by multi-member diagnostic teams. However, this is not always feasible and in some cases can be overwhelming for parents.[6] Instead, multidisciplinary should be interpreted to mean that multiple areas of functioning should be considered during a diagnostic evaluation.[15] Although a physician should always be available to provide a medical evaluation, it is most important that these multifaceted evaluations be completed by clinicians with extensive experience in the standardized testing of children with particular expertise in the assessment of ASD.

In addition to covering multiple domains, diagnostic evaluations should consider information from multiple sources. A comprehensive evaluation must, at minimum, include a parent interview and an observational assessment of the child's current functioning in a context in which social-communicative behavior and play or peer interaction can be observed by an experienced clinician. For the diagnosis of ASD, diagnostic specificity is much worse if only one or the other is performed.[16] The clinician's observation provides the opportunity to put the child's behavior into the context of knowledge about other children, but information from caregivers provides a broader context needed in understanding the child's day-to-day behavior in a wide range of situations, his or her history, as well as family expectations, resources, and experiences, and other important contextual factors. Thus, child testing and parent interviews should be viewed as complementary and necessary components of the diagnostic evaluation (**Fig. 1**).

It is the job of the clinician to integrate information across the various sources of information. No single result (eg, a borderline score on one instrument; a high score on another) is sufficient. A clinician can take into account that a caregiver was very uncomfortable saying anything negative about his or her child or, as a new parent, unfamiliar with typical development or that a child was so hyperactive or tired or shy that his or her behavior in the office was not likely representative of other times.

In some cases, diagnostic clarity is not easily obtained despite access to formal testing results. Research on the early diagnosis of ASD suggests that for diagnostically complex cases, best practices are to adapt a surveillance approach that is recursive, meaning repeated screening and assessment. Such a strategy may be particularly appropriate for very young children when formal estimates of functioning may not always remain stable,[17] for children with very difficult behaviors (eg, aggression, self-injury) for whom there are very pressing day-to-day concerns, and for children with the very mildest difficulties for whom the diagnosis may be less accurate.

When best practice evaluation results in a diagnosis of ASD, the referring physician should expect to receive specific details about the child's functioning that support the diagnosis from the evaluator. The evaluation report should explain why the child does or does not have autism. In addition, the report should include recommendations that are specific to the child's particular constellation of difficulties and the contexts in which they occur. Other important questions that should be answered by a diagnostic evaluation are given in **Box 1**.

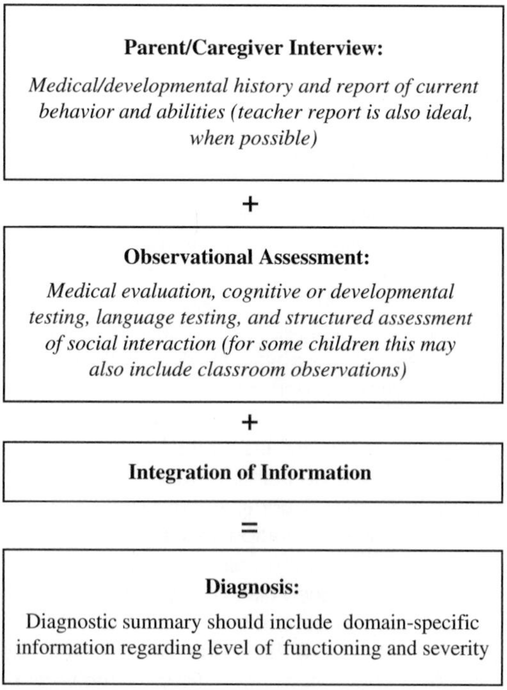

Parent/Caregiver Interview:

Medical/developmental history and report of current behavior and abilities (teacher report is also ideal, when possible)

+

Observational Assessment:

Medical evaluation, cognitive or developmental testing, language testing, and structured assessment of social interaction (for some children this may also include classroom observations)

+

Integration of Information

=

Diagnosis:

Diagnostic summary should include domain-specific information regarding level of functioning and severity

Fig. 1. Components of an ASD evaluation.

Box 1
Key questions for ASD diagnostic evaluations
1. What diagnostic classification best describes this child's pattern of behaviors and difficulties? If no diagnosis is confirmed, how often should this child continue to be monitored?
2. What is this child's overall level of functioning? Is cognitive functioning, language ability, or learning impaired? Or are results suspect?
3. Are there additional behaviors and/or diagnoses to consider for this child when planning treatment?
4. What behaviors/symptoms are most concerning to the family/caregivers? What role would they like to play in the child's treatment?
5. Given the current constellation of symptoms, what are the most important targets for intervention at this time?
6. Given family circumstances, community resources, and other contextual factors, what recommendations are most appropriate?
7. What is the prognosis for this child in the short term? Is there enough information to make predictions about prognosis over the long term?

Referrals for formal testing should not be limited to diagnostic evaluations. Children who have been diagnosed with ASD require reevaluations periodically, particularly at times of transition (eg, before the start of primary school). A child who receives a diagnosis of ASD at 2 or 3 years should receive testing the following year, sooner if any test results were suspect. Reevaluations need not be as comprehensive as the initial diagnostic testing but are important; over time, children with ASD change, not so much in diagnosis but in their needs, strengths, and difficulties.[18]

Diagnostic Instruments for ASD

A quick review of the current literature on ASD reveals an abundance of available diagnostic instruments. It may be difficult for clinicians to identify the standard instruments, but this becomes easier if one remembers the key elements set forth by the National Research Council Committee on Educational Interventions for Children With Autism[14]: best practice diagnostic tools should assess social functioning in a developmental context and should take into account the variability of behavior across settings. Following these criteria, a useful child testing tool in autism evaluations continues to be the Autism Diagnostic Observational Schedule (ADOS).[19] Recent revisions to the ADOS have improved its accuracy and expanded its clinical utility to include an indicator of severity.[20] Another development has been the toddler version of the ADOS, which uses a surveillance model of classification for very young children.[21] The Screening Tool for Autism in Toddlers and Young Children[22] and the Communication and Symbolic Behavior Scales[23] are also recommended for use in young children. A particular strength of all these instruments is that they are standardized in their administration and coding, ensuring careful assessment of something as complex as social behavior.[24]

For the parent interview, the Autism Diagnostic Interview-Revised (ADI-R) has been established as a useful diagnostic tool in the assessment of ASD. For use in very young children, toddler versions of the ADI-R diagnostic algorithm were recently created.[25] Although the ADI-R is useful for diagnosis, it is a lengthy instrument that requires significant training. Alternative methods of collecting parent report are needed. Currently, the use of the Social Communication Questionnaire[26] in conjunction with the ADOS seems to be a reasonable replacement when an ADI is not possible to perform.[27]

An emerging area of research involves validating ASD diagnostic instruments that have been translated into several different languages. However, the cultural equivalence of these translated instruments has not yet been established. In fact, for some instruments, there is emerging evidence that certain items function differently for non–English-speaking parents. For example, the restricted and repetitive behaviors on the ADI-R tend to be underendorsed by Spanish-speaking caregivers compared with their English-speaking counterparts.[28]

THE IMPORTANCE OF DIAGNOSTIC EVALUATIONS

Although time intensive, and often not adequately funded,[15] physicians must continue to refer children for formal diagnostic evaluations when ASD is suspected. Some school systems provide detailed assessments, but many do not. In addition, school assessments, although including parents and caregivers as informants, are not typically focused on helping families understand their children's difficulties and strengths and what families can do, but are necessarily oriented to educational services. Formal diagnostic testing is important for many reasons. First, although ASD very likely has genetic and neurobiological underpinnings, no accurate test based on biology exists. As a result, the diagnosis of ASD is based on behavior or, more accurately, on information about patterns of behavior and symptoms.[29] Second, estimates of functioning in key domains can also provide important prognostic information about the course of autism symptoms. For example, nonverbal cognitive skills at 2 years predict verbal ability at 5 years.[30] Poor adaptive skills coupled with repetitive behaviors at 2 years also predict more behavioral difficulties in older children with ASD; using any words at 2 years and having more expressive language at 3 years are predictors of more positive social outcomes.[31]

Third, even when diagnostic certainty is high, formal diagnostic assessment can contribute to treatment planning. The results obtained from a diagnostic evaluation can shed light on the function of behaviors and identify both near and eventual treatment targets, increasing the utility of interventions.[32] This does not always happen as the result of diagnostic assessments, but if not, the pediatrician should consider alternative referrals.

Several qualitative studies report that diagnostic evaluations also provide intangible benefits to the family of the child with ASD. Diagnostic confirmation, particularly for those with complex or atypical symptom presentations, often provides relief to the family.[33] Furthermore, formal testing is designed to provide additional information beyond diagnostic classification; a profile of a child's impairments and strengths satisfies many parents and caregivers who are trying to make sense of their child's behavior and ASD.[6] Moreover, when asked about their experiences with clinical providers, parents and caregivers frequently express a desire to be active participants in the process. Their feedback suggests that clinical best practices should include open communication with families about the suspected diagnoses and the procedures involved in evaluations.[34]

SUMMARY

Good diagnostic evaluations of ASD include the use of instruments designed to assess multiple domains of functioning and behavior, the inclusion of parents and caregivers as active partners, and the consideration of developmental factors throughout the diagnostic process. Physicians play a crucial role in ensuring best practices in autism evaluations through initial identification, selection of a referral, and discussions with parents and caregivers about what to expect and how to get the most from a diagnostic evaluation. Pediatricians in particular, given their more frequent contact with children compared with most specialists, are in the best position to monitor the needs of children with ASD over the course of development and within the context of their overall physical health. Pediatricians can also serve as very important advocates within the health care systems, with insurance companies and government agencies, to ensure all families have access to appropriate diagnostic and treatment services.

ACKNOWLEDGMENTS

The authors thank Sarah Butler for her assistance in the preparation of this manuscript.

REFERENCES

1. Lord C, Petkova E, Hus V, et al. A multi-site study of the clinical diagnosis of difference autism spectrum disorders. Arch Gen Psychiatry. In press.
2. Johnson CP, Myers SM, the Council on Children With Disabilities. Identification and evaluation of children with autism spectrum disorders. Pediatrics 2007; 120(5):1183–215. Available at: http://www.aap.org/pressroom/AutismID.pdf. Accessed July 25, 2007.
3. Filipek P, Accardo P, Ashwal S, et al. Practice parameter: screening and diagnosis of autism: report of the Quality Standards Subcommittee of the American Academy of Neurology and the Child Neurology Society. Neurology 2000;55(4): 468–79.
4. Jarquin VG, Wiggins LD, Schieve LA, et al. Racial disparities in community identification of autism spectrum disorders over time; Metropolitan Atlanta, Georgia, 2000–2006. J Dev Behav Pediatr 2011;32(3):179–87.
5. Yeargin-Allsop M, Rice C, Karapurkar T, et al. Prevalence of autism in a US metropolitan area. JAMA 2003;289(1):49–55.
6. Braiden HJ, Bothwell J, Duffy J. Parents' experience of the diagnostic process for autistic spectrum disorders. Child Care Pract 2010;16(4):377–89.
7. CDC. Prevalence of autism spectrum disorders—Autism and Developmental Disabilities Monitoring Network, 14 sites, United States, 2002. MMWR Surveill Summ 2007;56(1):12–28.
8. Sullivan M, Finelli J, Marvin A, et al. Response to joint attention in toddlers at risk for autism spectrum disorder: a prospective study. J Autism Dev Disord 2007; 37(1):37–48.
9. Chawarska K, Klin A, Paul R, et al. Autism spectrum disorder in the second year: stability and change in syndrome expression. J Child Psychol Psychiatry 2007; 48(2):128–38.
10. Richler J, Bishop SL, Kleinke JR, et al. Restricted and repetitive behaviors in young children autism spectrum disorders. J Autism Dev Disord 2007;37(1): 73–85.
11. Bishop SL, Richler J, Lord C. Association between restricted and repetitive behaviors and nonverbal IQ in children with autism spectrum disorders (ASD). Child Neuropsychology 2006;12(4–5):247–67.
12. Sigman M, McGovern CW. Improvement in cognitive and language skills from preschool to adolescence in autism. J Autism Dev Disord 2005;35(1):15–23.

13. Kim SK, Lord C. New Autism Diagnostic Interview-Revised algorithms for toddlers and preschoolers from 12 to 47 months of age. J Autism Dev Disord 2011. [Epub ahead of print].

14. National Research Council Committee on Educational Interventions for Children With Autism. Committee on Early Intervention for Children With Autism. Goals for children with autism and their families. In: Lord C, McGee J, editors. Educating children with autism spectrum disorders: report of the Committee on Early Intervention in Autism. Washington, DC: National Academy of Sciences; 2001. p. 21–44.

15. Lord C, Bishop SL. Autism spectrum disorders: diagnosis, prevalence and services for children and families. Society for Research in Child Development Public Policy Report 2010;24(2):1–21.

16. Risi S, Lord C, Gotham K, et al. Combining information from multiple sources in the diagnosis of autism spectrum disorders. J Am Acad Child Adolesc Psychiatry 2006;45(9):1094–103.

17. Charman T, Taylor E, Drew A, et al. Outcome at 7 years of children diagnosed with autism at age 2: predictive validity of assessments conducted at 2 and 3 years of age and pattern of symptom change over time. J Child Psychol Psychiatry 2005; 46(5):500–13.

18. Lord CL, Risi S, DiLavore PS, et al. Autism from 2 to 9 years of age. Arch Gen Psychiatry 2006;63(6):694–701.

19. Lord C, Rutter M, DiLavore PC, et al. Autism Diagnostic Observation Schedule. Los Angeles (CA): Western Psychological Services; 1999.

20. Gotham K, Risi S, Pickles A, et al. The Autism Diagnostic Observation Schedule (ADOS): revised algorithms for improved diagnostic validity. J Autism Dev Disord 2007;37(4):613–27.

21. Luyster R, Gotham K, Guthrie W, et al. The Autism Diagnostic Observation Schedule-Toddler Module: a new module of a standardized diagnostic measure for autism spectrum disorders. J Autism Dev Disord 2008;39:1305–20.

22. Stone WL, Coonrod EE, Ousley OY. Brief report: screening tool for autism in two-year-olds (STAT): development and preliminary data. J Autism Dev Disord 2000; 30(6):607–12.

23. Wetherby A, Allen L, Cleary J, et al. Validity and reliability of the communication and symbolic behavior scales developmental profile with very young children. J Speech Lang Hear Res 2002;45(6):1202–18.

24. Lord C, Risi S, Lambrecht L, et al. The ADOS-G (Autism Diagnostic Observation Schedule-Generic): a standard measure of social and communication deficits associated with autism spectrum disorder. J Autism Dev Disord 2000;30(3): 205–23.

25. Kim SH, Lord C. Restricted and repetitive behaviors in toddlers and preschoolers with autism spectrum disorders based on the Autism Diagnostic Observation Schedule (ADOS). Autism Res 2010;3(4):162–73.

26. Rutter M, Bailey A, Berument SK, et al. Social Communication Questionnaire (SCQ). Los Angeles (CA): Western Psychological Services; 2003.

27. Corsello C, Hus V, Pickles A, et al. Between a ROC and a hard place: decision making and making decisions about using the SCQ. J Child Psychol Psychiatry 2007;48(9):932–40.

28. Overton T, Fielding C, Garcia de Alba R. Differential diagnosis of Hispanic children referred for autism spectrum disorders: complex issues. J Autism Dev Disord 2007;37(10):1996–2007.

29. American Psychiatric Association. Diagnostic and statistical manual of mental disorders. 4th edition. Washington, DC: American Psychiatric Association; 1994.

30. Thurm A, Lord C, Lee LC, et al. Predictors of language acquisition in preschool children with autism spectrum disorders. J Autism Dev Disord 2007;37(9): 1721–31.
31. Anderson DK, Oti R, Lord C, et al. Patterns of growth in adaptive social abilities among children with autism spectrum disorder. J Abnorm Child Psychol 2009; 37(7):1019–34.
32. Turner M. Annotation: repetitive behaviour in autism: a review of psychological research. J Child Psychol Psychiatry 1999;40(6):839–49.
33. Midence K, O'Neill M. The experience of parents in the diagnosis of autism: a pilot study. Autism 1999;3(3):273–85.
34. Whitaker P. Supporting families of preschool children with autism: what parents want and what helps. Autism 2002;6(4):411–26.

Approach to the Genetic Evaluation of the Child with Autism

Helga V. Toriello, PhD[a,b,*]

KEYWORDS

- Syndrome • Diagnosis • Microarray
- Autism spectrum disorders • Family history

Autism is defined as a behavioral disorder, characterized by the triad of impaired social skills, delayed speech, and areas of intense focus.[1] In the past autism was thought to be relatively uncommon, with incidence figures of 1 in 2500 cited by various articles written in the 1980s.[2] Recently, however, the incidence of autism has increased, with figures as high as 1 in 110 published.[3] Two possible reasons, which may not necessarily be mutually exclusive, are increased exposure to environmental toxins and a broader definition of autism, so that it now comprises a spectrum (autism spectrum disorders [ASDs]) which also includes, for example, Asperger syndrome and pervasive developmental disorder.[2]

Autism is a heterogeneous entity that clearly has a substantial genetic component to its cause. This aspect is shown by a high concordance rate in monozygous twins, with approximately a 90% concordance for both twins having one of the ASDs. However, it is not uncommon for one twin to have autism and the other to have Asperger syndrome. As a result, the heritability is one of the highest cited for a psychiatric disorder, with a figure of 90% usually cited.[4] However, in fewer than half of the cases of autism can a cause be found, so the molecular basis of autism remains mostly unknown. Several epidemiologic studies have been done in an attempt to achieve a better understanding of potential mechanisms that might lead to autism. For example, Schendel and colleagues[5] examined the frequency of congenital anomalies in children with autism as well as the frequency of autism in children with congenital anomalies. The investigators found that children with a diagnosis of autism had an approximately twofold increased frequency of congenital anomalies (6% compared with a frequency of 3% in controls). In most of these children the anomaly was

The author has nothing to disclose regarding potential conflicts of interest.

[a] Department of Pediatrics and Human Development (MSU), Michigan State University, College of Human Medicine, Secchia Center, 15 Michigan Street, Room 363, Grand Rapids, MI 49503, USA
[b] Spectrum Health Hospitals, 25 Michigan Street, Suite 2000, Grand Rapids, MI 49503, USA
* Michigan State University, College of Human Medicine, Secchia Center, 15 Michigan Street, Room 363, Grand Rapids, MI 49503.
E-mail address: Toriello@msu.edu

Pediatr Clin N Am 59 (2012) 113–128
doi:10.1016/j.pcl.2011.10.014
0031-3955/12/$ – see front matter © 2012 Elsevier Inc. All rights reserved.

pediatric.theclinics.com

isolated, and in no case was a syndrome diagnosed. Similarly, the frequency of autism among children with congenital anomalies was double that of a control population, with frequencies of 0.43% and 0.22%, respectively. The autism frequency was not the same across all types of anomalies, but was greater in those with either a brain and/or eye anomaly.

Although it may be tempting to suggest that there are shared prenatal environmental factors responsible for the occurrence of both the anomaly and the autism, the investigators stated that "the pattern was indicative of neither a single etiology or pathogenetic mechanism nor a specific insult." However, they did stress that congenital anomalies could serve as indicators of central nervous system dysfunction, and thus the link to development of autism.

Another noteworthy association that has been described is the finding of a correlation between a family history of autoimmune disorders and ASDs.[6] This group found that among a group of 3325 children with a diagnosis of autism, with 1089 of those having infantile autism, there was a significantly greater frequency of maternal rheumatoid arthritis, maternal celiac disease, and both maternal and paternal type 1 diabetes (but only in the parents of those with infantile autism). One possible mechanism is via a genetic link to HLA system genes, some of which have been implicated in causing infantile autism.[7]

An association with increased paternal age has also been described by several groups.[8–10] This link has generally been attributed to increased mutation load in the sperm of older males; however, one group that studied families with more than one affected child[11] found that the often described male to female ratio of 4:1 diminished with increasing paternal age, so that among offspring born to men younger than 30 years, the sex ratio was 6.2:1 whereas among offspring born to men older than 45 years, the ratio was 1.2:1. Various mechanisms proposed to explain these findings included de novo copy number variant (CNV), new mutation, or chromosome anomalies, particularly involving the X chromosome.

Other studies have found a greater frequency of parental psychiatric disorders,[12] with such frequency approaching a twofold increase. Schizophrenia in both parents, and depression or personality disorders in mothers were more common in this study. The investigators noted that other studies had also found an association between parental psychiatric disorders and childhood autism, but differences existed among the various studies. Nonetheless, there is likely enough evidence to suggest that there are common genetic mechanisms that predispose to various psychiatric disorders.

More recent studies have attempted to identify the specific genes involved in predisposition to autism. One of the tools used by these studies is exome sequencing, in which all the coding regions of the human genome are simultaneously sequenced, searching for mutations that might be causative or contributory to the cause of an individual's disorder. O'Roak and colleagues,[13] using exome sequencing in 20 individuals with ASDs, found 21 de novo mutations, with 11 causing alterations in the gene product (protein). Therefore, in the not too distant future this technique will be applied clinically in an attempt to identify the causes of a particular child's autism.

Until that time, what should be done to evaluate the child for an identifiable genetic cause? Several studies have found that in a small subgroup of children with autism or ASD, there is an underlying genetic or chromosomal abnormality, with figures ranging between 10% and 41% for that proportion. **Table 1** summarizes some of these studies. It should be noted that some of these studies presented only genetic causes, whereas others attempted to identify all causes. The populations examined were also varied; some data were obtained from a group of children referred to a genetics clinic, whereas other data were from autism units or were recruited for the study.

Table 1
Results of investigative studies in children with autism

		Reference Investigation						
	Schaefer and Lutz[14]	Kosinovsky et al[15]	Roesser[16]	Benvenuto et al[17]	Shen et al[18]	Herman et al[19]	Battaglia and Carey[20]	Boddaert et al[21]
Source of patients	Genetics clinic	Autism centers	Autism centers	None (review article)	Recruited patients	Genetics clinic	Autism centers	Autism centers
Total N	32	132	207	NA	852	71	85	77 (8 unused)
Physical exam	2	—	13	3%–4%	—	—	—	—
Metabolic evaluation	0	0	—	—	—	0	0	—
Audiogram	1	—	—	—	—	—	1	—
Rubella titers	0	—	—	—	—	—	—	—
Karyotype	2	—	4	—	19	2	1	—
Fragile X	2	2	1	2%–5%	2	0	1	—
MRI	1	—	—	—	—	—	2	33/69
EEG	0	1	—	—	—	—	1	—
MECP2	2	—	0	—	—	3	—	—
22q11 FISH	0	—	0	—	—	—	—	—
15 interphase FISH	1	—	0	1%–2%	—	0	2	—
17p FISH	1	—	—	—	—	—	—	—
Uric acid	1	—	—	—	—	0	—	—
Microarray	—	—	—	1%–2%	154 CNV, 59 pathogenic	1	—	—
PTEN	—	—	—	—	—	2	—	—
Total	13/32 (41%)	1.5%	9%	7%–13%	9%–20%	11%	10.5%	48%

Dashes in cells indicate testing was not done.
Abbreviations: CNV, copy number variant; EEG, electroencephalography; FISH, fluorescence in situ hybridization; MRI, magnetic resonance imaging; NA, data not available; PTEN, phosphatase and tensin homolog.

Nevertheless, these data serve as starting points for providing guidelines for the evaluation of the child with autism.

What are these genetic conditions? In general, they can be subdivided into metabolic, mitochondrial, chromosomal, and monogenic (ie, caused by mutation in a single gene). An understanding of what these conditions are is useful in understanding the recommendations of the various specialty groups. Because there are good reviews of the various conditions associated with autism,[22,23] this article tries to answer the question, "what conditions should be considered in the child who does not appear to have a syndromic cause as the reason for the ASD phenotype?"

METABOLIC DISORDERS

Metabolic disorders are generally not considered to be a significant cause of autism, but because many are amenable to some form of treatment, it is important to recognize a metabolic disorder when it is present. The following is a brief review of some of these disorders that can be a cause of ASD.

Phenylketonuria

Phenylketonuria (PKU) is one of the more common disorders of amino acid metabolism, caused by homozygous or compound heterozygous mutation of the phenylalanine hydroxylase gene. PKU is one of the disorders for which newborn screening is done in the United States and several other countries; however, screening for PKU does not occur universally. In addition, if the screening is done too early (eg, first 12 hours of life), false-negative results can occur. Therefore, the physician needs to still consider PKU in the differential diagnosis in certain circumstances.

The phenotype of untreated PKU individuals includes cognitive impairment, seizures, microcephaly, decreased pigmentation, and a musty odor.[24] Among individuals with autism, PKU has been reported to occur more frequently than expected by chance[25]; however, the absolute frequency is still expected to be low, as demonstrated by the finding that autism in untreated PKU patients only occurs 5% of the time.[26] As already noted, if there is suspicion that the child may have PKU as the cause of the autism phenotype, diagnosis can easily be achieved by measurement of serum levels of phenylalanine.

Disorders of Purine Metabolism

Only one condition in this group is associated with the development of ASD, that being adenylosuccinate lyase (ADSL) deficiency. Phenotypic manifestations in this autosomal recessive condition include seizures, cognitive impairment, and hypotonia.[27] The frequency of autism as a component manifestation is unknown, although Jaeken and Van den Berghe[28] described autistic features in 3 of 8 children with this condition. Diagnosis is achieved by measurement of succinyladenosine and succinylamino imidazole carboxamide in cerebrospinal fluid, serum, or urine.

However, a second condition in this category deserves mention. Adenosine deaminase (ADA) deficiency can lead to severe combined immunodeficiency and, if untreated, early death.[27] Most untreated children die soon after birth, but in those who were treated by bone marrow transplantation, Rogers and colleagues[29] found behavioral abnormalities such as hyperactivity/attention-deficit disorder, aggressive behavior, and social problems. Autism was not described as occurring more frequently. This finding is relevant in that there are reports of children with autism having reduced levels of ADA in their sera,[30] leading some groups to search for mutations or polymorphisms in one ADA allele. Two Italian studies[31,32] did report a significantly increased relative risk for autism in patients with heterozygosity for an ADA allele (ADA2) associated with reduced catalytic activity, and suggested this variant might be associated with an increased risk of autism. Hettinger and colleagues[30] in a North American population did replicate these findings, so it was suggested that the ADA polymorphism may play a more significant role in Italian populations than in United States populations. In summary, ADA2, a variant form of the ADA gene, may be associated with an increased predisposition to develop autism, but having two mutations (pathogenic changes) causes a condition which is not associated with an increased risk of autism.

Succinic Semialdehyde Dehydrogenase Deficiency

This condition is a relatively rare (although the true prevalence is unknown) neurometabolic, autosomal recessive disorder that can be diagnosed by determination of succinic semialdehyde dehydrogenase (SSADH) enzymatic activity in leukocytes. The finding of elevated levels of 4-hydroxybutyric acid on urine organic acid screens often raises the suspicion that this is the underlying disorder. This condition is characterized by cognitive impairment, hypotonia of childhood onset, ataxia, and seizures. Behavioral disturbances include hyperkinesis, aggression, self-injury, and sleep disturbances.[33] Autistic features were described in 12% (4/33) of older individuals. Therefore, despite the unknown prevalence, it is likely that SSADH deficiency and autism affects fewer than 1 in several million. However, it is important to keep in mind that therapeutic decision making could be affected by knowledge that a patient has SSADH deficiency. For example, based on its pharmacologic properties, finasteride could prove to be a useful adjunctive therapy in those with SSADH deficiency.[34]

Disorders of Creatine Transport and Metabolism

Three different disorders have been identified as falling into this category. Deficiencies of arginine:glycine amidinotransferase (AGAT) and guanidinoacetate methyltransferase (GAMT) affect creatine metabolism, whereas deficiency of creatine transporter 1 (CT1) enzyme affects its transport into brain tissue. As a group, these conditions are termed the creatine deficiency syndromes (CDS).[35] AGAT and GAMT deficiencies are thought to be extremely rare, whereas CT1 is thought to account for as much as 1% to 4% of cases of X-linked cognitive impairment. Clinical manifestations in all include developmental delay, cognitive impairment, autistic manifestations, seizures, and hypotonia. Those with CT1 deficiency may also have the additional manifestations of midface hypoplasia and short stature.[36] In a review of CDS, Schulze[37] noted that two-thirds of those with a CDS had autism. Diagnosis of these conditions can be achieved by detection (or lack thereof) of the creatine peak on magnetic resonance spectroscopy, and confirmed by measurement of plasma and urine levels of creatine and guanidinoacetate. The pattern of results often points to the diagnosis (eg, in AGAT deficiency, plasma creatine is low/normal, whereas plasma and urine guanidinoacetate is low; in GAMT deficiency, plasma creatine is low, whereas plasma and urine guanidinoacetate are elevated).[36] It has been questioned whether children with autism should be screened for one of these disorders.[35] These conditions are admittedly rare; however, because therapeutic interventions can improve manifestations and, if given early enough, can prevent cognitive impairment and neurologic symptoms in some of these conditions,[36,38] consideration should be given to pursuing testing in children with consistent phenotypic manifestations. Unfortunately, treatment is less successful in the more common CT1.[38]

Cerebral Folate Deficiency

This group of conditions is defined as any one of the neurologic entities character-ized by low cerebrospinal fluid concentration of 5-methlyhydrofolate in the presence of normal serum folate levels. Cerebral folate deficiency comprises a heterogeneous group of conditions for which the molecular basis is incompletely understood, although disorders/genes identified to date include dihydrofolate reductase, α-5,10-methylene-tetrahydrofolate reductase, 3-phosphyglycerate dehydrogenase, or dihydropteridine reductase deficiencies; as well as Rett, Aicardi-Goutieres, or mito-chondrial syndromes.[39] Despite this heterogeneity, it has been suggested by some[40] but not others[41] that a clinical phenotype exists. This phenotype includes early normal development until approximately 4 to 6 months, with subsequent devel-opmental delay, agitation, sleep disturbances, deceleration of head growth, ataxia, hypotonia, and seizures.[40] However, Mangold and colleagues[41] did not find supportive evidence for this assertion, and cautioned against viewing this group of conditions as a distinct syndrome.

The diagnosis is achieved by measurement of cerebrospinal fluid 5-methyltetrahy-drofolate (5MTHF), and finding reduced levels. One group[41] recently described 103 patients with cerebral folate deficiency, although the frequency of autism in this cohort was not noted. Ramaekers and colleagues[42] described autism in 4 of 28 patients, whereas Moretti and colleagues[43] reported autism in 5 of 7 patients. Therefore, it is clear that autism is not a consistent finding in what is likely a rare group of disorders. Nonetheless, in a child with autistic manifestations with some of the other findings of this group of disorders, it may be worthwhile to pursue this diagnosis because there is some evidence that treatment with folinic acid may lead to improvement of some of the symptoms.[39]

Smith-Lemli-Opitz Syndrome

Smith-Lemli-Opitz syndrome (SLOS) is an autosomal recessive disorder of cholesterol metabolism characterized by a distinctive phenotype of physical, cognitive, and behavioral manifestations. The clinical findings include microcephaly, ptosis, ante-verted nares, micrognathia, and syndactyly between toes 2 and 3 (present in more than 90% of cases). Genital anomalies in males are also common. All have cognitive impairment, and at least 75% have autistic features.[44] The frequency of SLOS in the population is approximately 1 in 30,000 (but may be as high as 1 in 20,000) so a reason-able estimate for the prevalence of those with SLOS and autism is that 1 in 40,000, or 1 in 267 of those with autism will have SLOS. Therefore, screening all with autism for SLOS will have a very low yield; this was also found by Tierney and colleagues,[45] who did not find metabolic evidence for SLOS in those with autism, and suggested that the frequency of unrecognized SLOS among individuals with autism is less than 0.2%. However, targeted testing of those in whom there is clinical suspicion is worth-while. Diagnosis is accomplished by measurement of 7-dehydrocholesterol in serum. Benefits of diagnosis include the potential for amelioration of symptoms by treating with cholesterol; however, a recent prospective trial failed to identify a true effect on behavior.

Although Tierney and colleagues[45] did not identify individuals with SLOS in their study, they did find that abnormally low levels of cholesterol were found in almost 20% of children with autism, further supporting a role for reduced lipid levels in chil-dren with autism. This finding has potential for identification of possible interven-tional or preventive therapies[46] as well as for understanding additional causes of autism.

MITOCHONDRIAL DISORDERS

A study done in 2005 found that 7% of children with ASDs had evidence of a mitochondrial disorder, as demonstrated initially by elevated serum lactate, and subsequently by the demonstration in some of those of a mitochondrial respiratory chain disorder (n = 5/69). All 5 children were found to have moderate to severe cognitive impairment, and an autism diagnosis of severe autism.[47] A subsequent study evaluated 25 children with autism and confirmed mitochondrial disease, and pointed out that there were clinical characteristics that helped distinguish this group from nonmitochondrial autism. These children were more likely to have atypical developmental problems (eg, greatly delayed age at walking) and patterns of regression, and virtually all had nonneurologic disorders. One of the most common of these was gastrointestinal dysfunction, including cases with pancreatic and/or liver malfunction. Other non-neurologic anomalies included cardiac, hematologic, and growth involvement.[48] A good review of mitochondrial autism is provided by Haas,[49] and the reader is referred to that article for more detailed discussion on the topic. In summary, it is likely that a mitochondrial disorder is a rare, if ever, cause of autism without associated findings; however, a child with evidence of mitochondrial autism merits further evaluation. To that end, Frye and Rossignol[50] have suggested a protocol for determining the likelihood of mitochondrial disease in a child with ASD, with the so-called Morava protocol at least a starting point for considering the need for mitochondrial evaluation (which can often be extensive and costly). Although there are few, if any, proven therapies, there is some promise that in the future better interventions will become available.[51]

CHROMOSOME ANOMALIES

Several years ago, the only means of investigating a child for the presence of a chromosomal disorder was to do a karyotype, which identified an anomaly in a few percent of those with ASDs.[52] Recently developed techniques, termed chromosomal microarrays (CMAs), have been used to detect smaller deletions or duplications than could be found by karyotyping, and the yield in children with ASD has risen to 7% to 10%. In the vernacular, this is the proportion of children with a CNV. Among the numerous pathogenic CNVs that have been reported, several are found significantly more often in individuals with an ASD. These CNVs are briefly summarized below.

Dup 7q11.23

Williams syndrome is a common microdeletion syndrome characterized by (among other things) a characteristic facial phenotype, outgoing, sociable personality (often described as hypersocial), and mild cognitive impairment. More recently, microduplications of this region have been found in individuals with autistic-like features. Cognitive impairment may also be a component manifestation, although this is not a constant finding. There is said to also be a characteristic facial phenotype, although manifestations may be subtle. This phenotype includes prominent forehead, straight eyebrows, thin upper lip, and broad nose in older children.[53] It is noteworthy that haploinsufficiency of one of the genes in this region, Gtf2i, leads to increased social interaction in mice.[54] It is therefore not surprising that increased dosage of this gene could lead to decreased sociability.

Dup or Del 16p11.2

This anomaly is estimated to occur in up to 1% of all children with ASD. The phenotype in those with deletion or duplication may be dysmorphic, with deep-set appearing eyes, midface hypoplasia, and smooth philtrum as consistent findings. However, some individuals are described as nondysmorphic, thus an unremarkable phenotype does not exclude 16p11.2 CNV as the cause of ASD. The frequency of autism in 16p duplication is 75%, whereas it is 98% in those with deletions.[55]

Del 17q12

One study found this microdeletion in 24 of 23,271 patients with an ASD or schizophrenia, for a prevalence of approximately 0.1% of those tested. The phenotype is slightly dysmorphic, with macrocephaly, arched eyebrows, down-slanting palpebral fissures, epicanthal folds, and malar flattening the most common features. Although most had cognitive impairment, it was not a consistent finding. Most also had various neuropsychiatric comorbidities, including phobias, depression, mood lability, and bipolar disorder.[56] This deletion has also been found in individuals with schizophrenia, thus perhaps providing a reason for the observation that schizophrenia is more common in the parents of children with ASD described before. A similar observation has been made for duplication 16p11.2 (more common in those with schizophrenia).[57]

Del or dup 15q13

Individuals with deletions or duplications in this region have been reported to have autism or autistic manifestations. A recent study identified that 0.6% of children referred for microarray analysis for various indications (including developmental delay, cognitive impairment, learning disability, or ASD) were found to have CNVs at this locus.[58] The physical phenotype was described as nonspecific, and in a second study, some of these children were found to have inherited this CNV from a clinically unaffected parent.[59]

Many of these individuals have additional behavioral manifestations, including hyperactivity, aggression, and impulsive behavior. Other studies have also suggested a link with schizophrenia,[60] thus genes in this and previously described regions are likely responsible for alterations in brain function, which can lead to various behavioral, cognitive, and psychiatric manifestations.

Del 22q13

This underdiagnosed condition is likely secondary to the unremarkable phenotype. The described phenotype includes long eyelashes, bulbous nose, full cheeks, pointed chin, and large or unusual ears. The hands appear relatively large, and nails are dysplastic.[61] However, the recommendation for considering this diagnosis only includes hypotonia, absent speech, and global developmental delay. Most children with this condition are said to have autistic-like features. One of the relevant genes in this region is *SHANK3*, in which mutations have been found in autistic individuals.[62]

Therefore, as these pathogenic CNVs (microdeletions and duplications) are described in children with ASD, this will help to identify relevant genes for causing the ASD phenotype. CMAs are available at several laboratories throughout the United States, although in the author's experience insurance companies may not be willing to pay for this testing. It should also be emphasized that if a CNV is done, a karyotype should not be ordered at the same time, nor should specific fluorescence in situ hybridization probes be ordered. Based on the findings, the laboratory will direct the ordering physician as to which additional steps should be taken to clarify the result.

MONOGENIC DISORDERS

A few conditions that are associated with an increased frequency of ASD are described here. This list is not meant to be comprehensive (see Ref.[22] for a full list). However, the focus of this section is the conditions that may present with ASD but not be as readily apparent, at least physically. Therefore, conditions such as Cornelia de Lange, CHARGE, or Angelman syndromes, for example, are not discussed because the clinical diagnosis would likely precede the ASD diagnosis.

Neurofibromatosis Type 1

Neurofibromatosis type 1 (NF1) is an autosomal dominant condition that is relatively common, with an estimated frequency of 1 in 3000 to 1 in 4000.[63] A study done several years ago, likely using a narrower definition of ASD (using a frequency of 1 in 6000) found NF1 in 0.3% of patients with a diagnosis of autism. It is unknown whether using a broader definition of autism would increase or decrease that figure. Nonetheless, it is not unreasonable to search for manifestations of NF1 in a child with an ASD diagnosis.

The NF1 diagnosis is usually made on a clinical basis, using diagnostic criteria developed by the National Institutes of Health.[64] These criteria include 2 or more of the following manifestations:

1. Six or more café-au-lait macules
2. Two or more neurofibromas or 1 plexiform neurofibroma
3. Axillary or inguinal freckling
4. Optic glioma
5. Two or more Lisch nodules
6. Sphenoid dysplasia or tibial pseudarthrosis
7. First-degree relative (parent or sibling) with confirmed NF1.

All but the youngest children can be confidently diagnosed using these criteria; DeBella and colleagues[65] found that whereas only 54% of nonfamilial cases met diagnostic criteria by 1 year of age, almost all (97%) did so by 8 years of age. Molecular testing is available in ambiguous cases, but given that the average age of diagnosis for autism is 3.1 years,[66] the child with autism secondary to NF1 should have enough criteria for clinical suspicion, if not diagnosis. Therefore, use of a molecular test should be approached thoughtfully.

Tuberous Sclerosis

Tuberous sclerosis (TS) is another autosomal dominant condition in which autism is found more often. TS is caused by two different genes, so the condition is sometimes referred to as TS1 and TS2, depending on the gene involved. The frequency of TS in the population is 1 in 5800, with up to 45% of those having symptoms of ASD.[67,68] Conversely, the frequency of TS among children with ASD is 1.2%.[69] As in NF1, there are established diagnostic criteria[70] based on the presence of major and minor criteria. If a thorough evaluation is done on suspected cases, penetrance is thought to be 100%. Molecular testing is available at a limited number of laboratories, and detection rate is 80% (thus even with strong clinical suspicion, the diagnosis is unable to be confirmed in 20% of cases). Most individuals have TS2 mutations (60% vs 19%), so testing in a tiered fashion may be indicated. Although this is an expensive test (costing a few thousand dollars), it may be even more expensive to make the diagnosis clinically because such would involve magnetic resonance imaging, cardiac echocardiography, renal ultrasonography, and ophthalmologic examination.

Myotonic Dystrophy

Myotonic dystrophy is an autosomal dominant disorder that has a prevalence of approximately 1 in 20,000.[71] The cause is expansion of a trinucleotide repeat within the DM1 gene. The classic form has an age of onset of 10 to 30 years, and is characterized by the development of myotonia and relatively expressionless face. Additional manifestations that develop over time may include weakness (particularly distally), and cardiac, endocrine, and gastrointestinal dysfunction. The frequency of ASD in a group of children with myotonic dystrophy was reported as 49%, with age of onset of the myotonic dystrophy correlating with the presence and severity of ASD. In addition, 86% of this group had moderate to severe cognitive impairment.[72] This figure suggests that although children in this group who also have ASD are more likely to have cognitive impairment, this is not a consistent finding.[72,73] Although in the past it was necessary for electromyography and/or muscle biopsy to be done to make the diagnosis, molecular testing is 100% accurate and costs less than $300. Although myotonic dystrophy accounts for less than 0.2% of cases of ASD, in a child with evidence of myotonia, particularly when there is a positive family history that is supportive of this diagnosis, testing for myotonic dystrophy is a reasonable option.

Fragile X

Fragile X syndrome is another trinucleotide repeat disorder inherited as an X-linked trait. The population prevalence is estimated at approximately 1 in 5000.[74] The frequency among boys with ASD is estimated at 2.7%,[69] which is comparable with the frequency among children with developmental delay.[75,76] Autism is present in approximately 25% of those with fragile X[77]; pervasive developmental disorder is present in an additional 30%.[78] It has also been shown that among males with a pre-mutation (55–200 repeats, frequency 1/813 males and 1/259 females), autism is more common[78,79]; a second study found that 13% of premutation carrier males and 1% of premutation carrier females had ASD.[80] Testing is widely available for a few hundred dollars, and may be worth doing despite the anticipated relatively low yield.

Several single genes have also been identified as having a role to some extent in the cause of ASD. Here again, see Scherer and Dawson[81] for a more detailed review.

As a result of these and other studies, the American Academy of Neurology, the American Academy of Pediatrics, and the American College of Medical Genetics (ACMG) have developed guidelines for the investigation of autism (with the ACMG guidelines focusing on the genetic causes) (**Table 2**). Testing for some of these conditions has already been discussed in the context of the particular condition. It should not be understood from these guidelines that testing should be done on every child, nor should it be exhaustive. In a recent article on the topic of genetic testing in autism, Rapin[84] discussed that there are several reasons for testing, including:

1. Providing medical therapy for children with treatable manifestations
2. Providing information or recurrence risks for subsequent pregnancies or for other family members
3. Defining a specific etiology, even if therapy is not available.

Bockenhauer and colleagues[85] provide a similar discussion in their article on genetic testing in renal disease; they also examine reasons for genetic testing, and list as reasons:

1. Confirmation of diagnosis
2. Precise genetic counseling
3. Better understanding of pathophysiology
4. Supporting clinical management.

Genetic tests can be of different types, and include diagnostic, presymptomatic (testing done to determine if an individual has a gene for a disorder before the

Table 2
Recommendations of select professional societies

Evaluations	American Association of Pediatrics[82]	American Association of Neurology[83]	American College of Medical Genetics[a,4]
Physical exam	Yes, all children		First tier
Metabolic evaluations	Yes, if symptoms	Yes, if symptoms	First tier, but only if symptoms
Audiogram	Yes, all children	Yes	Preevaluation for autism
Rubella titers	NA	NA	First tier
Karyotype		If cognitive impairment	First tier
Fragile X	If cognitive impairment	If cognitive impairment	First tier
MRI	If tuberous sclerosis suspected	Not recommended	Third tier
EEG	History of seizures	Only if suspect seizures	Preevaluation
MECP2	Female with regression	NA	Females, second tier
Uric acid			Third tier
Microarray	If cognitive impairment	If cognitive impairment	Second tier
Mitochondrial evaluation	NA	Not recommended	First tier (lactate, pyruvate, acylcarnitines)
PTEN	NA	NA	If OFC >2.5 SD above mean, second tier
Fibroblast karyotype	NA	NA	If pigmentary anomaly, Second tier

Abbreviations: NA, not addressed; OFC, occipitofrontal circumference.
[a] Recommendations were allotted to tiers.

individual is showing any symptoms of that disease), or predispositional (testing to identify genetic changes that could increase the liability of an individual developing a particular disorder). When considering whether to order a genetic test, one needs to know some things about the test, including:

1. Sensitivity: how many individuals will be accurately diagnosed?
2. Specificity: how many gene changes are harmless (false positives)?
3. Ease of interpretation: will the specific genetic change assist with the prognosis? For example, there are several examples of mutations in the same gene causing different phenotypes
4. Cost and availability: most genetic tests are only done at a few laboratories, and are often expensive. Some insurance companies may not agree to pay for genetic testing, unless the results have an impact on management or treatment.[86]

In addition to testing for one specific disorder, some laboratories now offer panels of tests (in some cases, the so-called autism panel). The ordering physician needs to know whether these panels are for genetic changes of major effect (eg, monogenic conditions) or for changes that could be considered predispositional. Regardless, it is one thing to be able to tell a family that the child with ASD has a premutation in the fragile X gene, and quite another to inform the family that there are changes in one or more genes that are susceptibility loci for ASD.

At present newer tests are being developed for clinical use, which will likely be used fairly extensively in testing individuals for not only ASD but also a plethora of other conditions, be they syndromic or not. One such test is exome sequencing, which will be able to provide information on sequence variations in every coding region of an individual's genome. Although the test currently costs several thousand dollars, it is anticipated that such costs could come down to as much as $500, which is less than it currently costs to sequence one gene. Physicians will need to be able to explain to families what genetic testing will provide in terms of information and patient care.

REFERENCES

1. Bauman ML. Medical comorbidities in autism: Challenges to diagnosis and treatment. Neurotherapeutics 2010;7:320–7.
2. Bertoglio K, Hendren RL. New developments in autism. Psychiatr Clin North Am 2009;32:1–14.
3. Rice C. Prevalence of autism spectrum disorders—autism and developmental disabilities monitoring network, United States, 2006. MMWR Surveill Summ 2009;58(10):1–20.
4. Schaefer GB, Mendelsohn NJ, Professional Practice and Guidelines Committee. Clinical genetics evaluation in identifying the etiology of autism spectrum disorders. Genet Med 2008;10:301–5.
5. Schendel DE, Autry A, Wines R, et al. The co-occurrence of autism and birth defects: prevalence and risk in a population-based cohort. Dev Med Child Neurol 2009;51:779–86.
6. Atladottir HO, Pedersen MG, Scient C, et al. Association of family history of autoimmune diseases and autism spectrum disorders. Pediatrics 2009;124:687–94.
7. Warren RP, Odell JD, Warren WL, et al. Strong association of the third hypervariable region of the HLA-DR beta 1 with autism. J Neuroimmunol 1996;67:97–102.
8. Reichenberg A, Gross R, Weiser M, et al. Advancing paternal age and autism. Arch Gen Psychiatry 1996;63:1026–32.

9. Cantor RM, Yoon JL, Furr J, et al. Paternal age and autism are associated in a family-based sample. Mol Psychiatry 2007;12:419–21.

10. Croen LA, Najjar DV, Fireman B, et al. Maternal and paternal age and risk of autism spectrum disorders. Arch Pediatr Adolesc Med 2007;161:334–40.

11. Anello A, Reichenberg A, Luo X, et al. Brief report: parental age and sex ratio in autism. J Autism Dev Disord 2009;39:1487–92.

12. Daniels JL, Forssen U, Hultman CM, et al. Parental psychiatric disorders associated with autism spectrum disorders in offspring. Pediatrics 2008;121: 1357–62.

13. O'Roak BJ, Deriziotis P, Lee C, et al. Exome sequencing in sporadic autism spectrum disorders identifies severe de novo mutations. Nat Genet 2011;43:585–9.

14. Schaefer GB, Lutz RE. Diagnostic yield in the clinical genetic evaluation of autism spectrum disorders. Genet Med 2006;8:549–56.

15. Kosinovsky B, Hermon S, Yoran-Hegesh R, et al. The yield of laboratory investigations in children with infantile autism. J Neural Transm 2005;112:587–96.

16. Roesser J. Diagnostic yield of genetic testing in children diagnosed with autism spectrum disorders at a regional referral center. Clin Pediatr (Phila) 2011;50(9): 834–43. DOI: 10.1177/0009922811406261.

17. Benvenuto A, Manzi B, Alessandrelli R, et al. Recent advances in the pathogenesis of syndromic autisms. Int J Pediatr 2009;2009:198736.

18. Shen Y, Dies KA, Holm IA, et al. Clinical genetic testing for patients with autism spectrum disorders. Pediatrics 2010;125:727–35.

19. Herman GE, Henninger N, Ratliff-Schaul K, et al. Genetic testing in autism: how much is enough? Genet Med 2007;9:268–74.

20. Battaglia A, Carey JC. Etiologic yield of autistic spectrum disorders: a prospective study. Am J Med Genet 2006;142C:3–7.

21. Boddaert N, Zilbovicius M, Philipe A, et al. MRI findings in 77 children with non-syndromic autistic disorder. PLoS One 2009;4(2):e4415.

22. Betancur C. Etiologic heterogeneity in autism spectrum disorders: more than 100 genetic and genomic disorders and still counting. Brain Res 2011;1380:42–77.

23. Miles JH. Autism spectrum disorders—a genetics review. Genet Med 2011;13: 278–94.

24. Blau N, van Spronsen FJ, Levy HL. Phenylketonuria. Lancet 2010;376:1417–27.

25. Reiss AL, Feinstein C, Rosenbaum KN. Autism in genetic disorders. Schizophr Bull 1986;13:724–38.

26. Baieli S, Pavone L, Meli C, et al. Autism and phenylketonuria. J Autism Dev Disord 2003;33:201–4.

27. Camici M, Micheli V, Ipata PL, et al. Pediatric neurological syndromes and inborn errors of purine metabolism. Neurochem Int 2010;56:367–78.

28. Jaeken J, Van den Berghe G. An infantile autistic syndrome characterized by the presence of succinylpurines in body fluid. Lancet 1984;2:1058–61.

29. Rogers MH, Lwin R, Fairbanks L, et al. Cognitive and behavioral abnormalities in adenosine deaminase deficient severe combined immunodeficiency. J Pediatr 2001;139:44–50.

30. Hettinger JA, Liu X, Holden JJA. The G22A polymorphism of the ADA gene and susceptibility to autism spectrum disorders. J Autism Dev Disord 2008;38:14–9.

31. Bottini N, De Luca D, Saccucci P, et al. Autism: evidence of association with adenosine deaminase genetic polymorphism. Neurogenetics 2001;3:111–3.

32. Persico AM, Militerni R, Bravaccio C, et al. Adenosine deaminase alleles and autistic disorder: case-control and family-based association studies. Am J Med Genet 2000;96:784–90.

33. Knerr I, Gibson KM, Jakobs C, et al. Neuropsychiatric morbidity in adolescent and adult succinic semialdehyde dehydrogenase deficiency patients. CNS Spectr 2008;13:598–605.
34. Knerr I, Pearl PL, Bottiglieri T, et al. Therapeutic concepts in succinate semialdehyde dehydrogenase (SSADH; ALDH5a1) deficiency (γ-hydroxybutyric aciduria). Hypotheses evolved from 25 years of patient evaluation, studies in *Aldh5a1*$^{-/-}$ mice and characterization of γ-hydroxybutyric acid pharmacology. J Inherit Metab Dis 2007;30:279–94.
35. Wang L, Angley MT, Sorich MJ, et al. Is there a role for routinely screening children with autism spectrum disorder for creatine deficiency syndrome? Autism Res 2010;3:268–72.
36. Longo N, Ardon O, Vanzo R, et al. Disorders of creatine transport and metabolism. Am J Med Genet 2011;157:72–8.
37. Schulze A. Creatine deficiency syndromes. Mol Cell Biochem 2003;244:143–50.
38. Nasrallah F, Feki M, Kaabachi N. Creatine and creatine deficiency syndromes: biochemical and clinical aspects. Pediatr Neurol 2010;42:163–71.
39. Hyland K, Shoffner J, Heales SJ. Cerebral folate deficiency. J Inherit Metab Dis 2010;33:563–70.
40. Ramaekers VT, Hausler T, Opladen T, et al. Psychomotor retardation, spastic paraplegia, cerebellar ataxia and dyskinesia associated with low 5-methyltetrahydrofolate in cerebrospinal fluid: a novel neurometabolic condition responding to folinic acid substitution. Neuropediatrics 2002;33:301–8.
41. Mangold S, Blau N, Opladen T, et al. Cerebral folate deficiency: a neurometabolic syndrome? Mol Genet Metab 2011. [Epub ahead of print]. DOI: 10.1016/j.ymgme.2011.06.004.
42. Ramaekers VT, Rothenberg SP, Sequeira JM, et al. Autoantibodies to folate receptors in the cerebral folate deficiency syndrome. N Engl J Med 2005;352:1985–91.
43. Moretti P, Peters SU, del Gaudio D, et al. Brief report: autistic symptoms, developmental regression, mental retardation, epilepsy, and dyskinesias in CNS folate deficiency. J Autism Dev Disord 2008;38:1170–7.
44. Sikora DM, Pettit-Kekel K, Penfield J, et al. The near universal presence of autism spectrum disorders in children with Smith-Lemli-Opitz syndrome. Am J Med Genet A 2006;140:1511–8.
45. Tierney E, Bukelis I, Thompson RE, et al. Abnormalities of cholesterol metabolism in autism spectrum disorders. Am J Med Genet B Neuropsychiatr Genet 2006;141B:666–8.
46. Tamiji J, Crawford DA. The neurobiology of lipid metabolism in autism spectrum disorders. Neurosignals 2010;18:98–112.
47. Oliveira G, Diogo L, Grazina M, et al. Mitochondrial dysfunction in autism spectrum disorders: a population-based study. Dev Med Child Neurol 2005;47:185–9.
48. Weissman JR, Kelley RI, Bauman ML, et al. Mitochondrial disease in autism spectrum disorder patients: a cohort analysis. PLoS One 2008;11:e3815.
49. Haas RH. Autism and mitochondrial disease. Dev Disabil Res Rev 2010;16:144–53.
50. Frye RE, Rossignol DA. Mitochondrial dysfunction can connect the diverse medical symptoms associated with autism spectrum disorders. Pediatr Res 2011;69:41R–7R.
51. Suomalainen A. Therapy for mitochondrial disorders: little proof, high research activity, some promise. Sem Fetal Neonatal Med 2011;16:236–40.

52. Miller DT, Adam MP, Aradhya S, et al. Consensus statement: chromosomal micro-array is a first tier clinical diagnostic test for individuals with developmental disabilities or congenital anomalies. Am J Hum Genet 2010;86:749–64.
53. Van der Aa N, Rooms L, Vandeweyer G, et al. Fourteen new cases contribute to the characterization of the 7q11.23 microduplication syndrome. Eur J Med Genet 2009;52:94–100.
54. Sakurai T, Dorr NP, Takahashi N, et al. Haploinsufficiency of Gtf2i, a gene deleted in Williams syndrome, leads to increases in social interactions. Autism Res 2011; 4:28–39.
55. Sanders SJ, Ercan-Sencicek AG, Hus V, et al. Multiple recurrent de novo CNVs, including duplications of the 7q11.23 Williams syndrome region, are strongly associated with autism. Neuron 2011;70:863–85.
56. Moreno-De-Luca D, SGENE Consortium, Mulle JG, et al. Deletion 17q12 is a recurrent copy number variant that confers high risk of autism and schizo-phrenia. Am J Hum Genet 2010;87:618–30.
57. McCarthy SE, Makarov V, Kirov G, et al. Microduplications of 16p11.2 are asso-ciated with schizophrenia. Nat Genet 2009;41:1223–7.
58. Miller DT, Shen Y, Weiss LA, et al. Microdeletion duplication at 15q13.2q13.3 among individuals with features of autism and other neuropsychiatric disorders. J Med Genet 2009;46:242–8.
59. Van Bon BW, Mefford HC, Menten B, et al. Further delineation of the 15q13 micro-deletion and duplication syndromes: a clinical spectrum varying from non-pathogenic to a severe outcome. J Med Genet 2009;46:511–23.
60. Stefansson H, Rujescu D, Cichon S, et al. Large recurrent microdeletions associ-ated with schizophrenia. Nature 2008;455:178–9.
61. Cusmano-Ozog K, Manning MA, Hoyme HE. 22q13.3 deletion syndrome: a recognizable malformation syndrome associated with marked speech and language delay. Am J Med Genet C Semin Med Genet 2007;145C:393–8.
62. Dhar SU, del Gaudio D, German JR, et al. 22q13.3 deletion syndrome: clinical and molecular analysis using array CGH. Am J Med Genet A 2010;152A:573–81.
63. Friedman JM. Neurofibromatosis 1 (internet). In: Pagon RA, Bird TD, Dolan CR, et al, editors. Genereviews. Seattle (WA): University of WA; 2009.
64. National Institutes of Health Consensus Development Conference Statement: neuro-fibromatosis. Bethesda, MD, USA, July 13-15, 1987. Neurofibromatosis 1988;1:172–8.
65. DeBella K, Szudek J, Friedman JM. Use of the national institutes of health criteria for diagnosis of neurofibromatosis 1 in children. Pediatrics 2000;105:608–14.
66. Mandell DS, Novak MM, Zubritsky CD. Factors associated with age of diagnosis among children with autism spectrum disorders. Pediatrics 2005;116:1480–6.
67. Smalley SL. Autism and tuberous sclerosis. J Autism Dev Disord 1998;28:407–14.
68. Numis AL, Major P, Montenegro MA, et al. Identification of risk factors for autism spectrum disorders in tuberous sclerosis complex. Neurology 2011;76:981–7.
69. Fombonne E, Du Mazaubrun C, Cans C, et al. Autism and associated medical disorders in a French epidemiological survey. J Am Acad Child Adolesc Psychi-atry 1997;36:1561–9.
70. Roach ES, Sparagnana SP. Diagnosis of tuberous sclerosis complex. J Child Neurol 2004;19:643–9.
71. Bird TD. Myotonic dystrophy type 1 (internet). In: Pagon RA, Bird TD, Dolan CR, et al, editors. Genereviews. Seattle (WA): University of WA; 2011.
72. Ekstrom AB, Hakenas-Plate L, Samuelsson L, et al. Autism spectrum conditions in myotonic dystrophy type 1: a study on 57 individuals with congenital and child-hood forms. Am J Med Genet B Neuropsychiatr Genet 2008;147B:918–26.

73. Blondis TA, Cook E, Koza-Taylor P, et al. Asperger syndrome associated with Steinert's myotonic dystrophy. Dev Med Child Neurol 1996;38:840–7.

74. Coffee B, Keith K, Albizua I, et al. Incidence of fragile X syndrome by newborn screening for methylated FMR1 DNA. Am J Hum Genet 2009;85:503–14.

75. Curry CJ, Stevenson RE, Aughton D, et al. Evaluation of mental retardation: recommendations of a Consensus Conference: American College of Medical Genetics. Am J Med Genet 1997;12:468–77.

76. Rauch A, Hoyer J, Guth S, et al. Diagnostic yield of various genetic approaches in patients with unexplained developmental delay or mental retardation. Am J Med Genet A 2006;140:2063–74.

77. Hatton DD, Sideris J, Skinner M, et al. Autistic behavior in children with fragile X syndrome: prevalence, stability, and the impact of FMRP. Am J Med Genet A 2006;140:1804–13.

78. Hagerman R, Au J, Hagerman P. FMR1 premutation and full mutation molecular mechanisms related to autism. J Neurodev Disord 2011;3(3):211–24. DOI: 10.1007/s11689-011-9084-5.

79. Farzin F, Perry H, Hessl D, et al. Autism spectrum disorders and attention-deficit/hyperactivity disorder in boys with the fragile X premutation. J Dev Behav Pediatr 2006;27:S137–43.

80. Bailey DB Jr, Raspa M, Olmsted M, et al. Co-occurring conditions associated with FMR1 gene variations; findings from a national parent survey. Am J Med Genet A 2008;146:2060–9.

81. Scherer SW, Dawson G. Risk factors for autism: translating genomic discoveries into diagnostics. Hum Genet 2011;130:123–48.

82. Johnson CP, Myers SM. Council on Children with Disabilities. Identification and evaluation of children with autism spectrum disorders. Pediatrics 2007;120: 1183–215.

83. Filipek PA, Accardo PJ, Ashwal S, et al. Practice parameter: screening and diagnosis of autism: report of the quality standards subcommittee of the American Academy of Neurology and the Child Neurology Society. Neurology 2000;44: 468–79.

84. Rapin I. Appropriate investigations for clinical care versus research in children with autism. Brain Dev 1999;21:152–6.

85. Bockenhauer D, Medlar AJ, Ashton E, et al. Genetic testing in renal disease. Pediatr Nephrol 2011. [Epub ahead of print]. DOI: 10.1007/s00467-011-1865-2.

86. McPherson E. Genetic diagnosis and testing in clinical practice. Clin Med Res 2006;4:123–9.

Language and Communication in Autism: An Integrated View

Patricia J. Prelock, PhD, CCC-SLP[a],*,
Nickola Wolf Nelson, PhD, CCC-SLP[b]

KEYWORDS

• Language • Communication • Autism • Children

Children with autism face many developmental challenges. This article addresses difficulties related to the development of language and communication, which are related but not identical phenomena. Language and communication are best understood as complementary parts of an integrated social interaction system.

Language is a noun not a verb. People do not language; they speak, write, or sign to communicate using language. Language entails a set of abstract symbols, a lexicon, and a grammar that specifies syntax and discourse structures for combining symbols to represent an infinite variety of concrete and abstract meanings and to achieve communicative functions. Language must be encoded into and transmitted through physical symbols that can be understood by others who know the same language. Language may be expressed and understood phonologically through speech, orthographically through writing, or gesturally through sign language. Any form of symbolic communication that uses words is considered verbal, whether or not it is spoken. On the other hand, communication can be nonverbal as well as verbal. Communication involves co-construction of meaning by interacting partners who use gaze, nonsymbolic gestures, facial expression, physical proximity, tone of voice, and other forms of paralinguistic modulation (eg, intonation) to enrich linguistic meanings and convey the emotional tone of the message, or to communicate without verbal symbols. Children with autism may have varying degrees of difficulty acquiring speech and language, but social communication difficulties are a cardinal feature for diagnosing autism.

The authors have nothing to disclose.

[a] College of Nursing & Health Sciences, Department of Communication Sciences & Disorders, University of Vermont, 105 Rowell, 106 Carrigan Drive, Burlington, VT 05405, USA

[b] PhD program in Interdisciplinary Health Sciences, Department of Speech Pathology and Audiology, Western Michigan University, 1903 West Michigan, Kalamazoo, MI 49008-5379, USA

* Corresponding author.

E-mail address: patricia.prelock@uvm.edu

Pediatr Clin N Am 59 (2012) 129–145
doi:10.1016/j.pcl.2011.10.008
0031-3955/12/$ – see front matter © 2012 Elsevier Inc. All rights reserved.

The purpose of this article is to provide information about the language and communication challenges associated with autism spectrum disorders (ASDs) for physicians and other clinicians who work with children in this population. The article is organized to provide evidence-based answers (to the degree evidence is available) to questions about the role of communication and language across the core deficits of autism, ways to integrate assessment and intervention, and methods for supporting families to encourage their children's communication development.

INTEGRATED VIEW OF COMMUNICATION, LANGUAGE, AND AUTISM
What is the Role of Communication and Language Across the Core Deficits of Autism?

Communication impairment is one of 3 core deficit areas used to determine a diagnosis of autism in the *Diagnostic and Statistical Manual of Mental Disorders (4th edition)* (DSM-IV-TR).[1] Communication impairment is characterized by a delay or lack of communicative gesture use and spoken language development, challenges in the ability to initiate or maintain conversation, and unusual language use such as echolalia or idiosyncratic use of words. Unusual uses include private metaphors (eg, child says "ice cream trees" to refer to snow-covered trees, or "fix the alligator" to refer to fixing a tear on a book page that looks like an alligator); gestalt or unanalyzed phrases (eg, child repeats "Don't touch the pizza" whenever they see something hot); and video scripts (eg, using exact dialog from the *Cars* movie when playing with a friend). In addition, limitation of or a lack of symbolic or pretend play is associated with communication impairment.[1]

In the DSM-IV-TR,[1] autism was categorized as one of several types of pervasive developmental disorder (PDD). The new umbrella category label proposed for the *Diagnostic and Statistical Manual of Mental Disorders (5th edition)* (DSM-V) (http://www.dsm5.org) is ASD. The change from PDD to ASD as the overarching label is driven by identification of a common set of behaviors that characterize ASD as a single diagnostic category, with individual variability in severity, language level, intelligence, and change over time. Within the proposed DSM-V revision, language and communication remain critical to understanding ASD. However, the revision modifies the traditional triad of symptoms by integrating communication impairment with the social impairment that distinguishes children with ASD from those with other neurodevelopmental disabilities. This action is being taken to address the frequent overlaps and often indistinguishable boundaries between the social and communication difficulties that characterize autism. This change also recognizes the role of context in understanding the impact of social communication deficits. Further, because language deficits are not unique to autism, an integrated view of the role of language and communication within the social impairment in ASD more accurately reflects the clinical symptoms of this disorder.

The core deficits in the proposed DSM-V revision for ASD now include "persistent deficits in social communication and social interaction," with 3 specified criteria, all of which must be met for a diagnosis. In addition, the presence of "restricted, repetitive patterns of behaviors, interests or activities" must be documented about 4 criteria, 2 of which must be met for a diagnosis (http://www.dsm5.org). The social communication and social interaction deficits include challenges in social-emotional reciprocity, ranging from a lack of initiation, to an abnormal approach in a social context, to failure in back-and-forth conversational exchanges, including limited interest in sharing emotional and affective responses. Other symptoms include poorly integrated verbal and nonverbal communication abilities that contribute to social interactions, including abnormal eye contact and lack of gestures or facial expressions, as well as difficulties in developing and maintaining relationships. Relationship problems range from adjusting to a variety of social contexts, including sharing imaginative play with peers, to showing an interest in people and making friends. Considering the newly proposed social communication and social interaction criteria, the significant role language and communication play in the diagnosis becomes even clearer. Individuals must have an ability to understand the language that typically occurs in a social context (eg, how to interpret a joke, recognize tone of speech, or understand vocabulary used), as well as an ability to formulate a response (eg, answer questions, ask questions, or offer ideas).

The second core deficit area in the newly proposed diagnostic criteria for ASD is restricted, repetitive patterns of behavior (http://www.dsm5.org). These patterns of behavior include interests or activities that involve language and communication. For example, restrictive, repetitive behaviors may be characterized by stereotyped or repetitive speech (eg, idiosyncratic phrases or echolalia) and ritualized patterns of verbal behavior (eg, repetitive questioning) in addition to repetition or restricted patterns of nonverbal motor movements or object use; insistence on adherence to routines or resistance to change; restricted, fixated interests that are abnormal in intensity or focus (eg, perseverative interests); and overreactivity or underreactivity to sensory input or unusual sensory interests (eg, excessive smelling or object touching, fascination with lights or spinning objects).

Again, the role of language and communication becomes evident as verbal children with ASD use language in ways that are restricted, stereotyped, ritualized, and perseverative. Unconventional verbal behaviors such as echolalia, perseverative speech, and excessive questioning are common in autism.[2] Echolalia, which involves repeating exactly what is said or heard, can serve functional purposes, such as to request, label, maintain contact, or take a turn with a potential communicative partner.[3–5] These functions can be used as a bridge to more conventional communicative behavior. Perseverated speech involves imitated or self-generated utterances that are produced repeatedly with no real intent (eg, "Come on down" from a favorite TV program). It appears in contexts related to increased anxiety or language-processing difficulties.[2] A child or adolescent who exhibits excessive questioning may direct the same question to a communicative partner with an expectation for a response even although the answer has been provided previously, perhaps related to increased anxiety or language-processing difficulties. Talking about specific interests that may not be shared by the conversational partner is also a common social communication problem for this population, using language that interferes with the reciprocal nature of communication and social interaction. Each of these behaviors complicates the ability of an individual with ASD to engage fully in the give-and-take of conversational discourse expected during social exchanges and used for supporting the development of friendships.

What is the Role of Language and Communication Across the Subthreshold Diagnoses of ASD?

In DSM-IV-TR, autism is categorized under the umbrella label of PDD,[1] along with the subthreshold diagnoses of Rett disorder, childhood disintegrative disorder, Asperger disorder, and pervasive development disorder-not otherwise specified (PDD-NOS). The language and communication deficits across these disorders vary in severity and development, with associated implications for meaningful social communication. For example, Rett disorder is characterized by severe communication deficits, whereas childhood disintegrative disorder usually involves regression in receptive and expressive language skills and deficits in communication and social interaction typical of classic autism. With Asperger disorder, there is no significant delay in language development but frequent abnormalities in prosody,[6,7] speech that is considered pedantic or bookish,[8,9] deficits in conversation[10,11] and nonliteral language,[12,13] and a high incidence of faux pas in social contexts.[14] Individuals with Asperger disorder often have difficulty identifying another's attentional focus, emotional state and intentions, and selecting appropriate conversational topics based on context, the listener's perspective, and repairing communicative breakdowns.[15] In the proposed revisions for DSM-V, ASD is the umbrella label, and the category of ASD includes autistic disorder, Asperger disorder, childhood disintegrative disorder, and PDD-NOS.

What Developments During Infancy Contribute to Later Language and Communication?

Communicative behavior can be observed at birth in the intense mutual eye gaze that connects neonates to their parents, sealing the bond between them. Communication thus precedes language developmentally, and any difficulties can serve as early red flags so that preventative steps may be taken to engage the baby actively in reciprocal exchanges and shared attention. Early in infancy the establishment of joint attention is particularly important. It starts as mutual gaze between caregiver and infant and then proceeds to incorporate shared attention on a third object, person, or family pet, with the parent often commenting verbally as well as gesturally on the thing that is the focus of the child's attention. If development proceeds typically, the infant soon learns to recruit the attention of the caregiver by using body orientation, vocalization, and shifting gaze (ie, first looking at the parent and then the object of interest). The parent can use similar means to recruit the child's attention to new events or phenomena. The unfolding of this dance of social interaction requires the ability to coordinate visual attention around an object or activity and share an interest with another person.[16–22]

Research has shown that young children with ASD are less likely to use joint attention acts and gestures and are less able to coordinate their vocalizations, eye gaze, and gestures than typically developing peers and children with other developmental disabilities.[23] Poorly developed joint attention communicative acts are predictors of later language outcomes, and they have implications for development of conversational language.[18,23–25] The level of communicative competence achieved by individuals with ASD predicts their long-term positive outcomes.[26,27] These findings have led to a high interest in providing early interventions that teach parents to foster joint attention, with some promising results.[28–30]

What Roles are Played by Language and Communication in Later Academic and Social Learning?

The ability to decode verbal and nonverbal communication and then encode a response that is meaningful and socially relevant requires an intact language system. Wetherby and colleagues[22] reported that children with autism who can use fluent speech by age 5 years have a better prognosis for continued academic and social development. Some children and adolescents on the spectrum, especially those with Asperger disorder, have little difficulty learning language symbols and conventions for communicating and receiving literal messages. Some even show precocious reading without instruction, which is called hyperlexia.[31] However, all children and adolescents with ASD have social communication problems related to the inability to imagine what others think, know, and find interesting. This ability to imagine what is in another person's mind, which is termed having a theory of mind,[32] is critical for developing social relationships and responding appropriately to the social moves of others. Challenges experienced by children with high functioning autism for coping with the demands of school often relate to these difficulties, as well as to coping with anxiety about unpredictable routines, shifting schedules, and difficulty organizing their approaches to learning. Students on the autism spectrum who have the basic academic skills to be successful in postsecondary education may risk failure because of problems with executive functions and self-regulation rather than with the academic demands themselves.[33] Youth with ASD who have comorbid problems with cognition, speech, and language face challenges that may make it difficult for them to live independently.

INTEGRATED VIEW OF IDENTIFICATION AND ASSESSMENT
What is the Role of Physicians in Early Identification?

In providing early care, pediatricians play a critical role in the early detection of children with or at risk for ASD. Physicians are likely to see children during critical periods for identifying behaviors that differentiate children with ASD from children developing typically or showing other developmental disabilities. In recent years, clinical researchers have identified several early markers for ASD. Some researchers have used techniques such as retrospective video analysis of the social, communication, and play behaviors shown in the first 2 years of life by children later meeting diagnostic criteria for autism.[34–39] Other researchers have conducted prospective longitudinal studies in which children at risk for autism based on observation and screening results are followed over time to determine if hypothesized early markers are maintained and predictive of outcomes at 24 and 36 months of age.[40–44] Shumway and Wetherby[23] suggested that early identification of ASD is most often triggered by impairments in early social communication and repetitive behaviors. It is important, then, that primary care physicians follow the guidelines from the American Academy of Pediatrics for early screening and that they collaborate with families to identify those behaviors that place a child at risk for ASD. It is equally important that providers recognize the unique contribution of language understanding and use to the early markers for children with ASD. Early markers that research has shown to best differentiate children with ASD from those with other developmental disabilities are summarized in **Table 1**.

Ventola and colleagues[45] found children with ASD to score lower than children with developmental disabilities and other developmental language disorders in adaptive skills, expressive and receptive language, and fine motor and visual reception skills

Table 1
Cognitive-communicative abilities and problems that signal early red flags for ASD

Cognitive-Communicative Ability	Problems Observed Using the Ability
Mutual gaze	To establish intersubjective social contact
Shared gaze	To establish joint attention to another person, pet, or object
Pointing or showing	To express interest in objects or activities
Vocalizing	To gain attention
Responding to name attending to caregiver's voice	To show recognition of name or familiar voice
Showing interest in other children or people	To establish some early social interactions and communication exchanges
Pretending in play	To show symbol use and representation of objects, actions, characters, and so forth

on a screening measure for autism; further, deficits in joint attention and social interaction seemed to be particularly unique to autism. Considering a more integrated view of screening and assessment, it is important to consider all aspects of development when screening children with or at risk for autism and to recognize the likely delays in language understanding and expression as they relate to responding to and engaging with others to share experiences and interests.

Socially, toddlers with ASD have greater difficulty in joint attention, imitation, pointing to express interest, interest in other children, and displaying a range of facial expressions and empathic responses compared with other children with developmental disabilities.[44,46–48] This characteristic requires providers to have a clear understanding of typical development and developmental delays, and to use available developmental screenings tools (eg, Ages and Stages Questionnaire[49]), and autism-specific screening tools (eg, Modified Checklist for Autism in Toddlers [M-CHAT][50]) to facilitate earlier diagnosis of ASD. Children with a lack of appropriate gaze or warm, joyful expressions with eye gaze and alternating vocalization patterns as well as a failure to recognize familiar voices (eg, parents) and decreased use of gestures are red flags for a potential diagnosis of ASD.[51,52]

Understanding the developmental trajectory of communication is critical to the ability to make an early diagnosis. However, existing screening instruments have limitations ranging from methodological flaws to small samples, often missing children who are eventually diagnosed with ASD.[53] Another barrier to early diagnosis is that it is more difficult to make a diagnosis at 2 to 3 years because early delays in saying first words, establishing joint attention, and engaging socially may be attributed to normal variation, whereas at 5 to 6 years discrepancies from normal development are more obvious.[54] However, the evidence that early intervention is more effective than later is so compelling that health care providers must remain on high alert for early danger signs.[55–58] This challenge requires practitioners to have a developmental perspective on the assessment of language and communication difficulties and subsequent intervention in young children with ASD.[59,60] Vigilance also is required. Almost 30% of children with ASD present with periods of normal development followed by regression before 3 years.[61,62] Thus, any signs of language regression represent a serious concern that requires follow-up.[63]

To ensure effective assessment and intervention decision making, practitioners should engage family members in the process, and highly individualized profiles should be considered in program planning.[64] Social communication profiles can predict both developmental level and autism symptoms within 20-month-old children, who have a distinct social communication profile, with language understanding being a strong predictor of developmental level, and behavior regulation and gesture inventory being a strong predictor of autism diagnosis at age 3 years.[65] Programming is best supported by an integrated developmental framework that considers natural language samples, parental report, and standardized measures.[66] These are the types of assessments conducted by speech-language pathologists.

INTEGRATED VIEW OF HOW TO SUPPORT FAMILIES IN PROMOTING THEIR CHILDREN'S COMMUNICATION DEVELOPMENT

The past 15 years have seen a paradigm shift in which families are engaged actively as partners in the process of supporting their children's intervention programming.[67–69] This shift represents increased value placed on the combined expertise of providers and families as part of evidence-based practice[70] and offers promising outcomes for meeting the needs of children with neurodevelopmental disabilities.[71–76]

As a key component of the autism spectrum, communication has been an important intervention target for children with ASD. Several studies report positive results for the engagement of families as interventionists in facilitating language, communication, and social responsiveness.[77–81] Parents have been taught to facilitate response to and initiation of joint attention in their children with autism using contemporary behavioral approaches[28,82–84] as well as developmental and more naturalistic approaches.[29]

More than Words–The Hanen Program[85] is a family-based intervention designed for parents of children with ASD with the goal to integrate families' natural interaction skills with what is known about the communication and social challenges of children with ASD. This intervention provides numerous examples and opportunities for parents to practice what they learn in the context of everyday activities with their child. The first controlled trial of training effectiveness to facilitate parents' understanding of ASD and their support of social communication in their young children with ASD had a measurable effect on both the parents' and children's communication skills.[86] A second study examined the social interaction of 3 children with ASD (2.8–3.2 years of age) after their mother's participation in *More Than Words*, and found mothers increased their use of spontaneous interaction strategies whereas their children increased their vocabulary.[87] A recent multisite study[88] also revealed that children who played with a limited number of toys showed more improvement in their communication skills after their parents' participation in *More Than Words* training compared with children in community-based intervention only. Children showed progress in initiating joint attention, making behavioral requests, and communicating with intention. Parents also reported gains in nonverbal communication that were sustained 4 months after intervention.[88]

An integrated view for identification and assessment of children with ASD requires practitioners not only to understand the early markers for children with or at risk for ASD but also to engage families in the assessment process. Early identification and assessment can then lead to referral to speech-language pathologists and other specialists for early intervention and opportunities for families to engage their children and facilitate their communication.

INTEGRATED VIEW OF INTERVENTION APPROACHES FOR LANGUAGE, LITERACY, AND COMMUNICATION

Current evidence indicates that early intervention, and therefore identification, is a significant factor in long-term prognosis.[44,89,90] For example, children who receive early intervention are more likely to develop communication skills and fewer out-of-control behaviors,[91] and young children with ASD who develop language and symbolic play before age 5 years have better outcomes for educational placement and communication.[90] Furthermore, early intervention attenuates the severity of ASD-associated deficits (eg, impaired communication and deficits in social relatedness) that interfere with subsequent development.[92] Empirical studies of toddlers with ASD suggest that intensive, specialized early intervention has resulted in quantifiable gains and even children who are suspected of having ASD without a firm diagnosis should begin intervention services as early as possible.[27,52,93–95]

Over the last 10 years, there has been an evolution of thinking on the types of interventions most appropriate to support the communication and behavioral needs of children with ASD. Although traditional behavioral approaches have been plentiful and often the first choice for intervention in the psychology and education literature, other disciplines, such as speech-language pathology, have focused more on a social-pragmatic developmental approach. In the traditional behavioral approach, the adult interventionist uses a highly prescribed teaching structure to teach skills one-on-one with a predetermined correct response. Discrete trial training is an example of an applied behavioral analysis approach that has been used in classrooms, home-based programs and community-based programs to support communication, social, and adaptive skills in children with ASD.[96,97] In contrast, the adult interventionist using a social-pragmatic developmental approach follows the child's lead, emphasizing initiation and spontaneity, and delivers the intervention in the natural environment, reinforcing related responses. Floortime is an example of this type of approach. Caregivers learn to support and extend circles of communication (ie, reciprocal communicative exchanges) by joining a child's play and using playful obstruction to increase interaction with the interventionist.[98,99] Prizant and Wetherby[100] offered a middle-ground approach to intervention for children with ASD and suggested that both the behavioral and the developmental approaches make important contributions. These investigators described contemporary behavioral approaches that give children choices, share control of teaching opportunities, and use child-preferred activities and materials. An example of a contemporary behavioral approach is termed pivotal response training. It is an empirically validated play-based intervention, which uses both behavioral techniques and developmental principles to address the core deficits of autism, particularly communication and social interaction.[101,102]

Addressing questions about intervention effectiveness, the National Research Council (NRC)[103] convened clinical and applied researchers to examine the available intervention literature and determine best practices for children with ASD through the early childhood years. After their review, several guidelines emerged. First, it was determined that intervention should be initiated as early as possible and that active engagement in intensive instruction should occur within developmentally appropriate activities that are goal based and systematically planned. Second, planned teaching opportunities should occur throughout the day, including about 15-minute to 20-minute intervals for young children. Families and other communicative partners (eg, peers) should be included in the intervention to facilitate maintenance and generalization of skills being learned.

Shortly after the NRC document was published, Iovannone and colleagues[104] identified 6 core components that are considered effective educational practices for school-age children with ASD and their families. First, children with ASD require individualized supports and services that are matched to their profile through the individualized education program process. Second, systematic instruction is key to educational success and requires careful planning, valid goals, defined instructional procedures, and a process for evaluation and making needed changes. Third, a structured learning environment is critical so that the curriculum is clear to the students and staff. Fourth, specialized curriculum content should be added in the areas of social engagement, initiation and responding to social bids, and recreational and leisure skills. Fifth, a functional approach to problem behaviors is needed that focuses on replacing difficult behavior with appropriate behavior. Family involvement is crucial to the student's educational success.

Most recently, the National Autism Center (http://www.nationalautismcenter.org) published a report of the National Standards Project (NSP),[105] in which the current level of evidence for behavioral and educational interventions used for children and youth with ASD under age 22 years was identified. Based on a review and analysis of 775 peer-reviewed research studies in the previous 50 years, a classification system was developed categorizing treatments as established, emerging, unestablished, and ineffective/harmful. Eleven treatments were included in the established category, which means that there is sufficient evidence to conclude that these treatments

Table 2
Outline of established interventions for children with ASD

Established Treatment	Brief Description	Skills Taught	Behaviors Addressed	Age of Child (y)
Antecedent package (eg, time delay, reinforcement, fading, prompting, cueing)	Changing situational events that precede a behavior or lead to an increase in desired or a decrease in undesired behaviors	Communication, interpersonal, play, self-regulation, learning readiness, personal responsibility	Problem behaviors, sensory/ emotion regulation	3–18
Behavioral package (eg, chaining, contingency mapping, positive behavior supports, modeling, functional communication training)	Reducing difficult behaviors and teach meaningful alternatives	Academic, communication, interpersonal, learning readiness, personal responsibility, play, self	Problem behaviors, sensory/ emotion regulation, Restricted, repetitive behaviors	0–21
Comprehensive behavioral treatment of young children (eg, discrete trial, incidental teaching)	Using several different applied behavior analytical procedures usually delivered one-on-one; referred to as ABA programs	Communication, higher cognitive functions, interpersonal, motor, play, personal responsibility	Problem behaviors, general autism symptoms	0–8
Joint attention intervention	Teaching child to respond to or initiate social bids with another	Communication, interpersonal	None noted	0–5
Modeling (eg, live, self, and video modeling)	Showing a target behavior to facilitate imitation	Communication, cognition, social, play, personal responsibility	Problem behaviors, sensory/ emotion regulation	3–18
Naturalistic teaching strategies (eg, focused stimulation, milieu teaching)	Using child-directed interactions in the natural environment to support functional skills	Communication, interpersonal, learning readiness, play	None noted	0–9
Peer training package (eg, circle of friends, buddy skills, integrated play groups, peer mediation)	Teaching typically developing peers strategies to interact with children with ASD	Communication, social, play	Restricted, repetitive behaviors	3–14

(continued on next page)

Table 2
(continued)

Established Treatment	Brief Description	Skills Taught	Behaviors Addressed	Age of Child (y)
Pivotal response training	Teaching key behaviors like motivation, initiation, self-regulation to increase communication and social engagement	Communication, interpersonal, play	None noted	3–9
Schedules	Using visual supports to represent steps to complete tasks or activities	Self- regulation	None noted	3–14
Self-management	Teaching children to regulate their own behavior by identifying the behavior, recording it and reinforcing expected behavior	Interpersonal, self-regulation	Problem behaviors	3–18
Story-based intervention package (eg, social stories)	Describing situations in which expected behaviors are to occur using the written form	Interpersonal, self-regulation	None noted	6–14

Data from Randolph MA. National Standards Project: findings and conclusions–addressing the needs for evidence-based practice guidelines for autism spectrum disorders. Randolph, MA: National Autism Center; 2009. Available at: http://www.nationalautismcenter.org.

lead to favorable outcomes for children with ASD. Twenty-two treatments fell in the emerging category, which means that 1 or more studies have revealed positive outcomes for children with ASD but additional high-quality studies are needed to show the observed outcomes consistently. Five treatments were identified as unestablished, or as having little to no evidence, thus requiring additional research. A final classification category was established for treatments that were ineffective/harmful, but no specific treatments were identified in this category. **Table 2** summarizes the intervention treatments that were identified as established, brief descriptions of the treatments, and the skills being taught or the behaviors being addressed for children with ASD from birth to 21 years. Eight of the 11 established interventions have evidence for improving communication skills in children with ASD and 10 have evidence for supporting social or interpersonal skills. Overall, behavioral treatments had the strongest support in the NSP review although nonbehavioral approaches were identified as making a critical contribution requiring additional research.

SUMMARY

Children with ASD can vary widely in the expression of the disorder. Although there is no known cure for autism, the evidence is increasing that early and ongoing intervention can improve the prognosis for the development of language and communication skills that can support other learning and social interaction. Varied approaches have been found to be effective in engaging children with ASD, and many new possibilities could be explored. Intervention approaches with promise incorporate features of intensive, deliberate efforts to help children communicate socially by sharing attention with others, engaging in the imagination of play, and developing an understanding of how things function and how people think, feel, and imagine.

REFERENCES

1. American Psychiatric Association. Diagnostic and statistical manual of mental disorders, fourth edition (text revision) DSM-IV-TR. Washington, DC: American Psychiatric Association; 2000.
2. Prizant BM, Rydell PJ. Assessment and intervention considerations for unconventional verbal behavior. In: Warren SF, Reichle J, Wacker D, editors, Communicative alternatives to challenging behavior: integrating functional assessment and intervention strategies (communication and language intervention series), vol. 3. Baltimore (MD): Brookes; 1993. p. 263–97.
3. Prizant BM. Theoretical and clinical implications of echolalic behavior in autism. In: Layton T, editor. Language and treatment of autistic and developmentally disordered children. Springfield (MA): CC Thomas; 1987. p. 65–88.
4. Prizant BM, Wetherby AM, Rydell PJ. Communication intervention issues for young children with autism spectrum disorders. In: Wetherby AM, Prizant BM, editors, Autism spectrum disorders: a transactional developmental perspective (communication and language intervention series), vol. 9. Baltimore (MD): Brookes; 2000. p. 193–224.
5. Rydell PJ, Prizant BM. Assessment and intervention strategies for children who use echolalia. In: Quill KA, editor. Teaching children with autism: strategies to enhance communication and socialization. New York: Delmar; 1995. p. 105–32.
6. Eisenmajer R, Prior M, Leekam S, et al. Comparison of clinical symptoms in autism and Asperger's disorder. J Am Acad Child Adolesc Psychiatry 1996; 35:1523–31.

7. Shriberg LD, Paul R, McSweeney J, et al. Speech and prosody characteristics of adolescents and adults with high functioning autism and Asperger syndrome. J Speech Lang Hear Res 2001;44:1097–115.

8. Burgoine E, Wing L. Identical triplets with Asperger's syndrome. Br J Psychiatry 1983;143:261–5.

9. Ghaziuddin M, Gerstein L. Pedantic speaking style differentiates autism from Asperger syndrome. J Autism Dev Disord 1996;26:585–95.

10. Adams C, Green J, Gilchrist A, et al. Conversational behaviour of children with Asperger syndrome and conduct disorders. J Child Psychol Psychiatry 2002; 43:679–90.

11. Ramberg C, Ehlers S, Nyden A, et al. Language and pragmatic functions in school-age children on the autism spectrum. Eur J Disord Commun 1996;31: 387–414.

12. Kerbel D, Grunwell P. A study of idiom comprehension in children with semantic-pragmatic difficulties. Part I: task effects on the assessment of idiom comprehension in children. Int J Lang Commun Disord 1998;33:1–44.

13. Jolliffe T, Baron-Cohen S. Linguistic processing in high-functioning adults with autism or Asperger syndrome: can global coherence be achieved? A further test of central coherence theory. Psychol Med 2000;30:1169–87.

14. Baron-Cohen S, Ring H, Wheelwright S, et al. Social intelligence in the normal and autistic brain: an fMRI study. Eur J Neurosci 1999;11:1891–8.

15. Klin A, Volkmar FR, Sparrow SS. Asperger syndrome. New York: Guilford Press; 2000.

16. Carpenter M, Tomasello M. Joint attention, cultural learning, and language acquisition. In: Wetherby AM, Prizant BM, editors. Understanding the nature of communication and language impairments in autism spectrum disorders: a transactional developmental perspective. Baltimore (MD): Brookes; 2000. p. 31–54.

17. Charman T. Why is joint attention a pivotal skill in autism? Philos Trans R Soc Lond B Biol Sci 2003;358:315–24.

18. Mundy P, Sigman M, Kasari C. A longitudinal study of joint attention and language development in autistic children. J Autism Dev Disord 1990;20: 115–28.

19. Mundy P, Stella J. Joint attention, social orienting, and nonverbal communication in autism. In: Wetherby AM, Prizant BM, editors, Autism spectrum disorders: a transactional developmental perspective (communication and language intervention series), vol. 9. Baltimore (MD): Brookes; 2000. p. 55–77.

20. Wetherby AM, Prizant BM. Profiling young children's communicative competence. In: Warren SF, Reichle J, editors, Communication and language intervention series: causes and effects in communication and language intervention, vol. 1. Baltimore (MD): Brookes; 1992. p. 217–53.

21. Wetherby AM, Prizant BM, Hutchinson TA. Communicative, social/affective, and symbolic profiles of young children with autism and pervasive developmental disorders. Am J Speech Lang Pathol 1998;7:79–91.

22. Wetherby AM, Prizant BM, Schuler AL. Understanding the nature of communication and language impairments. In: Wetherby AM, Prizant BM, editors, Autism spectrum disorders: a transactional developmental perspective (communication and language intervention series), vol. 9. Baltimore (MD): Brookes; 2000. p. 109–41.

23. Shumway S, Wetherby AM. Communicative acts of children with ASD in the second year of life. J Speech Lang Hear Res 2009;52:1139–56.

24. Charman T, Howlin P, Aldred C, et al. Research into early intervention for children with autism and related disorders: methodological and design issues. Autism 2003;7:217–25.

25. Dawson G, Toth K, Abbott R, et al. Early social attention impairments in autism: social orienting, joint attention, and attention to distress. Dev Psychol 2004;40: 271–83.

26. Grafin D, Lord C. Communication as a social problem in autism. In: Schopler E, Mesibov G, editors. Social behavior in autism. New York: Plenum Press; 1986. p. 237–61.

27. McEachin J, Smith T, Lovaas OI. Long-term outcome for children with autism who received early intensive behavioral treatment. Am J Ment Retard 1993;97: 359–72.

28. Rocha ML, Schreibman L, Stahmer AC. Effectiveness of training parents to teach joint attention in children with autism. J Early Interv 2007;29:154–73.

29. Schertz HH, Odom SL. Promoting joint attention in toddlers with autism: a parent-mediated developmental model. J Autism Dev Disord 2007;37: 1562–75.

30. Woods JJ, Brown JA. Integrating family capacity building and child outcomes to support social communication development in young children with ASD. Topics Lang Disord 2011;31:235–46.

31. Mirenda P. "He's not really a reader....": perspectives on supporting literacy development in individuals with autism. Top Lang Disord 2003;23:271–82.

32. Baron-Cohen S. Mindblindness: an essay on autism and theory of mind. Cambridge (United Kingdom): The MIT Press; 1995.

33. Hewitt LE. Perspectives on support needs of individuals with autism spectrum disorders: transition to college. Top Lang Disord 2011;31:273–85.

34. Adrien JL, Perror A, Sauvage D, et al. Early symptoms in autism from family home movies: evaluation and comparison between 1st and 2nd year of life using I.B.S.E. Scale. Acta Paedopsychiatr 1992;55:71–5.

35. Baranek GT. Autism during infancy: a retrospective video analysis of sensory-motor and social behaviors at 9-12 months of age. J Autism Dev Disord 1999; 29:213–24.

36. Clifford S, Young R, Williamson P. Assessing the early characteristics of autistic disorder using video analysis. J Autism Dev Disord 2007;37:301–13.

37. Mars AE, Maujk JE, Dowrick PW. Symptoms of pervasive developmental disorders as observed in prediagnostic home videos of infants and toddlers. J Pediatr 1998;132:5000–4.

38. Osterling J, Dawson G. Early recognition of children with autism: a study of first birthday home videotapes. J Autism Dev Disord 1994;24:247–58.

39. Werner E, Dawson G, Osterling J, et al. Brief report: recognition of autism spectrum disorder before one year of age: a retrospective study based on home videotapes. J Autism Dev Disord 2000;30:157–8.

40. Baird G, Charman T, Baron-Cohen S, et al. A screening instrument for autism at 18 months of age: a six-year follow-up study. J Am Acad Child Adolesc Psychiatry 2000;39:694–702.

41. Baron-Cohen S, Allen J, Gillberg C. Can autism be detected at 18 months? The needle, the haystack, and the CHAT. Br J Psychiatry 1992;161:839–43.

42. Baron-Cohen S, Cox A, Baird G, et al. Psychological markers in the detection of autism in infancy in a large population. Br J Psychiatry 1996;168:138–63.

43. Dietz C, Swinkels S, van Daalen E, et al. Screening for autistic spectrum disorder in children aged 14-15 months II: population screening with the Early

Screening of Autistic Traits Questionnaire (ESAT). Design and general findings. J Autism Dev Disord 2006;36:713–22.

44. Lord C. Follow-up of two-year-olds referred for possible autism. J Child Psychol Psychiatry 1995;36:1365–82.

45. Ventoloa P, Kleinman J, Pandey J, et al. Differentiating between ASD and other developmental disabilities in children who failed a screening instrument for ASD. J Autism Dev Disord 2007;37:425–36.

46. Charman T, Swettenham J, Baron-Cohen S, et al. An experimental investigation of social-cognitive abilities in infants with autism: clinical implications. J Infant Mental Health 1998;19:1–26.

47. Landry SH, Loveland KA. Communication behaviors in autism and developmental language delay. J Child Psychol Psychiatry 1988;29:621–34.

48. Trillingsgaard A, Sorensen EU, Nemec G, et al. What distinguishes autism spectrum disorders from other developmental disorders before the age of four years. Eur Child Adolesc Psychiatry 2005;14:65–72.

49. Bricker D, Squires J. Ages and stages questionnaires: a parent-completed child-monitoring system. 2nd edition. Baltimore (MD): Brookes; 1999.

50. Robins DL, Fein D, Barton ML, et al. The modified checklist for autism in toddlers: an initial study investigating the early detection of autism and pervasive developmental disorders. J Autism Dev Disord 2001;31:131–44.

51. Johnson CP. Recognition of autism before age 2 years. Pediatr Rev 2008;29:86–96.

52. Johnson CP, Myers SM, Council on Children with Disabilities. Identification and evaluation of children with autism spectrum disorders. Pediatrics 2007;120:1183–93.

53. Bryson SE, Rogers SJ, Fombonne E. Autism spectrum disorders: early detection, intervention, education, and psychopharmacological management. Can J Psychiatry 2003;48:506–16.

54. Lord C, Risi S. Early diagnosis in children with autism spectrum disorders. Advocate 2000;33:23–6.

55. Boyd BA, Odom SL, Humphreys BP. Infants and toddlers with autism spectrum disorder: early identification and intervention. J Early Interv 2010;32:75–98.

56. Reznick JJ, Baranek G, Reavis S, et al. A parent-report instrument for identifying one-year-olds at risk for an eventual diagnosis of autism: the first year inventory. J Autism Dev Disord 2007;37:1691–710.

57. Wetherby AM, Woods JJ. Effectiveness of early intervention for children with autism spectrum disorders beginning in the second year of life. Topics Early Child Spec Educ 2006;26:67–82.

58. Zwaigenbaum L, Bryson S, Rogers T, et al. Behavioral manifestations of autism in the first year of life. Int J Dev Neurosci 2005;23:143–52.

59. Prelock PA. Communication assessment and intervention in autism spectrum disorders. Austin (TX): Pro-Ed; 2006.

60. Watson LR, Baranek G, Crais ER, et al. The first year inventory: retrospective parent responses to a questionnaire designed to identify one-year-olds at risk for autism. J Autism Dev Disord 2007;37:49–61.

61. Chawarska K, Klin A, Paul R, et al. Autism spectrum disorder in the second year: stability and change in syndrome expression. J Child Psychol Psychiatry 2007;48:128–38.

62. Tuchman RF, Rapin I. Regression in pervasive developmental disorders: seizures and epileptiform electroencephalogram correlates. Pediatrics 1997;99:560–6.

63. Wilson S, Djukic A, Shinnar S, et al. Clinical characteristics of language regression in children. Dev Med Child Neurol 2003;45:508–14.
64. Fernell E, Hedvall A, Norrelgen F, et al. Developmental profiles in preschool children with ASD referred for intervention. Res Dev Disabil 2010;31:790–9.
65. Wetherby AM, Watt N, Morgan L, et al. Social communication profiles of children with autism spectrum disorders late in the second year of life. J Autism Dev Disord 2007;37:960–75.
66. Tager-Flusberg H, Rogers S, Cooper J, et al. Defining spoken language benchmarks and selecting measures of expressive language development for young children with ASD. J Speech Lang Hear Res 2009;52:643–52.
67. Prelock PA, Beatson J, Contompasis S, et al. A model for family-centered interdisciplinary practice. Top Lang Disord 1999;19:36–51.
68. Shelton TL, Jeppson ES, Johnson BH. Family-centered care for children with special health care needs. Bethesda (MD): Association for the Care of Children's Health; 1987.
69. Vincent LJ. Family relationships. Equals in this partnership: parents of disabled and at-risk infants and toddlers speak to professionals. Washington, DC: National Center for Clinical Infant Programs; 1985. p. 33–41.
70. Straus SE, Sackett DL. Using research findings in clinical practice. BMJ 1998; 317:339–43.
71. Andrews J, Andrews A. Family-based treatment in communicative disorders. Sandwich (IL): Janelle Publications; 1990.
72. Brewer EJ, McPherson M, Magrab PR, et al. Family-centered, community-based, coordinated care for children with special health care needs. Pediatrics 1989;83:1055–60.
73. Dunst CJ, Trivette CM, Deal A. Enabling and empowering families. Cambridge (United Kingdom): Brookline Books; 1988.
74. Roberts-DeGennaro M. An interdisciplinary training model in the field of early intervention. J Soc Work Educ 1996;18:20–9.
75. Shelton TL, Stepanek JS. Family-centered care for children needing specialized health and developmental services. Bethesda (MD): Association for the Care of Children's Health; 1994.
76. Vig S, Kaminer R. Comprehensive interdisciplinary evaluation as intervention for young children. Infants Young Child 2003;16:342–53.
77. Aldred C, Green J, Adams C. A new social communication intervention for children with autism: pilot randomized controlled treatment study suggesting effectiveness. J Child Psychol Psychiatry 2004;45:1420–30.
78. Delaney EM, Kaiser AP. The effects of teaching parents blended communication and behavior support strategies. Behav Disord 2001;26:93–116.
79. Mahoney G, Perales F. Using relationship-focused intervention to enhance the social-emotional functioning of your children with autism spectrum disorders. Top Early Child Spec Educ 2003;23:77–89.
80. Moes DR, Frea WD. Contextualized behavioral support in early intervention for children with autism and their families. J Autism Dev Disord 2002;32: 519–33.
81. Siller M, Sigman M. The behaviors of parents of children with autism predict the subsequent development of their children's communication. J Autism Dev Disord 2002;32:77–89.
82. Kasari C, Freeman S, Paparella T. Joint attention and symbolic play in young children with autism: a randomized controlled intervention study. J Child Psychol Psychiatry 2006;47:611–20.

83. Kasari C, Paparella T, Freeman S, et al. Language outcome in autism: randomized comparison of joint attention and play interventions. J Consult Clin Psychol 2008;76:125–37.

84. Whalen C, Schreibman L, Ingersoll B. The collateral effects of joint attention training on social initiations, positive affect, imitation, and spontaneous speech for young children with autism. J Autism Dev Disord 2006;36:655–64.

85. Sussman F. More than words: helping parents promote communication and social skills in children with autism spectrum disorders. Toronto: A Hanen Centre Publication; 1999.

86. McConachie H, Val Randle V, Hammal D, et al. A controlled trial of a training course for parents of children with suspected autism spectrum disorders. J Pediatr 2005;147:335–40.

87. Girolametto L, Sussman F, Weitzman E. Using case study methods to investigate the effects of interactive intervention for children with autism spectrum disorders. J Commun Dis 2007;40:470–92.

88. Carter AS, Messinger DS, Stone WL, et al. A randomized controlled trial of Hanen's 'More Than Words' in toddlers with early autism symptoms. J Child Psychol Psychiatry 2011. DOI: 10.1111/j.1469-7610.2011.02395.x.

89. Prizant BM, Wetherby AM. Providing services to children with autism (ages 0-2 years) and their families. Top Lang Disord 1988;9:1–2.

90. Mays RM, Gillon JE. Autism in young children: an update. J Pediatr Health Care 1993;7:17–23.

91. Siegel B, Pliner C, Eschler J, et al. How children with autism are diagnosed: difficulties in identification of children with multiple developmental delays, 1988 children with multiple developmental delays. J Dev Behav Pediatr 1988;9:199–204.

92. Robins D, Dumont-Mathieu T. Early screening for autism spectrum disorders: update on the modified checklist for autism in toddlers and other measures. J Dev Behav Pediatr 2006;27(Suppl 2):S111–9.

93. Horner R, Carr E, Strain P, et al. Problem behavior interventions for young children with autism: a research synthesis. J Autism Dev Disord 2002;32:423–46.

94. Sallows G, Graupner T. Intensive behavioral treatment for children with autism: four-year outcome and predictors. Am J Ment Retard 2005;110:417–38.

95. Schreibman L. Intensive behavioral/psychoeducational treatments for autism: research needs and future directions. J Autism Dev Disord 2000;30:373–8.

96. Karsten AM, Carr JE. The effects of differential reinforcement of unprompted responding on the skill acquisition of children with autism. J Appl Behav Anal 2009;42:327–34.

97. Newman B, Reinecke D, Ramos M. Is a reasonable attempt reasonable? Shaping versus reinforcing verbal attempts of preschoolers with autism. Analysis of Verbal Behavior 2009;25:67–72.

98. Greenspan SI, Weider S. Developmental patterns and outcomes in infants and children with disorders in relating and communicating: a chart review of 200 cases of children with autistic spectrum disorder. Journal of Developmental Learning Disabilities 1997;1:87–141.

99. Greenspan SI, Wieder S. The child with special needs: encouraging intellectual and emotional growth. Reading (MA): Perseus Books; 1998.

100. Prizant BM, Wetherby AM. Understanding the continuum of discrete-trial traditional behavioral to social-pragmatic developmental approaches in communication enhancement for young children with autism/PDD. Semin Speech Lang 1998;19:329–52.

101. Koegel LK, Koegel R, Harrower J, et al. Pivotal response intervention I: overview of approach. J Assoc Pers Sev Handicaps 1999;24:174–85.
102. Koegel LK, Koegel RL, Shoshan Y, et al. Pivotal response intervention II: preliminary long-term outcomes data. J Assoc Pers Sev Handicaps 1999;24:186–98.
103. National Research Council. Educating children with autism. Washington, DC: National Academy Press; 2001.
104. Iovannone R, Dunlap G, Huber H, et al. Effective educational practices for students with autism spectrum disorders. Focus on Autism Other Dev Disable 2003;18:150–65.
105. National Autism Center. National Standards Project: findings and conclusions–addressing the needs for evidence-based practice guidelines for autism spectrum disorders. Randolph (MA): National Autism Center; 2009. Available at: http://www.nationalautismcenter.org. Accessed May 1, 2011.

Behavioral Interventions for Children with Autism Spectrum Disorders

Linda A. LeBlanc, PhD, BCBA-D*, Jennifer M. Gillis, PhD, BCBA-D

KEYWORDS

- Autism • Behavioral intervention • Consultation
- Evidence-based practice • Families

Pediatricians are now equipped with excellent tools and guidelines for screening young children for autism spectrum disorders (ASDs) as part of standard pediatric care (see the article by Patel and Pratt elsewhere in this issue).[1,2] When those screenings suggest that a referral for a comprehensive evaluation is warranted, clinicians have psychometrically sound tools to assist with diagnosing a growing number of children with ASDs at early ages (see the article by Huerta and Lord elsewhere in this issue).[3] Early identification is critically important to ensure that families have the opportunity to reap the many unique benefits that may arise from early intervention efforts. For example, intervention efforts that occur early during a child's development may have the advantage of increased brain plasticity, which may enhance outcomes.[4] Intervention efforts that are designed to have both sustained and developmental trajectory-altering impacts have the greatest likelihood of eliminating developmental delays when they occur earlier in the developmental course.[5] In addition, earlier intervention and family supports decrease the likelihood of the development of severe problem behaviors that often arise and negatively affect family functioning.[6,7]

As the primary care provider, pediatricians are the first and best source of guidance for families who are seeking treatment services after the initial diagnosis of an ASD and as new problems arise throughout childhood and adolescence. Although excellent resources and practice guidelines have been disseminated to facilitate surveillance and screening of ASDs,[1,8] fewer comprehensive resources exist to guide treatment selection. The currently available treatments for ASDs vary greatly with respect to the degree of dissemination and the degree to which their effectiveness is supported by well-controlled research.[9] The only psychoeducational treatment that meets the

The authors have nothing to disclose.
Department of Psychology, 226 Thach Hall, Auburn University, Auburn, AL 36849-5214, USA
* Corresponding author.
E-mail address: leblanc@auburn.edu

criteria as a well-established and efficacious intervention for ASD is behavioral treatment,[10–12] which is often referred to as applied behavior analysis (ABA). In the National Autism Center guidelines, virtually all of the 11 interventions identified as established treatments are components of applied behavior analysis.[13] However, families may be unaware of the existence of ABA services, unsure how to find a qualified provider to access the services, or may mistakenly think that there is only 1 version of ABA services (early intensive behavioral intervention [EIBI]) when other forms of behavioral treatment have proved effective for concerns across the lifespan and at lower intensities.[12,14]

Families are likely to turn to their pediatrician for guidance about what sources are useful and trustworthy and what information should guide their selection of treatments and providers. This article provides information to guide recommendations to families in seeking behavioral treatment. The appendices are useful resources for pediatricians and are appropriate for distribution to families. Information is provided about the different models of behavioral intervention along with a review of the evidence for their effectiveness, including information about dosage effects and predictors of response to intervention, where available. In addition, this article provides information about what families should look for when seeking a provider of behavioral treatment services (ie, qualifications and credentials, indicators of quality programming), and recommendations about the types of collaboration and assistance pediatricians might expect from a behavior analyst who is serving one of their patients.

BEHAVIORAL TREATMENT

There are at least 3 critical features of all behavioral treatments. First, the procedures are derived directly from behavioral theory and research. Second, there is an emphasis on frequent measurement of observable indicators of progress. Third, all aspects of the child's functioning (eg, skills, deficits, problem behavior) are considered products of the interaction between children and influential aspects of their environments. After a careful examination of the interplay between the child and the environment (eg, people, events) reveals important interaction patterns, problematic interactions can be directly targeted using behavioral treatment procedures. Sometimes the interaction pattern is changed by teaching the child important new functional skills (ie, requests) and sometimes the interaction pattern is changed by altering some aspect of the environment (eg, availability of certain interactions, adult responses to problem behaviors). However, substantial differences exist in behavioral treatments related to the scope and goals of the therapy, the venue for delivering the services, and unique client characteristics (eg, age, clinical presentation). For example, a recently diagnosed 2.5-year-old with limited language, social, and cognitive skills may be a prime candidate for intensive instructional services. In contrast, an 8-year-old who attends general educational classes in school but has substantial anxiety and social skills deficits might benefit from behavioral consultation and less intensive outpatient services.

The terms commonly used for these different varieties of behavioral treatment are often foreign to families. For example, Ivar Lovaas coined the phrase discrete trial training (DTT) to refer to the first brand of intensive behavioral intervention for ASD, and that version of behavioral treatment is sometimes referred to as DTT, Lovaas therapy, or UCLA (University of California, Los Angeles) model behavioral treatment. Other terms for this specific application of ABA might be used depending on regional influences and provider preferences. Appendix 1 provides a list of common terms and definitions that a pediatrician might find useful or that could be directly disseminated to parents as they prepare to seek treatment services.

EIBI

The purpose of EIBI is to increase intellectual (ie, communication, cognitive, academic) skills and adaptive functioning (ie, social skills, self-care skills, safety) to prepare children with ASD to learn from, and succeed in, typical home and school environments with the fewest possible supports.[15–18] These goals are achieved by creating a precise and sophisticated instructional environment for as many of the child's waking hours as possible, at the youngest age possible, to alter the developmental trajectory in all areas of functioning. Perhaps the most critical repertoires targeted are the learning-to-learn skills (eg, imitation, following instructions, initiating interactions) that allow children to learn from more typical environments in ways that are similar to their peers.[17,18] Large and sustained improvements in specific skills and in overall functioning increase the likelihood that a child will continue to be able to succeed throughout life with less intensive behavioral supports.[16]

EIBI has several characteristic features that are critical to producing successful outcomes regardless of whether the services are provided in the family home or in a center-based clinic program. Families should be encouraged to evaluate their potential service options to determine the extent to which these characteristics are readily evident.[17] First, the intervention model should focus on teaching small units of learning systematically and the targeted skills should be arranged in a carefully constructed behavior analytical curriculum. Children with ASDs do not readily learn complex skills from typical environments; thus, EIBI is designed to establish all of the component skills that evolve into complex skills.[18] Any EIBI program should be using a well-established behavior analytical curriculum to guide programming, and several excellent ones have been published.[19–22] Some provider agencies develop their own excellent proprietary curricula rather than using one that is commercially available; however, the agency should be willing and prepared to show that curriculum to a family that is considering their services. Second, the teaching procedures should be specified in great detail with respect to precise behavioral instructional procedures (ie, prompting strategies along with powerful rewards for every success). Third, the learning opportunities are repeated many times and in many environments until the child can perform all the skills independently across all natural settings (ie, generalized skills with all people, in all places, and in play contexts). Fourth, data are collected on performance during virtually all learning opportunities to examine progress in each area so that instruction can be modified as quickly as possible to ensure rapid progress. Furthermore, parents should expect a quality behavioral provider to collect data, to show them graphs of performance frequently, and to teach them how to collect data.

In addition to the characteristics of EIBI listed earlier, effective programs always include a substantial component of parent support and training designed to assist families in crafting a home environment that promotes optimal functioning for their child and minimize the likelihood of development of severe problem behavior.[18] Providers teach parents how to play with their children in ways that feel natural, but are likely to promote better social interactions and more meaningful and appropriate play.[18,23,24] They also learn how to prevent problem behavior or how to change their interactions with the child if problem behavior emerges, and how to teach daily living skills, communication, and social skills using behavioral instructional procedures.[18,25]

Since the publication of the findings of the American Psychological Association's task force on empirically supported treatments for children and adolescents, the

Chambliss Criteria have been used to evaluate the degree of published empirical support for psychosocial interventions.[26] The category with the most stringent criteria and greatest evidence is Well-established and Efficacious, which requires multiple controlled trials of the intervention compared with various reasonable controls. Other categories include Probably Efficacious, Promising, and Not Supported, based on less rigorous evaluations, fewer evaluations, or lack of evidence of demonstrated effectiveness. Based on multiple meta-analyses and systematic reviews, EIBI is the only intervention for ASD that meets the criteria for the category Well-established and Efficacious.[11,12,27,28]

The initial demonstration of the effectiveness of comprehensive EIBI indicated that about 40 hours per week of intervention at very young ages resulted in 47% of participants achieving best outcome, as opposed to 2% of participants in a treatment-as-usual control group.[15] Best outcome was defined as an intelligence quotient (IQ) in the normal range and a full-inclusion first grade placement with ameliorated symptoms of ASD such that these children were indistinguishable from their peers. Although the common vernacular of recovered or recovery has been used with regard to this outcome, we do not recommended using this term with families because ASD is a life-long neurobiological disorder rather than a fluctuating disease state.[29,30] These individuals typically continue to experience some characteristic features of the ASD although their functioning is substantially improved, they are able to participate more fully in society, and they may be indistinguishable from their nonaffected peers. Families that view ASD as a lifelong serious condition tend to have better adjustment outcomes and are more likely to pursue scientifically validated treatments than families who view it as having an unpredictable timeline or course.[31] Encourage families to view the goal of EIBI as producing the best possible functionality and happiness in life for their children with ASD, exactly as they would hope for any of their children who do not have ASD.

Using this best outcome standard, the effectiveness of EIBI for young children with ASD has been shown in several replications and extensions in the past decade.[12,32–35] Recent research has identified important parameters of EIBI, including the level of intensity and duration of services, the age for which EIBI is most effective, and the qualifications of the most effective providers. The most positive child outcomes have been documented when EIBI is consistently delivered at a high dosage or intensity (ie, at least 25–40 hours per week and for a duration of 2–3 years).[18,33–35] However, it is critical that the high volume of services consist of EIBI because, compared with equally intensive traditional or eclectic model special education services, EIBI consistently produces better outcomes.[33,34,36] In addition, when the intensity of EIBI decreases to approximately 12 to 20 hours per week, children with ASDs show only modest gains in functioning, although these outcomes are better than those achieved with the other types of treatment discussed earlier.[37,38]

Common to most replication studies is the young age at which children with ASDs receive EIBI: compared with children who entered EIBI programs after the age of 5 years, younger children are more likely to experience greater positive outcomes (eg, public school classroom placement).[39,40] Older children (ie, 7 years old) do respond positively to intensive behavioral interventions, although to a limited degree compared with younger children.[32,41] Smith and colleagues[42] reported that EIBI was not effective with 3 girls initially diagnosed with autism and later identified as having Rett disorder, even though the services were provided at a young age and intensively. Rett disorder is slated to be removed from the category that will be referred to as ASD in the new diagnostic classification system, and these girls should not be considered exceptional candidates for EIBI as children with ASD are. Based on the available literature, children should begin EIBI programs before the age of 5 years,[12] preferably before the age of 3 years[43]; however, this will only occur if ASD screening occurs at recommended well-child visits.[1]

In addition to starting an EIBI program at the youngest possible age, it is also important to have the services provided and supervised by quality behavior analytical professionals.[12,18,44] In replication studies on the effects of EIBI, the training model and credentials of the supervisors was one of the few variables that predicted differential outcomes (ie, supervisors with higher credentials and certification produced better outcomes).[12,27] One UK study found significantly poorer outcomes for children served in home-based EIBI programs coordinated by their parents and supervised intermittently by providers with varying degrees of training, compared with the published studies in which programming was coordinated and supervised by certified providers.[44]

The international credentialing body for certifying behavior analysts is the Behavior Analyst Certification Board, which was established at the international level in 1998 and evolved from a previously established credentialing program in Florida.[45] The Behavior Analyst Certification Board (BACB) is accredited by the National Council for Certifying Agencies and is endorsed by the national and international professional organizations of behavior analysis in the United States and Europe.[45] This certification requires a passing score on an international content examination, documentation of supervised practical training, required coursework in behavior analysis, and ongoing continuing education in behavior analysis.[45,46]

The BACB certifies 3 levels of providers and maintains an online directory of all currently certified behavior analysts by state and country.[45] The highest level of credential, the Board Certified Behavior Analyst-Doctoral (BCBA-D) requires a doctorate degree. The most common credential for direct providers and EIBI program supervisors is the Board Certified Behavior Analyst (BCBA) credential, which requires a minimum of a Master's degree. The Board Certified Assistant Behavior Analyst (BCaBA) is the credential for individuals with a Bachelor's degree and this credential requires ongoing supervision by a BCBA or BCBA-D during practice. Certification is considered the practice credential for individuals practicing behavior analysis, similar to the medical license for a physician. In addition to certification, some qualified providers have credentials pertinent to their degree specialization (eg, licensed psychologist, licensed social worker, certified teacher, certified speech-language pathologist) or for specific models of EIBI intervention programming (eg, UCLA model certification) in addition to the broader discipline of behavior analysis. Families seeking EIBI services should seek a provider with the BCBA practice credential because this is the basic standard for behavior analysis. Families are also encouraged to check the BACB Web site (www.bacb.com), which provides information for consumers about the guidelines for professional conduct for the field and about any prior or outstanding complaints and sanctions against credentialed providers.[46] In addition, most states or regions have an organization or association for behavior analysis that may be a good source of information about potential providers and statewide intervention resources.

As a family seeks EIBI services, they need to identify a qualified provider and determine how to manage the finances associated with pursuing this intervention. The costs of EIBI can be substantial over the course of 2 to 3 years of treatment, although the savings accrued by avoiding 16 to 18 years of special education costs and adult support services costs are substantial.[47,48] In spite of the potential savings to government agencies, not all states have legislated funding mechanisms to cover these costs. In some states and Canadian provinces,[49,50] the costs of EIBI services are covered by governmental entities or are mandated as part of health insurance coverage up to a certain dollar amount. In other states, no such legislation and funding streams exist and families may encounter tens of thousands of dollars of out-of-pocket expenses per year. The advocacy organization, Autism Speaks, maintains an up-to-date accounting of the states that have mandated insurance coverage, which increased from 1 state to more than 25 states in just 5 years (see www.autismspeaks.org for current information).

In summary, EIBI is the treatment of choice for young children identified with ASDs. This form of behavioral treatment involves a highly structured curriculum and precise teaching methodologies to target skills that allow children to learn more effectively from typical environments. Multiple studies show the robust effects of EIBI for children with ASDs, particularly when services are provided at young ages, at a substantial level of intensity, and by highly qualified providers. Meta-analyses of these findings have confirmed that approximately 30% to 50% of children who receive EIBI achieve outcomes such as improved global functioning (eg, cognitive or intellectual functioning, adaptive behaviors, language) along with placement in regular education classrooms. The remaining children typically experience moderate to substantial increases in functioning compared with before treatment, but may not achieve typical intellectual functioning and full integration in subsequent schooling.[27,28] Appendix 2 includes common questions of parents about behavioral treatment services and answers that could be directly distributed to families. Appendix 2 also includes a list of recommended books and Web site resources that could be distributed directly to families.

PROBLEM-FOCUSED OUTPATIENT AND CONSULTATIVE SERVICES

Similar to EIBI, behavioral outpatient or consultation services typically focus on decreasing problematic behaviors or developing specific skill sets or behavioral repertoires; however, the purpose and model of implementation differ from EIBI. Outpatient and consultative behavioral treatment services are typically short-term, focused interventions requiring less intensive contact with the provider (ie, 1–2 hours per week). The typical course of services involves targeted assessment of a few specific problems followed by development of a specific intervention plan. Subsequent implementation occurs either directly by the outpatient therapist or by the family or school personnel who have been trained by the therapist to provide the intervention.[51,52] This model is appropriate for children or adolescents with milder forms of ASD such as Asperger disorder with no concomitant intellectual impairment, for children who have completed EIBI and are experiencing new clinical issues throughout their development, or when EIBI services or funding are unavailable.

Characteristics of behavioral consultation and therapy significantly overlap with those of EIBI, because the same theoretic approach is used for both forms of behavioral treatment. There are several critical features of successful behavioral consultation and outpatient therapy. First, the provider should be a qualified behavior analyst, psychologist, or member of another discipline (eg, speech-language pathologist, special educator, social worker) with appropriate training and expertise in the areas of behavioral treatment and ASD.[53] Second, the services should begin with well-validated behavioral assessment procedures (eg, functional analysis, preference assessment, skills assessments) that involve direct observation.[54] Third, the targets should be limited to 2 or 3 at any given time because of the limited hours of service, and interventions should focus on altering aspects of the environment that may maintain the problems and teaching functional skills using reinforcement-based procedures. Fourth, there should be an emphasis on the importance of consistent and frequent implementation across all people and settings that are likely to affect the child or adolescent (eg, teachers, parents). Fifth, as in EIBI, regularly scheduled data collection should occur to facilitate clinical decision making regarding progress and intervention revision.

Behavioral consultation and outpatient therapy services are usually provided in the community (eg, private practice office, school) and often involve the development of a behavioral intervention plan for both home and school settings. Often the consultant or outpatient provider serve, as a member of a multidisciplinary team that establishes and implements the child's individualized education plan (IEP).[53] Some of the most common targeted skills for acquisition in this model include social skills, emotion regulation skills, and self-management skills.[55–57] Common problematic behaviors referred for treatment include self-injury, noncompliance, tantrums and disruptive behavior,[54] and regulatory issues (eg, sleeping, feeding, and toileting issues),[52,58,59] particularly for young children on the autism spectrum. Before and during adolescence, individuals with an ASD become increasingly affected by social difficulties including teasing and bullying, and present with an unusually high rate of comorbid mental health concerns such as anxiety[60] and depression.[61]

The same level of experimental rigor evident in the literature on EIBI has yet to be applied to the myriad of behavioral treatments listed in the appendices for children and adolescents with ASDs. However, several behavioral treatments listed do meet the criteria for established treatments according to the National Autism Center's National Standards Report.[13] Research efforts to show the efficacy and effectiveness of behavioral treatments continues and most behavioral treatments show positive outcomes for children and adolescents with ASDs.[13,62] The literature is too expansive for a comprehensive review of all areas in the current article, but the evidence for 2 clinical concerns is reviewed later to illustrate the general structure and components of behavioral interventions for concerns with older children and adolescents (eg, anxiety) and with younger children through adolescence (eg, sleep problems).

Mental health problems such as anxiety and depression are typically addressed using manualized cognitive behavior therapy (CBT) interventions delivered in an individual or group context or individual exposure therapy to address specific fears. Several case studies and small sample group designs have evaluated the effectiveness of CBT interventions for children and adolescents with ASD and comorbid anxiety disorders, with most of these studies documenting significant reduction of anxiety symptoms per parent report.[63,64] These behavioral interventions can be delivered in individual or group therapy formats with positive outcomes.[65,66] Usually these interventions are offered in outpatient settings and are delivered on a weekly basis for approximately 11 to 16 weeks and include substantial components of social skills training, self-management skills training, and interventions to target emotion regulation (eg, Multimodal Anxiety and Social Skills Intervention [MASSI]).[62,63,65] Families and teachers are often involved to foster generalization of the treatment effects across settings. Moreover, it is generally recommended to incorporate specific interventions shown to be effective for individuals with ASDs, such as those grounded in ABA, in combination with the available evidence-based interventions shown to be effective for the comorbid disorder in child or adolescent populations.[62,65–68] A similar approached would likely be used for depression, with or without medication, using modified manualized treatments developed for children or adolescents,[69,70] although no clinical outcome studies have been conducted with individuals with ASD.

Behavioral treatment is likely to take a different form for targeted concerns that are common in early childhood and can persist into adolescence (eg, toileting, sleep, feeding, problem behavior). With each of these concerns, there are multiple behavioral treatments with evidence to support their effectiveness and therapists use assessment procedures to determine which of those interventions are appropriate for the individual case. For example, children who exhibit tantrums, aggression, and self-injury need a functional assessment to indicate what environmental events are exacerbating the problem behavior.[54] That information is used to design the specific changes that are needed for the environment to decrease problem behavior and usually to increase some functional communication skill at the same time.[71]

Behavioral treatment of sleep difficulties provides an example of this process with a clinical problem that is prevalent in individuals with ASD and is often resistant to pharmacologic interventions. Children and adolescents with ASDs often experience sleep difficulties, with estimates of disordered sleep in 40% to 80% of the population with ASD.[72-75] Common concerns include long latencies to sleep onset accompanied by bedtime resistance (ie, tantrums, refusal to stay in the bed) and poor sleep maintenance, which can be accompanied by safety issues caused by the lack of monitoring during the night.[72] After a pediatrician has ruled out underlying medical conditions, a behavioral treatment provider typically assesses the pattern of sleep and wakefulness, any related problem behaviors, and the environmental events that could be changed to establish healthy sleep patterns, which often results in improvements in other daytime behaviors (eg, social skills, academic skills, mood, and emotionality) as overall sleep increases.[76]

In the past decade, there has been more than a twofold increase in the number of behavioral sleep interventions for children with ASDs.[77] These behavioral interventions all include a component to promote a regular sleep/wake cycle by improving sleep hygiene. A recent review of the literature indicates that this is an effective intervention for children with ASDs.[72] Sleep hygiene interventions usually include establishing a set bedtime with a positive bedtime routine that reduces environmental stimulation in the evening during the 20 minutes before the desired sleep time and altering various factors that can lead to wakefulness (eg, room temperature, diet and caffeine intake, sounds).[78-80] Sleep hygiene is often supplemented with other behavioral interventions that have shown positive outcomes if it does not produce sufficient improvement as a solitary intervention.[80] Although no single or multicomponent behavioral intervention has met the criteria to be considered well established, 2 are considered possibly efficacious: (1) scheduled awakening for decreasing night terrors, and (2) extinction (ie, no longer responding as the parent used to respond) for decreasing night waking.[78]

Families find the process of accessing outpatient and consultation services similar to the process for any other outpatient psychological services. That is, qualified providers hold the appropriate license or certification for their profession (eg, licensed psychologist, licensed social worker). In addition to requesting recommendations from the pediatrician, families should be encouraged to check with national and state professional organizations to obtain more information about behavioral treatment providers in their state who have expertise in ASD.[53] For example, the Association for Behavioral and Cognitive Therapies (www.abct.org) maintains a list of CBT therapists by geographic location and areas of specialization. Each profession's national organization provides public information about professional codes of conduct and ethical guidelines (eg, American Psychological Association, www.apa.org). The state board for the various service providers (eg, Psychology Licensure Board) maintains information about the current status of an individual provider's credentials, any ethical violations, and, at times, the area(s) of the provider's expertise. Funding for outpatient and consultation services is typically covered to some extent as part of a family's mental health benefits in their health insurance plan and may also be funded by state agencies (eg, Medicaid, public school system) if the child qualifies under the pertinent guidelines.

COLLABORATION AND COORDINATION WITH BEHAVIORAL TREATMENT PROVIDERS

Child with ASD and their families are likely to benefit most when the pediatrician and behavioral treatment provider are able to communicate regularly and collaborate in ongoing interdisciplinary care.[81,82] Behavioral treatment providers are often well situated to provide some potentially useful information for pediatricians as they provide ongoing pediatric medical care. Myers and Johnson[83] identify common areas that often require medical management (eg, tissue damage from self-injury, severe aggression, feeding problems, and failure to thrive) and often result in costs of care that are 4 times higher for children with ASD than other children.[84] A behavioral treatment provider often sees the child and family more frequently than a pediatrician and is usually already collecting data or asking the family to collect data that could be useful in evaluating medical interventions. The behavioral treatment provider may be able to track important indicators such as hours of sleep per night, daily rate of problem behavior, or total daily food consumption to inform the standard course of medical treatment.[85] In addition, the behavioral treatment provider may also be able to investigate whether presenting medical concerns are particularly susceptible to environmental influences with accompanying intervention recommendations. For example, Arvans and LeBlanc[86] describe an adolescent with ASD who presented with frequent and increasing complaints of severe migraines, particularly on school days. A functional assessment of school refusal and careful tracking of migraine complaints revealed that the adolescent frequently stayed home or returned home from school based on his complaints, with sudden remission of pain on departure from school. They were able to design a token economy-based incentive system for attending school for progressively longer periods each day and virtually eliminated migraine complaints.

Research suggests that behavioral treatment may be warranted either in place of or in conjunction with medical treatment of certain problems such as sleep disturbances and aggressive behavior, particularly when the adverse side effects of psychopharmacologic interventions are prohibitive (ie, agitation, weight gain).[87–89] Behavioral interventions may also be used to address the side effects from medication (eg, an exercise program to address weight gain). As Myers and Johnson[83] point out, aggressive behavior that immediately increases in frequency or severity may be related to an underlying medication condition (eg, otitis media); however, if no underlying medical condition is identified or aggression continues after the medical condition is treated, consultation and referral for behavioral treatment might be warranted. In addition, behavioral treatment may prove useful in pediatric care settings if extreme behavior or noncompliance with medical procedures is interfering with the pediatrician's ability to provide care. For example, several studies with children with various disabilities and medical conditions show that behavioral treatments can be used to increase compliance with electroencephalographic procedures,[90] invasive medical procedures such as venipuncture,[91] and neuroimaging procedures.[92]

SUMMARY

Behavioral treatment in the form of EIBI is currently the only well-established treatment of young children with ASD.[11,12,27,28] In addition to EIBI for young children, many other behavioral interventions are available in outpatient treatment and consultation services that are effective for targeted concerns of children and adolescents with ASD.[52,57,65,66,71,77,78,80,85,86,93,94] This article provides an overview of models of behavioral treatment and appendices that will prove useful to pediatricians in guiding families as they seek providers and participate in behavioral treatment services. We offer 4 specific recommendations for pediatricians as they interface with their patients about behavioral treatments. First, encourage families to pursue evidence-based practices such as those described in this article rather than treatments that have not been shown to produce powerful and replicable gains for children with ASD. Second, guide families to seek highly qualified providers of services using the information sources outlined in this article,[45,46] because the skills and qualifications of the provider make an important difference in treatment outcomes.[27,44,53] Third, help families to maintain optimistic but realistic expectations for outcomes for their children (ie, important skill improvements rather than recovery) and to have appropriate expectations about their role in achieving those outcomes (ie, importance of parent training, long-term planning, and consistent responding). Fourth, be creative about collaborations with your patients' behavioral treatment providers and ask them to assist with tasks such as evaluating the effects of medication trials, increasing compliance with necessary medical procedures, or determining whether seemingly medical issues might have mitigating environmental determinants, among others.

REFERENCES

1. Johnson CP, Myers SM. Identification and evaluation of children with autism spectrum disorders. Pediatrics 2007;120:1183–215.
2. Gura GF, Champagne MT, Blood-Siegfried JE. Autism spectrum disorder screening in primary care. J Dev Behav Pediatr 2011;32:48–51.
3. Luyster R, Gotham K, Guthrie W, et al. The autism diagnostic observation schedule – toddler module: a new module of a standardized diagnostic measure for autism spectrum disorders. J Autism Dev Disord 2009;39:1305–20.
4. Dawson G. Early behavioral intervention, brain plasticity, and the prevention of autism spectrum disorder. Dev Psychopathol 2008;20:775–803.
5. Guralnick MJ. Effectiveness of early intervention for vulnerable children: a developmental perspective. Am J Ment Retard 1997;102:319–45.
6. Hastings RP, Kovshoff H, Ward NJ, et al. Systems analysis of stress and positive perceptions in mothers and fathers of pre-school children with autism. J Autism Dev Disord 2005;35:635–44.
7. Davis NO, Carter AS. Parenting stress in mothers and fathers of toddlers with autism spectrum disorders: associations with child characteristics. J Autism Dev Disord 2008;38:1278–91.
8. Filipek PA, Accardo PJ, Ashwal S, et al. Practice parameter: screening and diagnosis of autism: report on the Quality Standards Subcommittee of the American Academy of Neurology and the Child Neurology Society. Neurology 2000;55: 468–79.
9. Reichow B, Doehring P, Cicchetti DV, et al. Evidence-based practices and treatments for children with autism. New York: Springer; 2011.
10. US Department of Health and Human Services. Mental health: a report of the surgeon general. Rockville (MD): US Department of Health and Human Services, Substance Abuse and Mental Health Services Administration, Center for Mental Health Services, National Institutes of Health, National Institute of Mental Health; 1999.

11. Eldevik S, Hastings RP, Hughes JC, et al. Meta-analysis of early intensive behavioral intervention for children with autism. J Clin Child Adolesc Psychol 2009;38: 439–50.

12. Rogers SJ, Vismara LA. Evidence-based comprehensive treatments for early autism. J Clin Child Adolesc Psychol 2008;37:8–38.

13. National Autism Center. National Standards Report: The National Standards Project: addressing the need for evidence-based practice guidelines for autism spectrum disorders. National Autism Center website. November, 2009. Available at: http://www.nationalautismcenter.org/pdf/NAC%20Standards%20Report.pdf. Accessed July 11, 2011.

14. Vismara LA, Rogers SJ. Behavioral treatments in autism spectrum disorders: what do we know? Rev Clin Psychol 2010;6:447–68.

15. Lovaas OI. Behavioral treatment and normal educational and intellectual functioning in young autistic children. J Consult Clin Psychol 1987;55:3–9.

16. McEachin JJ, Smith T, Lovaas OI. Long-term outcome for children with autism who received early intensive behavioral treatment. Am J Ment Retard 1993;97: 359–72.

17. Green G. Early behavioral intervention for autism: what does the research tell us? In: Maurice C, Green G, Luce S, editors. Behavioral interventions for young children with autism: a manual for parents and professionals. Austin (TX): Pro-Ed; 1996. p. 29–44.

18. Lovaas OI, Smith T. Early and intensive behavioral intervention in autism. In: Kazdin AE, Weisz JR, editors. Evidence-based psychotherapies for children and adolescents. New York: Guilford Press; 2003. p. 325–40.

19. Lovaas OI. Teaching individuals with developmental delays: basic intervention techniques. Austin (TX): Pro-Ed; 2003.

20. Leaf R, McEachin J. A work in progress: behavior management strategies and a curriculum for intensive behavioral treatment of autism. New York: DRL Books; 1999.

21. Romanczyk RG, Lockshin S, Matey L. Individualized goal selection curriculum. 9th edition. Apalachin (NY): CBTA; 1996.

22. Koegel RL, Koegel LK. Pivotal response treatments for autism: communication, social, and academic development. Baltimore (MD): Paul H Brookes; 2006.

23. Koegel RL, O'Dell MC, Koegel LK. A natural language teaching paradigm for nonverbal autistic children. J Autism Dev Disord 1987;17:187–200.

24. Gillett JN, LeBlanc LA. Parent implemented natural language paradigm to increase language and play in children with autism. Res Autism Spectr Disord 2007;3:247–55.

25. Symon JBG, Boettcher MA. Family support and participation. In: Luiselli JK, Russo DC, Christian WP, et al, editors. Effective practices for children with autism: educational and behavioral support interventions that work. New York: Oxford University Press; 2008. p. 455–90.

26. Chambliss DL, Hollon SD. Defining empirically supported therapies. J Consult Clin Psychol 1998;66:7–18.

27. Reichow BR, Woolery M. Comprehensive synthesis of early intensive behavioral interventions for young children with autism based on the UCLA Young Autism Project model. J Autism Dev Disord 2009;39:23–41.

28. Eikeseth S. Outcome of comprehensive psycho-educational interventions for young children with autism. Res Dev Disabil 2009;30:158–78.

29. Minshew NJ, Sweeney JA, Bauman ML, et al. Neurologic aspects of autism. In: Volkmar FR, Paul R, Klin A, et al, editors. Handbook of autism and pervasive

developmental disorders: volume one diagnosis, development, neurobiology and behavior. Hoboken (NJ): John Wiley; 2005. p. 473–514.

30. Seltzer MM, Shattuck P, Abbeduto L, et al. Trajectory of development in adolescents and adults with autism. Ment Retard Dev Disabil Res Rev 2004;10: 234–47.

31. Al Anbar NN, Dardennes RM, Prado-Netto A, et al. Treatment choice in autism spectrum disorder: the role of parental illness perceptions. Res Dev Disabil 2010;31:817–28.

32. Eikeseth S, Smith T, Jahr E, et al. Intensive behavioral treatment at school for 4- to 7-year-old children with autism: a 1-year comparison controlled study. Behav Modif 2002;26:49–68.

33. Howard JS, Sparkman CR, Cohen HG, et al. Comparison of intensive behavior analytic and eclectic treatments for young children with autism. Res Dev Disabil 2005;26:359–83.

34. Smith T, Groen AD, Wynn JW. Randomized trial of intensive early intervention for children with pervasive developmental disorder. Am J Ment Retard 2000;105: 269–85.

35. Sallows GO, Graupner TD. Intensive behavioral treatment for children with autism: four year outcome and predictors. Am J Ment Retard 2005;110: 417–38.

36. Cohen H, Amerine-Dickens M, Smith T. Early intensive behavioral treatment: replication of the UCLA model in a community setting. J Dev Behav Pediatr 2006;27: S145–55.

37. Reed P, Osborne LA, Corness M. Relative effectiveness of different home-based behavioral approaches to early teaching intervention. J Autism Dev Disord 2007; 37:1815–21.

38. Eldevik S, Eikeseth S, Jahr E, et al. Effects of low-intensity behavioral treatment for children with autism and mental retardation. J Autism Dev Disord 2006;36: 211–24.

39. Fenske EC, Zalenski S, Krantz PJ, et al. Age at intervention and treatment outcome for autistic children in a comprehensive intervention program. Anal Interv Dev Disabil 1985;3:49–58.

40. Harris SL, Handleman JS. Age and IQ at intake as predictors of placement for young children with autism: a four- to six-year follow-up. J Autism Dev Disord 2000;30:137–42.

41. Granpeeshah D, Dixon DR, Tarbox J, et al. The effects of age and treatment intensity on behavioral intervention outcomes for children with autism spectrum disorders. Res Autism Spectr Disord 2009;3:1014–22.

42. Smith T, Klevstrand M, Lovaas OI. Behavioral treatment of Rett's disorder: ineffectiveness in three cases. Am J Ment Retard 1995;100:317–22.

43. Howlin P, Magiati I, Charman T, et al. Systematic review of early intensive behavioral interventions for children with autism. Am J Intellect Dev Disabil 2009;114: 23–41.

44. Bibby P, Eikeseth S, Martin NT, et al. Progress and outcomes for children with autism receiving parent-managed intensive interventions. Res Dev Disabil 2002;22:425–47.

45. Shook GL, Johnston JM. Training and professional certification in applied behavior analysis. In: Fisher WW, Piazza CC, Roane HS, editors. Handbook of applied behavior analysis. New York: Guilford Press; 2011. p. 498–510.

46. Shook GL, Favell JE. The Behavior Analyst Certification Board and the profession of behavior analysis. Behav Anal Pract 2008;1:44–8.

47. Chasson GS, Harris GE, Neely WJ. Cost comparison of early intensive behavioral intervention and special education for children with autism. J Child Fam Stud 2007;16:401–13.
48. Jacobson JW, Mulick JA, Green G. Cost-benefit estimates for early intensive behavioral intervention for young children with autism—general model and single state case. Behav Interv 1998;13:201–26.
49. Perry A, Cummings A, Geier JD, et al. Predictors of outcome for children receiving intensive behavioral intervention in a large, community-based program. Res Autism Spectr Disord 2011;5:592–603.
50. Perry A, Cummings A, Geier JD, et al. Effectiveness of intensive behavioral intervention in a large, community-based program. Res Autism Spectr Disord 2008;2: 621–42.
51. Stewart KK, Carr JE, LeBlanc LA. Evaluation of family-implemented behavioral skills training for teaching social skills to a child with Asperger's disorder. Clin Case Stud 2007;6:252–62.
52. LeBlanc LA, Carr JE, Crossett SE, et al. Intensive outpatient behavioral treatment of primary urinary incontinence of children with autism. Focus Autism Other Dev Disabl 2005;20:98–105.
53. Gillis JM, Beights R. New and familiar roles for clinical psychologists in the effective treatment for children for children with autism spectrum disorder. Cogn Behav Pract 2011. DOI: 10.1016/j.cbpra.2011.02.007.
54. Love JR, Carr JE, LeBlanc LA. Functional assessment of problem behavior in children with autism spectrum disorders: a summary of 32 outpatient cases. J Autism Dev Disord 2009;39:363–72.
55. White SW, Keonig K, Schaill L. Social skills development in children with autism spectrum disorders: a review of the intervention research. J Autism Dev Disord 2007;37:1858–68.
56. Loveland KA. Social-emotional impairment and self-regulation in autism spectrum disorders. In: Nadel J, Muir D, editors. Emotional development. New York: Oxford University Press; 2005. p. 365–82.
57. Sofronoff K, Attwood T, Hinton S, et al. A randomized controlled trial of a cognitive behavioural intervention for anger management in children diagnosed with Asperger syndrome. J Autism Dev Disord 2007;37:1203–14.
58. Southall CM, Gast DL. Self-management procedures: a comparison across the autism spectrum. Educ Train Autism Disabil 2011;46:155–61.
59. Polimeni MA, Richdale AL, Francis AJ. A survey of sleep problems in autism, Asperger's disorder and typically developing children. J Intellect Disabil Res 2005;49:260–8.
60. Martins Y, Young RL, Robson DC. Feeding and eating behaviors in children with autism and typically developing children. J Autism Dev Disord 2008;38:1878–87.
61. Leyfer OT, Folstein SE, Bacalman S, et al. Comorbid psychiatric disorders in children with autism: interview development and rates of disorders. J Autism Dev Disord 2006;36:849–61.
62. White SW, Albano AM, Johnson CR, et al. Development of a cognitive-behavioral intervention program to treat anxiety and social deficits in teens with high-functioning autism. Clin Child Fam Psychol Rev 2010;13:77–90.
63. White SW, Ollendick T, Scahill L, et al. Preliminary efficacy of a cognitive-behavioral treatment program for anxious youth with autism spectrum disorders. J Autism Dev Disord 2009;39:1652–62.
64. Wood JJ, Fujii C, Renno P. Cognitive behavioral therapy in high-functioning autism: review and recommendations for treatment development. In: Reichow B,

Doehring P, Cicchetti DV, et al, editors. Evidence-based practices and treatments for children with autism. New York: Springer; 2011. p. 197–230.

65. Wood JJ, Drahota A, Sze K, et al. Cognitive behavioral therapy for anxiety in children with autism spectrum disorders: a randomized, controlled trial. J Child Psychol Psychiatry 2009;50:224–34.

66. Jennett H, Hagopian LP. Identifying empirically supported treatments for phobic avoidance in individuals with intellectual disabilities. Behav Ther 2008; 39:151–61.

67. Sze KM, Wood JJ. Cognitive behavioral treatment of comorbid anxiety disorders and social difficulties in children with high-functioning autism: a case report. J Contemp Psychother 2009;37:133–43.

68. El-Ghoroury NH, Krackow E. A developmental-behavioral approach to outpatient therapy with children with autism spectrum disorders. J Contemp Psychother 2011;41:11–7.

69. Lusk P, Melnyk BM. The brief cognitive-behavioral COPE intervention for depressed adolescents: outcomes and feasibility of delivery in 30-minute outpatient visits. J Am Psychiatr Nurses Assoc 2011;17:226–36.

70. Treatment for Adolescents With Depression Study (TADS) Team. The Treatment for Adolescents with Depression Study (TADS): outcomes over 1 year of naturalistic follow-up. Am J Psychiatry 2009;166:1141–9.

71. Durand VM, Merges E. Functional communication training to treat challenging behavior. In: O'Donohue WO, Fisher J, editors. Cognitive behavior therapy: applying empirically supported techniques in your practice. 2nd edition. Hoboken (NJ): John Wiley; 2008. p. 222–9.

72. Cortesi F, Giannotti F, Ivanenko A, et al. Sleep in children with autistic spectrum disorder. Sleep Med 2010;11:659–64.

73. Malow BA, Marzec ML, McGrew SG, et al. Characterizing sleep in children with autism spectrum disorders: a multidimensional approach. Sleep 2006;29:1563–71.

74. Richdale AL. Sleep problems in autism: prevalence, cause and intervention. Dev Med Child Neurol 1999;41:60–6.

75. Ming X, Brimacombe M, Chaaban J, et al. Autism spectrum disorders: concurrent clinical disorders. J Child Neurol 2008;23:6–13.

76. Schreck KA, Mulick JA, Smith A. Sleep problems as possible predictors of intensified symptoms of autism. Res Dev Disabil 2004;24:57–66.

77. Vriend JL, Corkum PV, Moon EC, et al. Behavioral interventions for sleep problems in children with autism spectrum disorders: current findings and future directions. J Pediatr Psychol 2011;36(9):1017–29. DOI: 10.1093/jpepsy/jsr044.

78. Richdale A, Wiggs L. Behavioral approaches to the treatment of sleep problems in children with developmental disorders. What is the state of the art? Int J Behav Consult Ther 2005;1:165–89.

79. Wiggs L, Stores G. Sleep patterns and sleep disorders in children with autistic spectrum disorders: insights using parent report and actigraphy. Dev Med Child Neurol 2004;46:372–80.

80. Durand VM. Sleep better: a guide to improving sleep for children with special needs. Baltimore (MD): Paul H Brookes; 1998.

81. Carbone PS, Behl DD, Murphy NA. The medical home for children with autism spectrum disorders: parent and pediatrician perspectives. J Autism Dev Disord 2010;40:317–24.

82. Vargas CM, Prelock PA. Caring for children with neurodevelopmental disabilities and their families: an innovative approach to interdisciplinary practice. Mahwah (NJ): Lawrence Erlbaum Associates; 2004.

83. Myers SM, Johnson CP. Management of children with autism spectrum disorders. Pediatrics 2007;120:1162–82.

84. Flanders SC, Engelhart L, Pandina GJ, et al. Direct health care costs for children with pervasive developmental disorders: 1996-2002. Adm Policy Ment Health Ment Health Serv Res 2007;34:213–20.

85. Tang B, Piazza C, Dolezal D, et al. Severe feeding disorder and malnutrition in 2 children with autism. J Dev Behav Pediatr 2011;32:264–7.

86. Arvans RK, LeBlanc LA. Functional assessment and treatment of migraine reports and school absences in an adolescent with Asperger's disorder. Educ Treat Children 2009;32:151–66.

87. Matson JL, Hess JA. Psychotropic drug efficacy and side effects for persons with autism spectrum disorders. Res Autism Spectr Disord 2011;5:230–6.

88. Hoekstra PJ, Troost PW, Lahuis BE, et al. Risperidone-induced weight gain in referred children with autism spectrum disorders is associated with a common polymorphism in the 5-hydrosyryptamine 2C receptor gene. J Child Adolesc Psychopharmacol 2010;20:473–7.

89. Nickels KC, Katusic SK, Colligan RC. Stimulant medication treatment of target behavior in children with autism: a population-based study. J Dev Behav Pediatr 2008;29:75–81.

90. Slifer KJ, Avis KT, Frutchey RA. Behavioral intervention to increase compliance with electroencephalographic procedures in children with developmental disabilities. Epilepsy Behav 2008;13:189–95.

91. Slifer KJ, Babbitt RL, Cataldo MD. Simulation and counterconditioning as adjuncts to pharmacotherapy for invasive pediatric procedures. J Dev Behav Pediatr 1995;16:133–41.

92. Slifer K, Cataldo M, Cataldo M, et al. Behavior analysis of motion control for pediatric neuroimaging. J Appl Behav Anal 1993;26:469–70.

93. Green G. Early intensive behavior analytic intervention for autism spectrum disorders. In: Mayville EA, Mulick JA, editors. Behavioral foundations of autism treatment. Cornwall-on-Hudson (NY): Sloan Publishing; 2011. p. 183–200.

94. Laud RB, Girolami PA, Boscoe JH, et al. Treatment outcomes for severe feeding problems in children with autism spectrum disorders. Behav Modif 2009;33:520–36.

APPENDIX 1: COMMON TERMS USED IN BEHAVIORAL TREATMENT OF ASDs

Term	Definition
ABA	The application of the principles and procedures from the science of behavior analysis (learning) to socially significant behavior
BCBA	The standard practice credential for direct providers of EIBI and ABA
CBT and behavior therapy	Short-term outpatient therapies designed to teach specific skills or change specific behaviors to lead to improvements in many areas, such as sleep, anxiety, depression, feeding, toilet training, and social skills
DTT	A highly structured teaching strategy commonly used in EIBI. DTT is implemented in a 1-to-1 setting and often is used to teach specific behaviors or skills necessary for learning more complex ones
EIBI	A behavioral treatment based on the principles of ABA that is delivered early (before age 5 years) and intensively (25–40 hours per week) usually over a span of 2–3 years. Currently, EIBI is the only current well-established treatment that produces positive outcomes for children with ASDs
Functional assessment	Various different assessment strategies that are initially used to determine the functions of a child's behavior (ie, why the behavior is occurring). Interviews, behavioral observations, checklists, and functional analyses are often used as part of a functional assessment
Functional analysis	A strategy used in functional assessment. It involves direct observation of behaviors in specific conditions created to test whether the suspected functions identified in other types of functional assessment are contributing to problem behavior
Lovaas/UCLA model	Originally developed by O. Ivar Lovaas at UCLA and referred to as the Young Autism Project. The UCLA model is a comprehensive behavioral treatment that has the most research evidence of all the EIBI or ABA treatment models
Parent training	An important component of behavioral intervention in which parents become actively involved in their child's intervention by learning to implement interventions consistently. Leads to more effective interactions with their child and increased learning opportunities for their child

APPENDIX 2: FREQUENTLY ASKED QUESTIONS ABOUT BEHAVIOR TREATMENT OF ASD AND RESOURCES FOR FAMILIES

Q: What is EIBI? A: EIBI is a behavioral treatment based on the principles of ABA that is delivered early (before age 5 years) and intensively (25–40 hours per week) usually over a span of 2–3 years. EIBI is designed to teach children how to learn and to equip them to be able to benefit from school-based services. To date, EIBI is the intervention with the most evidence of positive outcomes (improvement in IQ, adaptive behavior, best chance for regular education placements) for children with ASDs.

Q: When should I start EIBI? A: The optimal age to begin EIBI is shortly after your child is diagnosed with an ASD. Your child could begin as early as 18 months of age. When children begin before the age of 5 years, they are likely to experience positive outcomes.

Q: I have heard that EIBI involves parent training. What does that mean? A: Quality EIBI programs include both parent support and parent training designed to improve your child's quality of life at home.

Q: Are special education services or eclectic interventions the same as EIBI? A: No. Even when some behavioral programming is included as part of special education or autism-specific educational programming (ie, eclectic treatment approach), the services are typically less structured and less intensive and do not have the same level of documented outcomes compared with early and intensive services in multiple research studies.

Q: Who pays for EIBI? A: Some states have mandated health insurance companies to pay for EIBI treatment. In some states, governmental entities might also help to pay for EIBI services, such as county early intervention programs (for children <3 years of age) or local school districts (beginning at 3 years of age). It is important to contact your case coordinator (if your child is in early intervention) or school district representative for more information and seek information from your local or state article of the Autism Society of America. Autism Speaks (www.autismspeaks.org) maintains a list of states that have health insurance coverage for ABA services.

Q: Who is qualified to provide EIBI services and how do I find them? A: Seek services from a behavior analyst who is certified by the BACB, the national credentialing organization for this profession. You will want to find a BCBA-D or BCBA to coordinate your program, if possible. The BACB maintains a Certificant Registry on its Web site (www.bacb.com) to allow you to search for certified professionals in your area.

Q: Will an EIBI program be stressful to me as a parent? A: Parents of children with ASDs experience higher levels of stress overall compared with parents of children with various other special concerns; however, studies indicate that parents do not report increased stress caused by EIBI. However, the commitment to EIBI is important and should be carefully considered because of the effort involved; any family member experiencing stress or other difficulties associated with any aspect of managing an ASD should contact the primary care physician, a licensed psychologist, or mental health professional for screening and potential services.

Q: What are outpatient behavioral treatment services and for what types of problems would that option be good for my child? A: Outpatient services are usually more limited in scope. Your family might see a therapist once or twice a week for an hour to target specific concern such as problem behavior, social skills deficits, or anxiety or depression. These services are usually provided by a licensed psychologist under the mental health benefits of your insurance plan or by a school psychologist as part of your IEP and are sometimes called CBT or behavioral consultation.

BEHAVIORAL TREATMENT RESOURCES FOR FAMILIES

If you already have behavioral treatment provider, they can assist you with finding many of these resources. If you do not already have a provider, seek information from resources available to families in the local and national community, such as the Autism Society (local and national articles), Autism Speaks, and Web sites of behavioral organizations, as listed later.

Information about the Behavioral Treatment of ASD and Qualified Providers on the Web:

Several associations and organizations maintain up-to-date information on the behavioral treatment of ASD. We recommend these because not all Web sites have information that is equally science based. You are encouraged to check the following Web sites for accurate information about treatment and providers:

Association for Behavior Analysis: International (ABAI): www.abainternational.org
Association for Behavioral and Cognitive Therapies (ABCT): www.abct.org
Association of Professional Behavior Analysts (APBA): www.apbahome.net
Association for Science in Autism Treatment (ASAT): www.asatonline.org
Autism Society: www.autism-society.org/
Autism Speaks: www.autismspeaks.org
BACB: www.bacb.com
Organization for Autism Research (OAR): www.researchautism.org

Resource Books for Parents:

1. Baker BL, Brightman AJ. Steps to independence: Teaching everyday skills to children with special needs (fourth edition). Baltimore: Paul Brookes; 2004.
2. Durand VM. Sleep better: a guide to improving sleep for children with special needs. Baltimore: Paul Brookes; 1998.
3. Freeman S. The complete guide to autism treatments. A parent's handbook: make sure your child gets what works! Langley, BC: SKF Books; 2011.
4. Harris SL, Weiss MJ. Right from the start: behavioral intervention for young children with autism. A guide for parents and professionals. Bethesda: Woodbine House; 1998.
5. Harris SL, Glasberg, BA. Siblings of children with autism: a guide for families. Bethesda: Woodbine House; 2003.
6. Maurice C, Green G. Luce SC. Behavioral intervention for young children with Autism. Austin: Pro-Ed; 1996.
7. Powers MP. Children with autism: a parent's guide, 2nd edition. Bethesda: Woodbine House; 2000.
8. Weiss MJ. Harris SL. Reaching out, joining in: teaching social skills to young children with autism. Bethesda: Woodbine House; 2001.
9. Luiselli JK, Russo DC, Christian WP, et al, eds. Effective practices for children with autism: educational and behavior support interventions that work. New York, NY: Oxford University Press; 2008.
10. Leaf R, McEachin J, Taubman M. Sense and nonsense in the behavioral treatment of autism: it has to be said. New York, NY: DRL Books; 2008.
11. Offit PA. Autism's false prophets: Bad science, risky medicine, and the search for a cure. New York: Columbia University Press; 2008.
12. Lovaas OI. Teaching individuals with developmental delays: basic intervention techniques. Austin: Pro-Ed; 2003.
13. Maurice C, Green G, Foxx RM, eds. Making a difference: behavioral intervention for Autism. Austin: Pro-Ed; 2001.

Social Skills Training for Children with Autism

Amy J. Bohlander, PhD[a],*, Felice Orlich, PhD[a],
Christopher K. Varley, MD[b]

KEYWORDS

- Social skills • Autism • Asperger • Intervention • Training
- High-functioning autism

Autism spectrum disorders (ASD) are developmental disabilities characterized by difficulties in social communication, along with restricted interests or repetitive behaviors. The term includes the current *Diagnostic and Statistical Manual of Mental Disorders, Fourth Edition (Text Revision)* (DSM-IV) diagnoses of autism, Asperger syndrome, and pervasive developmental disorder not otherwise specified.[1] The prevalence of ASD has increased steadily in the past several decades, partly because of the increasingly broad criteria for diagnosis, as well increased awareness by health care providers and by families, and earlier case finding. Current estimates are that 1 in approximately 110 children in the United States meet criteria for ASD,[2,3] with similar prevalence across different racial, ethnic, and socioeconomic groups,[4] making intervention for this population an important and timely issue. The range of abilities of individuals within the autism spectrum is broad, ranging from individuals with co-occurring intellectual disability (ie, low-functioning autism) to those with milder symptoms who have average or higher intelligence (ie, high-functioning autism). What these diverse individuals have in common is a core deficit in the area of social skills.

SOCIAL SKILLS DEFICITS IN ASD

Difficulties with social skills and social interactions are a hallmark of ASD, although how these difficulties manifest differs from child to child and depends to some extent on age and functioning level of the child. Examples of social skills include making eye

---

The authors have nothing to disclose.

[a] Department of Psychiatry, Seattle Children's Hospital, Autism Clinic, M/S CAC, 4909 25th Avenue NE, Seattle, WA 98105, USA

[b] Division of Child and Adolescent Psychiatry, Department of Psychiatry and Behavioral Sciences, University of Washington School of Medicine, Box 359300/W-3636, Seattle, WA 98195-0371, USA

* Corresponding author.

E-mail address: amy.bohlander@seattlechildrens.org

contact, initiating interactions with others, understanding and using nonverbal communication such as gestures and facial expressions, and maintaining reciprocal conversations. Young children with autism may show social skills delays in terms of limited eye contact, social smiling, joint attention, and pointing, whereas older children and adolescents may show difficulties maintaining conversations, taking another's point of view, initiating social interactions, reading nonverbal body cues, and making and keeping friends.

Helping youth with ASD to improve their social skills is an important goal because this population reports having fewer friends, less satisfying friendships and relationships, and more feelings of loneliness than their typically developing peers, despite desiring more peer interactions and friendships.[5] Furthermore, they report lower rates of self-esteem and higher rates of bullying and teasing than typically developing children and adolescents.[6,7] In addition, improving the social skills of youth with ASD is important because research has found that the social skills impairments in individuals with ASD contribute to underachievement at school and at work.[8]

Given the growing awareness of ASD, pediatricians are increasingly called on to assess children and adolescents for ASD and to guide families to the most appropriate services. This article describes some of the most frequently used social skill interventions and what is known about their effectiveness. It concludes with future directions and recommendations for pediatricians.

SOCIAL SKILLS INTERVENTIONS

Many interventions have been designed to address the social skills deficits of children and adolescents with ASD. The types of appropriate social skills training vary with the age of the child or adolescent and functioning level. Typically, social skills interventions are facilitated by a therapist or teacher and may involve training peers, siblings, or parents to interact with youth with ASD in ways that increase their social skills, or may involve direct teaching of social skills to individuals with ASD. Social skills training may be individual or group based, may incorporate visuals such as videos or pictures, and usually takes place within school or clinic settings.

Although empirical support is still in the early stages, there is a growing body of evidence to support the effectiveness of different types of social skills training for youth with ASD.[9] In particular, several types of social skills interventions are emerging as evidence based, including peer mentoring,[10] social skills groups,[11] and video modeling.[12] Other types of social skills training, such as social stories, have shown preliminary evidence of efficacy[13] but require additional research, whereas others, such as some of the commercially available social skills group curricula, are popular but have not yet undergone trials to measure effectiveness. **Table 1** gives a description of these types of social skills training, as well as recommended resources for parents or practitioners who would like to learn more about implementing these interventions.

Peer Mentoring

Peer mentoring is a type of social skills intervention traditionally used with preschool-aged children within the regular classroom. In this model, typically developing peers are taught how to interact with children with autism to encourage the development of their social skills. In a peer-mentoring model, peers may be taught, for example, how to be a good buddy, which may include staying with an assigned child with ASD, playing with him or her, and talking with the child even if the child with ASD does not respond.[14] This model is especially appropriate now that many children

Table 1
Types of social skills training and recommended resources

Types of Interventions	Recommended Resources
Peer mentoring	
Typically developing peers are trained to interact with children with ASD in ways that promote positive development of social skills, within a regular classroom setting	*Peer Play and the Autism Spectrum: The Art of Guiding Children's Socialization and Imagination* by Wolfberg[42] is a manual for practitioners and caregivers that describes techniques for integrating play groups of typically developing peers and those with ASD
Social skills groups	
4–5 students with ASD participate in lessons about various social skills topics, within school or clinic settings. Groups may also include typical peers as models/mentors	*Social STAR: Peer Interaction Skills* by Gajewski et al[24] *Think Social! A Social Thinking Curriculum for School-Age Students* by Winner[23] *Navigating the Social World: A Curriculum for Individuals with Asperger's Syndrome, High Functioning Autism, and Related Disorders* by McAfee[25] These 3 curricula are designed to be presented in group format to school-aged children with ASD and include fun and interactive lessons about various social skills topics
Video modeling	
Children with ASD watch videos showing themselves or peers demonstrating specific social skills, and then practice the skills	*Seeing is Believing: Video Self-Modeling for People with Autism and Other Developmental Disabilities* by Buggey[43] describes how to create and use video self-modeling to teach social and other skills to individuals with ASD
Social stories	
Children with ASD read short stories written in the first person, in which they use an appropriate social skill	*The New Social Stories Book* by Gray[37] describes how to write social stories and includes many examples that can be used as templates and individualized to specific children's needs
Picture books	
Children with ASD look at photographic sequences of social skills to learn how and why to perform the skill	*The Social Skills Picture Book: Teaching Communication, Play and Emotion* by Baker[39] contains step-by-step comic-strip illustrations of children performing social skills, along with thought bubbles explaining how the children perform the skill, and why

with ASD participate in general education classrooms alongside typically developing peers. Furthermore, merely participating in an inclusive classroom setting is not sufficient to increase social interactions and improve social skills for children with autism[15] because, without intervention, typically developing children choose to play with other typically developing peers rather than with children with autism.[16] However, with training, typically developing children are able and willing to interact with children with ASD. Training typical peers and siblings to model and reinforce appropriate social skills for preschool children with ASD within an inclusive classroom setting has been shown to be one of the most effective strategies for increasing the early social communication skills of preschool children with ASD, and children with ASD seem to generalize and maintain the gains over time and across other settings and children.[10,14,17,18]

Pivotal Response Training (PRT) is a behaviorally-based intervention for children with autism.[19] One application of PRT is as a peer-delivered model to teach social reinforcement (eg, paying attention to the child with ASD), to follow the lead of the child with ASD (eg, allowing the child with ASD choose the activity to play), and to model appropriate social behaviors such as turn taking and conversation. Although much training is required, this model is found to be effective when implemented.[3] Peer-mediated PRT has also been used with school-aged children. For example, one study found that using peer-mediated PRT techniques with elementary school–aged children with ASD resulted in an increase in social skills including initiations and turn taking.[20]

Social Skills Groups

One of the most commonly used interventions for school-aged children and adolescents on the autism spectrum is social skills groups. In a traditional social skills group, approximately 4 or 5 children with ASD participate in social skills lessons taught by a teacher or therapist. These groups usually meet at the child's school along with other classmates, or in an outpatient clinic setting with other youth with ASD from the broader community. Session topics might include greeting others, being friendly, joining or initiating play with others, reading nonverbal cues, and starting and maintaining conversations. See **Table 2** for examples of topics taught in social skills groups for school-aged children and adolescents with ASD.[21,22]

Several commercially available curricula for social skills groups for youth with ASD have enjoyed a great deal of clinical success, although their effectiveness has not yet been fully evaluated through research. Some of these programs include Winner's[23] *Think Social!*, Gajewski and colleagues'[24] *Social STAR*, and McAfee's[25] *Navigating the Social World*. These curricula are created for teachers and therapists to deliver within schools or clinics to school-age students with ASD or related difficulties in social skills. They include fun and interactive lessons on topics such as greeting others, starting and ending a conversation, being a friend, dealing with teasing, recognizing emotions, asking for help, giving and receiving compliments, and reading other people's body cues.

In addition to lesson-based groups such as those described earlier, social skills groups can also be activity based to foster social interactions between members. One such social skills group model that has shown effectiveness was one in which

Table 2
Examples of lesson topics for social skills groups

Elementary School Age Group[22]	Adolescent Social Skills Group[21]
Getting to know someone	Meeting new people/asking questions
Body talk (nonverbals)	Using body talk
Dealing with emotions	Using body signals to express and understand emotions
Conversation	Being positive
Making impressions	Keeping the conversation going/active listening
Teasing vs humor	Teen obstacles
Friendship tips	Sharing opinions

elementary school–aged children were split into groups of 3 for Lego therapy; 1 child in each group was designated the engineer, supplier, and builder, and had to work together to build different Lego projects while following certain rules such as working together, being polite, and sharing. Results showed improvements in social skills compared with a more traditional lesson-based social skills group.[26] This concept could be applied to other social skills groups with themes such as cooking, in which students might be split into groups of 3, with recipes being chosen and explained by the teacher or therapist, and each group having a head chef, sous chef, and ingredient gatherer.

Several recent summary papers and meta-analyses on social skills groups for school-aged youth with ASD have found emerging evidence of effectiveness, although it is unclear how well participants generalize the new skills and maintain them over time.[11,27–29] Several factors have been identified that may improve the effects, generalization, and maintenance of social skills groups. These factors include having at least 30 hours of group time, implementing the group within the natural setting (ie, the child's classroom, rather than a pullout model), matching the strategies and skills taught to the individual participants' specific social skills difficulties, and ensuring implementation fidelity of the interventions.[29]

Another factor that may aide in the generalization and maintenance of the skills learned in social skills groups is the inclusion of opportunities to interact with typical peers who are trained to promote and encourage social skills of peers with ASD.[30] Some newer models of social skills groups that are currently undergoing randomized, controlled trials are those that include typical peers from the child's school and take place within the classroom setting. In this model, typically developing peers with strong social skills and interest in helping peers with social challenges volunteer to serve as peer mentors in the group and receive training before participation. See **Box 1** for an example of peer training information used in a social skills group model; the efficacy of this information is currently being investigated in a multisite research project.[21] Preliminary evidence is showing that this may be an effective strategy.

Another component that has recently begun to be incorporated into social skills groups is mindfulness and relaxation training. Mindfulness refers to the practice of being aware of and focusing on the present moment and is taught using meditation exercises.[31,32] Mindfulness training is used in dialectical behavior therapy[33] to treat individuals with borderline personality disorder, and it has also been used successfully to treat other conditions, including anxiety and chronic pain.[32] Previous research has shown the effectiveness of mindfulness practices on reducing anxiety and improving social skills in other populations, including individuals with learning disabilities.[34] In social skills groups for ASD, mindfulness may help group members focus on the group and lessen distractions from the school day. See **Box 2** for an example of a mindfulness exercise that may be used at the start of an adolescent social skills group.

Video Modeling

Video modeling is a type of social skills intervention in which children with ASD watch video demonstrations of themselves or other children successfully performing appropriate social skills, and then imitate the skills modeled in the video. Research has widely supported video modeling as an effective intervention for children and adolescents with ASD to learn many types of skills, including social skills.[11,12,35] Skills learned through video modeling tend to be maintained over time and generalized to other people and settings.[12] Video modeling seems to be most effective when it is combined with other interventions to teach social skills.[36]

Box 1
Example of peer mentor training information for adolescent social skills groups

10 tips for working with students in the group

10. Be as concrete as possible. Explain sarcasm, double meanings in jokes, and idioms.

9. Remember that facial expressions and body language cues may not work. Be direct.

8. Avoid verbal overload. Be clear and use short sentences. These students often struggle to find the main point.

7. If a student does something that hurts your feelings, say "When you did ___, it made me feel ___. Next time, can you please try ___."

6. Planning activities may be particularly difficult for students in this group because making changes from daily routines can be a challenge. Reminders and preparation for the activity are helpful.

5. If students insist that they are correct and get into repetitive verbal arguments, have them write down the statement.

4. Be aware that these students may be sensitive to noises, smells, sights, or other senses that can make it virtually impossible to concentrate on anything else.

3. Do not take anything personally. Sometimes they may say things that are inappropriate; help to guide them towards an understanding of why it hurts your feelings. Perspective taking is hard for these students and they need practice.

2. Involve the students as much as possible, cueing them what to say if they seem at a loss during group activities or conversations (both inside and outside the group).

1. Most of all: have fun!! You will learn as much from these students as they will learn from you.

Adapted from Christy Bateman, Mark Sands. Newport High School, Bellevue (WA); and *From* Gerdts J, Oti R, Orlich F, et al. School-based social skills curriculum for adolescents: ENGAGE manual: Seattle Children's Hospital Research Institute; 2009; with permission.

Social Stories and Picture Books

Social stories are brief, individualized stories written to teach a social skill or behavior, or about a concept or event. Specific procedures for creating social stories are described by Gray[37] and involve a parent or teacher writing a short story about the child with ASD, in the first person, about a skill, activity, or event, and lets the child know what, when, where, and

---

Box 2
A mindfulness exercise for a social skills group

"Imagine yourself sitting inside an invisible egg. There is an invisible eggshell, a big circle all around you, front, back, up, down, and sideways. Close your eyes and stay very still. Relax into the quiet, not moving. Just rest there in the peaceful stillness, imagining yourself completely at ease. Expand into this space, as far as your mind can go, including the whole universe." (Ring a bell.) "Now, see if you can hear the sound of the bell all the way to the end." (Pause until the sound stops. Ring the bell at intervals of 30–60 seconds, over a period of ~4–5 minutes).

From Gerdts J, Oti R, Orlich F, et al. School-based social skills curriculum for adolescents: ENGAGE manual: Seattle Children's Hospital Research Institute; 2009; with permission.

why the situation, skill, or event will happen, along with the expected behavior or response of the child with ASD. For example, a parent or teacher may write a social story about a specific social skill such as greeting others, joining an activity, or giving a compliment. A social story about greeting others may describe the child going up to another child, saying hello, and asking how the other child is doing, and would explain why the child does this and the result. Studies have found some evidence of effectiveness for social stories when used as part of a more comprehensive social skills program.[13,38]

In a similar way to social stories, picture books can be used to teach social skills. Baker's[39] *Social Skills Picture Book* is an example of a picture book that is used for this purpose. This book has a collection of comic-strip photographs of children demonstrating various social skills and explaining why they are using those skills. Each set of pictures breaks up the social skill into several different components and the pictures are narrated using thought bubbles to show what the people depicted are thinking and feeling to make the social skills explicit.

ACCESS TO SERVICES

Recognition of the disorder and accurate diagnoses are the first steps in the provision of appropriate services. The resources available to children and adolescents with ASD are increasing, but parents often struggle with access to effective services. Information regarding social skill training services is available through local and national organizations, with the Internet being one of the most effective ways to access information about specific opportunities in the child's community. For example, pediatricians or parents may visit the Web site for the national advocacy group Autism Speaks (www.autismspeaks.org) and search for local social skills training opportunities under the Family Services tab. In addition, many large cities have Web sites designed to provide information about accessing local services. For instance, in the Seattle (WA) area, the Web site of the Asperger Support Network (www.seattleaspergers.org) provides information about social skills training opportunities in the area. The interventions described on these Web sites are typically social skills groups provided by speech therapists, occupational therapists, Board-certified Behavior Analysts, or mental health therapists in the area. In addition, many different social skills curricula can be found by searching online book retailers, as well as through local libraries and bookstores.

Another good way to access services is through the schools of children and adolescent with ASD. As schools are becoming more familiar with the needs of this population, they are more commonly offering social skills groups for these children through their individualized education programs (IEPs). Parents and pediatricians may request social skills groups as a part of the IEP for any child on the autism spectrum if this is not already being provided. As with all school-based services provided through an IEP, this service is free of charge to parents and is considered part of the child's education.

FUTURE DIRECTIONS

There are many different strategies to teach social skills to youth with ASD, and social skills training is an important component of intervention for this population. As a result of several recent calls for more multisite, randomized, controlled trials to determine the essential ingredients of effective programs,[29,40,41] additional research is being conducted on manualized interventions and the literature body is expected to increase substantially in the next decade. Currently, specific research questions include pinpointing what works for which types of children and adolescents with ASD and designing effective programs that can be implemented at schools across the country.

We expect that social skills interventions will continue to improve and that including typical peers in social skills training will become standard in most interventions to increase the generalization of skills. We also believe that mindfulness training will be an important component of social skills training for adolescents with ASD. As is the case across interventions for ASD and other developmental disabilities, interventions will be most effective when they are tailored to the specific needs of the children receiving the training.

SUMMARY, CLINICAL IMPLICATIONS, AND RECOMMENDATIONS FOR PEDIATRICIANS

Social skills deficits are a core feature of ASD and are amenable to treatment. Evidence is emerging for the effectiveness of social skills training for youth with ASD, with treatment options including social skills groups at school or in the community, peer training or mentoring, social stories, and video modeling. We recommend that social skills training should be included as a part of any comprehensive intervention program for youth with ASD.

Given the increasing prevalence of ASD, it is likely the pediatricians will encounter youth with ASD in their practices. Pediatricians are strongly encouraged to recommend social skills training as a part of routine care for this population. Pediatricians should consider asking parents of children with ASD about their children's intervention programs (eg, speech therapy, occupational therapy, social skills training) and should recommend social skills training to those who are not already receiving it. Pediatricians may encourage parents to ask (and advocate, when needed) for these groups at their schools (typically through their child's IEP), outpatient mental health centers, or developmental disability clinics, as well as through their speech and occupational therapists. Pediatricians may also recommend to parents and teachers the social skills training resources listed in **Table 1**.

REFERENCES

1. American Psychiatric Association. Diagnostic and statistical manual of mental disorders, fourth edition (text revision). Washington, DC: APA; 2000.
2. Autism and Developmental Disabilities Monitoring Network Surveillance Year 2006 Principal Investigators. Prevalence of autism spectrum disorders. Autism and Developmental Disabilities Monitoring Network, United States, 2006. Morb and Mort Wkly Rpt 2009;58(SS10):1–20.
3. Pierce K, Schreibman L. Using peer trainers to promote social behavior in autism: are they effective at enhancing multiple social modalities? J Appl Behav Anal 1997;12:207–18.
4. Autism and Developmental Disabilities Monitoring Network Surveillance Year 2000 Principal Investigators. Prevalence of autism spectrum disorders - Autism and Developmental Disabilities Monitoring Network. Morb and Mort Wkly Rpt 2007;56(SS01):1–11.
5. Bauminger N, Kasari C. Loneliness and friendship in high-functioning children with autism. Child Dev 2000;71:447–56.
6. Humphrey N, Symes W. Perceptions of social support and experience of bullying among pupils with autistic spectrum disorders in mainstream secondary schools. Eur J Spec Needs Educ 2010;25:77–91.
7. Carter S. Bullying of students with Asperger syndrome. Issues Compr Pediatr Nurs 2009;32:145–54.

8. Howlin P, Goode S. Outcome in adult life for people with autism, Asperger syndrome. In: Volkmar F, editor. Autism and pervasive developmental disorders. New York: Cambridge University Press; 1998. p. 209–41.

9. McConnell S. Interventions to facilitate social interaction in young children with autism: review of available research and recommendations for educational intervention and future research. J Autism Dev Disord 2002;32:351–72.

10. Bass J, Mulick J. Social play skill enhancement of children with autism using peers and siblings as therapists. Psychol Schools 2007;44:727–35.

11. Reichow B, Volkmar F. Social skills interventions for individuals with autism: evaluation for evidence-based practices within a best evidence synthesis framework. J Autism Dev Disord 2010;40:149–66.

12. Bellini S, Akullian J. A meta-analysis of video modeling and video self-modeling interventions for children and adolescents with autism spectrum disorders. Coun Exc Child 2007;73:264–87.

13. Scattone D, Tingstrom D, Wilczynski S. Increasing appropriate social interactions of children with autism spectrum disorders using social stories. Focus Autism Other Dev Disabl 2006;21:211–22.

14. Laushey K, Heflin L. Enhancing social skills of kindergarten children with autism through the training of multiple peers as tutors. J Autism Dev Disord 2000;30: 183–93.

15. Gresham F. Social skills and self-efficacy for exceptional children. Except Child 1984;51:253–61.

16. Strain P. Social behavior patterns of nonhandicapped and developmentally disabled friend pairs in mainstream preschools. Anal Interv Dev Disabl 1984;4: 15–28.

17. DiSalvo C, Oswald D. Peer-mediated interventions to increase the social interaction of children with autism: consideration of peer expectancies. Focus Autism Other Dev Disabl 2002;17:198–207.

18. Rogers S. Interventions that facilitate socialization in children with autism. J Autism Dev Disord 2000;30:399–409.

19. Pierce K, Schreibman L. Increasing complex social behaviors in children with autism: effects of peer-implemented pivotal response training. J Appl Behav Anal 1995;28(3):285–95.

20. Harper C, Symon J, Frea W. Recess is time-in: using peers to improve social skills of children with autism. J Autism Dev Disord 2008;38:815–26.

21. Gerdts J, Oti R, Orlich F, et al. School-based social skills curriculum for adolescents: ENGAGE manual. Seattle (WA): Seattle Children's Hospital Research Institute; 2009.

22. Toth K, Orlich F. Social skills interventions in children and teens with HFA, in Intervention Manual. Seattle (WA): Seattle Children's Research Foundation; 2009.

23. Garcia Winner M. Think social! A social thinking curriculum for school-age students. San Jose (CA): Think Social Publishing; 2008.

24. Gajewski N, Hirn P, Mayo P. Social STAR: peer interaction skills. Greenville (SC): Super Duper Publications; 2008.

25. McAfee J. Navigating the social world: a curriculum for individuals with Asperger's syndrome, high functioning autism, and related disorders. Arlington (TX): Future Horizons; 2002.

26. Owens G, Granader Y, Humphrey A, et al. LEGO therapy and the social use of language programme: an evaluation of two social skills interventions for children with high functioning autism and Asperger syndrome. J Autism Dev Disord 2008; 38:1944–57.

27. White S, Keonig K, Scahill L. Social skills development in children with autism spectrum disorders: a review of the intervention research. J Autism Dev Disord 2007;37:1858–68.
28. Rao P, Beidel D, Murray M. Social skills intervention for children with Asperger's syndrome or high-functioning autism: a review and recommendations. J Autism Dev Disord 2008;38:353–61.
29. Bellini S, Peters J, Benner L, et al. A meta-analysis of school-based social skills interventions for children with autism spectrum disorders. Remedial and Spec Ed 2007;28:153–62.
30. Barry T, Klinger L, Lee J, et al. Examining the effectiveness of an outpatient clinic-based social skills group for high-functioning children with autism. J Autism Dev Disord 2003;33:685–701.
31. Kabat-Zinn J. Wherever you go, there you are: mindfulness meditation in everyday life. New York: Hyperion; 1994.
32. Baer R. Mindfulness training as a clinical intervention: a conceptual and empirical review. Clin Psychol Sci Pract 2003;10:125–43.
33. Linehan M. Cognitive-behavioral treatment of borderline personality disorder. New York: Guilford Press; 1993.
34. Beauchemin J, Hutchins T, Patterson F. Mindfulness meditation may lessen anxiety, promote social skills, and improve academic performance among adolescents with learning disabilities. Complement Health Pract Rev 2008;13: 34–45.
35. Kroeger K, Schultz J, Newsom C. A comparison of two group-delivered social skills programs for young children with autism. J Autism Dev Disord 2007;37: 808–17.
36. Taylor B, Levin L, Jasper S. Increasing play-related statements in children with autism toward their siblings: effects of video modeling. J Dev Phys Disabil 1999;11.
37. Gray C. The new social stories book. Arlington (TX): Future Horizons; 2000.
38. Thiemann K, Goldstein H. Social stories, written text cues, and video feedback: effects on social communication of children with autism. J Appl Behav Anal 2001;34:425–46.
39. Baker J. The social skills picture book: teaching communication, play and emotion. Arlington (TX): Future Horizons; 2001.
40. Kasari C. Assessing change in early intervention programs for children with autism. J Autism Dev Disord 2002;32:447–61.
41. Lord C, Wagner A, Rogers S, et al. Challenges in evaluating psychosocial interventions for autistic spectrum disorders. J Autism Dev Disord 2005;35:695–708.
42. Wolfberg P. Peer play and the autism spectrum: the art of guiding children's socialization and imagination. Shawnee Mission (KS): Autism Asperger Publishing; 2003.
43. Buggey T. Seeing is believing: video self-modeling for people with autism and other developmental disabilities. Bethesda (MD): Woodbine House; 2009.

Psychopharmacology of Autism Spectrum Disorders

Gabriel Kaplan, MD[a,b,*], James T. McCracken, MD[c]

KEYWORDS

- Autism spectrum disorders • Autism • Stimulants • Irritability
- Repetitive behaviors • Hyperactivity • Antipsychotics
- Psychopharmacology

Readers of this issue of *Pediatric Clinics* will become aware that autism spectrum disorders (ASDs) comprise a very heterogeneous group of illnesses that present with a wide range of impairments, from moderate to catastrophic. According to the *Diagnostic and Statistical Manual of Mental Disorders* (Fourth Edition, Text Revised) (DSM-IV-TR),[1] ASDs are diagnosed in the presence of 3 core deficits: (1) impairment of social interactions, (2) impaired communication, and (3) repetitive and stereotyped patterns of behavior, interests, and activities. Though not required to make a diagnosis, frequent associated/comorbid symptoms are observed such as aggression, self-injury, impulsivity, decreased attention, anxiety, depression, and sleep disruption,[2] which can become a major source of additional distress and interference in functioning. While advances in the field of psychopharmacology have led to significant improvement in the symptoms and outcomes of many psychiatric diseases, unfortunately this has been less true for treating core symptoms of ASD. Regarding medications, Sir Michael Rutter recently wrote "...studies have been striking (and surprising) in their evidence on no clinically meaningful benefits with respect to the core symptoms of autism."[3] Therefore, an array of behavioral and educational approaches, reviewed elsewhere in this issue, is the cornerstone of a comprehensive treatment plan for ASD core symptoms and delays. Because such therapies are intensive and require the cooperation of the patient, the development of the aforementioned severe and challenging behaviors can threaten overall treatment success. Fortunately, progress has been made in the use of psychotropic medications to manage these common and often impairing associated features. Medications can be beneficial in reducing the

[a] Department of Psychiatry, Hoboken University Medical Center, 308 Willow Avenue, Hoboken, NJ 07030, USA
[b] Department of Psychiatry, University of Medicine and Dentistry of New Jersey, 65 Bergen Street, Newark, NJ 07107, USA
[c] Department of Psychiatry and Biobehavioral Sciences, David Geffen School of Medicine at UCLA, 760 Westwood Plaza, Los Angeles, CA 90024, USA
* Corresponding author. 535 Morris Avenue, Springfield, NJ 07081.
E-mail address: drgkaplan@gmail.com

Pediatr Clin N Am 59 (2012) 175–187
doi:10.1016/j.pcl.2011.10.005
0031-3955/12/$ – see front matter © 2012 Elsevier Inc. All rights reserved.

severity of disruptive behaviors and other problems that interfere with psychosocial and educational interventions, impair social functioning and learning, and result in safety risks to self or others.

Pediatricians are often the first professionals to start the ASD diagnostic process, although patients are usually later referred to specialist care for more comprehensive evaluations. However, families continue consulting with their primary doctor to obtain advice on the benefits of the multiple available ASD-specific treatment options, as well as medical monitoring and follow-up care. This course of action is in line with The American Academy of Pediatrics' recommendation that encourages physicians to take on guiding and supportive roles, as ASD are chronic syndromes that will persist, often with significant deficits, into adulthood.[4] Therefore, understanding the role of psychopharmacologic treatments in ASD, usual dosing, side effects, and monitoring guidelines has become important to primary care pediatrics.

It should be noted that most psychotropic use in ASD is off-label, as there are currently just two medications approved by the Food and Drug Administration (FDA), and only for the treatment of associated behaviors. Because ASDs are chronic, markedly impairing in many cases, and of poorly understood etiology, there is justifiably a high desire for effective treatments. This desire sometimes leads to premature enthusiasm for agents and interventions that appear promising in early reports but later do not withstand the rigor of evidence-based research methods.[5] Consequently, this article principally discusses information supplied by randomized controlled trials (RCTs), universally accepted as the primary source of evidence-based data. Other types of studies are mentioned only if they provide noteworthy, clinically relevant information.

Regarding this article's organization, rather than reviewing medications class by class, it addresses the most commonly associated behaviors separately; namely, aggression, repetitive behaviors, hyperactivity, depression and anxiety, and sleep disorders. Study results, benefits, and potential adverse effects of agents recommended for specific maladaptive conditions are described under distinct headings. Because the lack of biological markers to assess treatment progress has led researchers to develop sophisticated, psychometrically valid rating scales to evaluate outcomes, a section is dedicated to review tools frequently used to determine outcomes. In addition, paragraphs throughout the article on clinical implications provide a bridge between research and clinic. By offering information that is current, relevant, and organized in a user-friendly manner, the aim is to form a concise but informative reference guide for primary pediatric clinicians, who are often asked by caretakers to provide input in the selection of appropriate and efficacious agents for an ASD patient.

TOOLS USED TO MEASURE OUTCOMES
Clinical Global Impression Scale

The Clinical Global Impressions (CGI) Scale[6] is a standardized assessment tool used by clinicians to rate the severity of illness, change over time, and efficacy of medication. It is not ASD specific but is one of the most well-known and widely used scales in psychopharmacology studies, and is brief and convenient to use. It consists of 3 subscales. The first one, Severity of Illness, which is often used both before and after treatment, is a 7-point scale that rates the severity of the patient's mental illness at the time of assessment as: 1, normal, not at all ill; 2, borderline mentally ill; 3, mildly ill; 4, moderately ill; 5, markedly ill; 6, severely ill; or 7, extremely ill. The second subscale, Clinical Global Impression-Improvement (CGI-I), is also a 7-point scale that assesses how much the patient's illness has improved or worsened relative to a baseline state at the beginning of the intervention, and rated as: 1, very much improved; 2, much improved; 3, minimally improved; 4, no change; 5, minimally worse; 6, much worse; or 7, very much worse. The third subscale, Clinical Global Impression-Efficacy Index, which attempts to integrate benefits against side effects, does not appear in the studies reviewed here.

Aberrant Behavior Checklist

The Aberrant Behavior Checklist (ABC) is a 58-item caregiver report checklist developed specifically to assess maladaptive behaviors in individuals with developmental disabilities, using a simple 4-point rating scale (0–3) with higher scores reflecting more problems. ABC items are grouped into 5 subscales: (1) Irritability (ABC-I), agitation, crying (15 items); (2) Lethargy, social withdrawal (16 items); (3) Stereotypic behavior (7 items); (4) Hyperactivity, noncompliance (ABC-H) (16 items); and (5) Inappropriate speech (4 items). The ABC is frequently used in pharmacologic trials in autism as one of the main end points for treatment evaluation.[7] Most studies reviewed in this article have used ABC-I and ABC-H as outcome measures.

Children's Psychiatric Rating Scale

The Children's Psychiatric Rating Scale (CPRS)[8] is a 63-item scale developed by the Psychopharmacology Branch of the National Institute of Mental Health (NIMH) to rate childhood psychopathology. Each item is rated from 1 (not present) to 7 (extremely severe). Four factors have been derived from these items: Autism Factor (social withdrawal, rhythmic motions/stereotype, abnormal object relations, unspontaneous relation to examiner, underproductive speech), Anger/Uncooperativeness Factor (angry affect, labile affect, negative and uncooperative), Hyperactivity Factor (fidgetiness, hyperactivity, hypoactivity), and Speech Deviance Factor (speech deviance, low voice).

Children's Yale-Brown Obsessive Compulsive Scale Modified for Pervasive Developmental Disorder

The Children's Yale-Brown Obsessive Compulsive Scale (CY-BOCS) is a semistructured clinician rating that measures the current severity of obsessions and compulsions in youth with obsessive-compulsive disorder. Obsessions and compulsions are then each rated on a 0 to 4 scale across 5 severity items: Time Spent, Interference, Distress, Resistance, and Degree of Control. The modified CY-BOCS[9] for use in children with pervasive developmental disorder (PDD) eliminates the obsessions checklist and severity scales while retaining the compulsions checklist, which was expanded to include repetitive behaviors commonly seen in children with PDD. Furthermore, the modified version relies more on parental input rather than the child's input.

TREATMENT OF ASD-ASSOCIATED/COMORBID SYMPTOMS
Aggression, Irritability, and Self-Injury

Aggression and related symptoms are the associated problems that often elicit the most concern in ASD. Although behavioral and environmental approaches are recommended as the initial treatment, more severe or even dangerous behaviors usually result in requests for urgent pharmacologic intervention. Such behaviors can lead to injury, removal from less-restrictive classrooms or placements, and hospitalization. Patients can present with a variety of aggressive acts directed to self, others, and property. The prevalence of such acts is high. For instance, in a study of 1380 subjects with ASD, 68% demonstrated aggression to a caregiver and 49% to noncaregivers.[10] The following classes of medications are used to treat aggressive behaviors.

Antipsychotics

The efficacy of these agents was first documented in the 1970s by Magda Campbell at NY Bellevue Hospital. In her now classic studies,[11] Campbell pioneered the use of RCTs in child psychopharmacology, a field that had been largely dominated up to that point by case reports and naturalistic studies. Antipsychotics have now become commonly used agents in ASD,[12] perhaps influenced by observations of possible benefits on a variety of commonly associated behaviors and the fact that the only two FDA-approved agents for the condition are aripiprazole and risperidone.

Haloperidol Campbell and colleagues[11] studied ASD children with severe aggression aged 2.6 to 7.2 years and randomized them to haloperidol or placebo in combination with language training. Haloperidol at an average dose of 1.7 mg/d resulted in significant improvement in withdrawal and stereotypy in children 4.5 years and older, as assessed by the CPRS. In addition, there were beneficial effects on learning when the antipsychotic was combined with behavioral treatment. Later studies[13] confirmed the initial beneficial findings, including an improvement in aggression, as haloperidol was shown to be more effective than placebo for negativism, angry affect, and lability of affect. However, sedation was common, and about one-third of children developed motor symptoms such as dystonias and withdrawal dyskinesias. As a result, concern over the possible high risk of tardive dyskinesia emerged,[14] and the potential for these side effects made haloperidol a less favored option once atypical antipsychotics became available.[15]

Risperidone Dissatisfaction with conventional antipsychotics, due to extrapyramidal side effects and lack of efficacy in negative symptoms of schizophrenia, led to intense efforts to find alternatives. Risperidone, the first in a new class of agents termed atypical antipsychotics, was approved for schizophrenia in adults by the FDA in 1993. Given the expectation of improved efficacy and lower rates of adverse effects, atypicals became first-line agents for many conditions requiring neuroleptics, including ASD. Following the Campbell tradition, risperidone was rigorously studied by the NIMH Research Units on Pediatric Psychopharmacology (RUPP) Autism Network. RUPP conducted a multiphase trial comparing the effects of risperidone in comparison with placebo for the treatment of aggressive behaviors in patients aged 5 to 17 years with ASD. There was an initial double-blind, 8-week RCT study[16] with 101 participants, followed by a 4-month open-label trial ending in an 8-week randomized, double-blind, placebo-substitution study of risperidone withdrawal.[17] The studies found that risperidone, in mean doses of 2.08 mg/d, was effective for reducing moderate to severe tantrums, aggression, and self-injurious behavior in children with autism. Outcomes were assessed by the ABC-I and CGI-I. These gains were stable over time and did not necessitate dose increases, but relapse was seen in the majority if the medication was withdrawn at 6 months. The investigators found no evidence of dyskinesia or dystonia. However, the observed weight gain of 5.6 kg for the risperidone group was more than twice the expected weight gain over a 6-month period. The FDA approved risperidone in 2006 for the treatment of irritability associated with autistic disorder, including symptoms of aggression, deliberate self-injury, temper tantrums, and quickly changing moods, in children and adolescents aged 5 to 16 years, with a maximum recommended dose of 3 mg/d. A meta-analysis that reviewed all risperidone RCT studies for subjects with ASD published after 2000 found that the agent yielded a large mean effect size of 1.21.[18]

Aripiprazole Two large controlled studies documented the short-term efficacy of aripiprazole for severe aggression and irritability in subjects 6 to 17 years old with autistic disorder. A fixed-dose 8-week study[19] found that the agent at 5, 10, or 15 mg/d was superior to placebo. The second RCT[20] was also 8 weeks long but used flexible doses reaching a mean of 8.6 mg/d by the end of the study. Symptoms in both studies were rated with the ABC-I and the CGI-I. The most commonly reported adverse events associated with aripiprazole treatment were sedation and weight gain in both studies, and extrapyramidal symptoms mostly in the fixed-dose study, but these events rarely led to treatment discontinuation. Aripiprazole was approved by the FDA for the treatment of irritability associated with autistic disorder in patients aged 6 to 17 years in 2009. Aripiprazole dosing and response can vary considerably; the usual recommended clinical dose for maintenance is between 5 and 15 mg/d.

Other antipsychotics Other agents in this class lack large-scale controlled studies. Small open-label reports suggest variable benefits of olanzapine[21] and ziprasidone,[22] which have possible support, versus quetiapine,[23] which has not appeared to be beneficial.

Adverse effects All antipsychotics in children carry the risk of potentially serious side effects such as neuroleptic malignant syndrome, galactorrhea, dyskinesias, cardiovascular changes, and allergic reactions. Fortunately, these serious adverse events are estimated to be rare or uncommon; a large review estimated the annualized risk for tardive dyskinesia to be less than 0.5%, and remission of the disorder after drug discontinuation is a common observation.[24] Nevertheless, it is of obvious importance to systematically monitor for the appearance of such untoward effects and develop strategies to minimize them. Although a comprehensive discussion of this topic is beyond the scope of this article, an excellent review is available elsewhere.[25] **Box 1** lists common adverse effects and suggestions for monitoring adverse effects including observation, laboratory tests, and specific rating scales such as the Abnormal Involuntary Movement Scale (AIMS).[26]

Methylphenidate

The role of methylphenidate (MPH) in treating attentional problems in typically developing children is well documented.[27] Two RCTs examined MPH's potential benefit for the treatment of aggression in ASD[28,29] in subjects 5 to 11 years old. Although the results showed superiority over placebo on the ABC-I, the trials were small and of short duration, and one study[28] had a high percentage of children with intolerable side effects, often including agitation, mood changes, and abnormal movements. Overall, MPH is less commonly used for the treatment of aggression.

Box 1
Antipsychotic side effects and monitoring strategies

Side Effect	Monitor Frequency	Monitor Strategy
Sedation, lethargy	Each visit	Observation, caretaker report
Parkinsonism	Each visit	Observation, caretaker report
Tardive dyskinesia	Every 6 months	(AIMS)
Weight increase	Each visit	Monthly weight measures
Hyperglycemia	Every 6 months	Laboratory
Hyperlipidemia	Every 6 months	Laboratory
Hyperprolactinemia	Every few visits	If symptoms reported, obtain level

Divalproex

A 12-week randomized double-blind, placebo-controlled study[30] evaluated the use of divalproex sodium for aggression in 55 children aged 5 to 17 years, in which the agent demonstrated modest superiority to placebo. The primary outcome measures were the ABC-I and CGI. There was a trend for responders to have higher valproate blood levels compared with nonresponders. Adverse effects reported in the study were minimal.

Other agents

Naltrexone, an opioid receptor antagonist, and clonidine, an α2-adrenergic agonist, were studied in RCTs and showed superiority to placebo.[31] However, small samples and other study limitations made the findings difficult to generalize, so these agents are not considered a first choice for treating aggression.

Clinical implications

Aggressive behaviors toward self and others displayed by some ASD children result in grave concern, possibly more restrictive placements, and are significant predictors of inpatient treatment.[32] Consequently, many of the pharmacologic investigations in this population are geared toward addressing this potentially dangerous set of behaviors. The atypical antipsychotics risperidone and aripiprazole are the most studied agents in ASD, are approved by the FDA for treating irritability (not ASD per se), and have shown solid evidence of effectiveness. Older haloperidol studies also provide favorable evidence for its off-label use. However, the level of evidence is also high for the risk of developing clinically limiting side effects for all antipsychotics, such as the extrapyramidal effects of conventional agents or the metabolic changes of atypical neuroleptics.[11,16,20] Close monitoring of patients using these agents is essential. Divalproex and MPH are off-label options with modest evidence of effectiveness. The decision to initiate pharmacologic treatment should be based on severity of symptomatology, degree of impairment, risk to self or others, and prevention of hospitalization. While no widely endorsed clinical algorithms for treatment of aggression exist, clinicians generally attempt initial treatment with lower-risk alternatives to antipsychotics. However, in the context of poor response or tolerability, or severe and dangerous symptoms, such agents are often replaced by one of the two FDA-approved antipsychotics for rapid management and stabilization. Length of recommended treatment is difficult to derive from published evidence, but treatment benefits appear to be durable for up to 6 to 12 months. Efforts to reduce and possibly discontinue such treatment at the end of this period should be strongly considered.

Repetitive Behaviors

Restricted repetitive and stereotyped patterns of behavior, interests, and activities (RRBs) have been described since the work of Kanner[33] as core features of ASD, and their presence is also currently necessary to meet DSM-IV-TR[1] diagnostic criteria. RRBs can be classified into lower-level repetitive motor behaviors such as rocking and limb movements, and higher-level routines and rituals such as the classically described insistence on sameness. RRBs and stereotypies are not unique to ASD and can be found in many other developmental disorders, although researchers agree that these tend to be more frequent in ASD.[34] Behavioral therapies are the first line for RRBs but the behaviors can be quite difficult to manage; because of the major challenges that uncontrolled RRBs can pose to educational and social performance, and risks of danger and actual harm to self or others, pharmacologic treatment is often considered. The following agents have been evaluated and are often prescribed for the target of RRBs.

Selective serotonin reuptake inhibitors

Researchers reasoned that selective serotonin reuptake inhibitors (SSRIs) could be effective for RRBs, because of the consistent reports of serotoninergic dysfunction in ASD and because such symptoms share aspects of the phenomenology of obsessions and compulsions known to respond to SSRIs. Antidepressants are the most common class of psychotropics prescribed for individuals with ASD,[12] and although their benefits have been described in many case reports and uncontrolled studies,[35] such benefits have not been confirmed in large RCTs. Rigorous studies were conducted in youth with ASD only for fluoxetine and citalopram. Fluoxetine at a mean dose of 9.9 mg/d was better than placebo for RRBs according to the CY-BOCS in a study of 39 children aged 5 to 16 years.[36] On the other hand, a later study of 158 subjects with autism 5 to 17 years old[37] compared fluoxetine with placebo; using the CY-BOCS-PDD measure of repetitive behaviors during a 14-week treatment period, no fluoxetine benefit was observed. In addition, a 12-week RCT of citalopram studied 149 children aged 5 to 17 years with ASD and high levels of RRBs, who were begun on 2.5 mg of citalopram daily with weekly increases up to a maximum dose of 20 mg/d (mean dose 16 mg/d). The outcome was evaluated by CY-BOCS and again, no significant differences were found between the placebo and citalopram groups.[38] One-third of children in these studies were reported to experience serotoninergic activation type side effects, specifically increased activity, mood changes, and insomnia. On the other hand, open label studies of escitalopram have been more positive on benefits for irritability.[39] Therefore, taken together, the literature on the benefits and safety of SSRIs in ASD is quite mixed, despite the high frequency of their community use.

Atypical antipsychotics

RRBs were examined as secondary outcomes in the same studies mentioned in the aggression section. For instance, in the RUPP studies, risperidone achieved significantly greater reduction of repetitive behavior than did placebo (35% vs 15% reductions from baseline respectively), as reflected in scores on the compulsion subscale of the CY-BOCS modified for ASD.[40] Similarly, both aforementioned aripiprazole studies[19,20] showed that the agent significantly improved RRBs over placebo as measured by CY-BOCS when secondary analyses were conducted.

Divalproex

In a small study of 13 individuals with ASD who participated in an 8-week double-blind, placebo-controlled trial of divalproex sodium versus placebo, a significant group difference for divalproex on improvement in repetitive behaviors as measured by the CY-BOCS was noted.[41]

Clinical implications

RRBs constitute a frequent problematic behavior in children with ASD but treatment choices are difficult given the relative absence of support for efficacy of a particular medication class. Adverse effects of medications used for this target are commonplace and can be difficult to tolerate. Clinicians are advised to recognize current treatment limitations and to restrict drug therapy to those patients who display clear anxiety or distress associated with RRBs, or where RRBs are severe.

Hyperactivity

Clinicians have long noted the high prevalence of inattentive and hyperactive symptoms in children with ASD, and research has found that 28% to 78% of children with ASD meet diagnostic criteria for attention-deficit/hyperactivity disorder (ADHD).[42,43] Furthermore, children who meet both diagnostic criteria have more severe clinical difficulties than children with ASD alone.[44] Although current DSM-IV criteria do not allow the comorbid coding of both diagnoses,[1] it seems that DSM-V, scheduled to appear in 2013, will resolve this dilemma.[45] Multiple agents have been investigated to treat hyperactivity.

Stimulants

Amphetamines and MPH are the options of choice to treat attentional hyperactive problems in typically developing children.[27] Stimulants are the third most common class of drug prescribed in ASD.[12] MPH has been used preferentially in this population. A retrospective chart review of 195 subjects aged 2 to 19 years found that stimulants appeared to be ineffective and poorly tolerated for the majority of patients with ASD. There is only one published large MPH RCT study, which was conducted by the NIMH RUPP Autism Network.[46] The study of 72 children aged 5 to 13 years was designed to evaluate the efficacy and safety of multiple daily doses of immediate release MPH. Three strengths were used of about 0.15 mg/kg, 0.25 mg/kg, and 0.5 mg/kg. These doses, lower than those recommended for typically developing children, were used to minimize the possibility of side effects. All doses were superior to placebo in reducing hyperactivity and impulsiveness as measured by the ABC hyperactivity subscale, the primary outcome measure. However, even the highest effect size of 0.54 in this study was much lower than that usually achieved in typically developing children.[47] Irritability was a common complaint and overall, 18% of subjects discontinued the trial because of adverse effects, at least double the intolerance seen in typically developing children with ADHD.

Atomoxetine

Atomoxetine is a selective norepinephrine reuptake inhibitor, approved by the FDA for treatment of ADHD symptoms in typically developing children and adults. Atomoxetine was examined in a small placebo-controlled, crossover pilot trial[48] for the treatment of hyperactivity of children with ASD. In this study, there were 16 children aged 5 to 15 years treated for 6 weeks at doses of 1.2 to 1.4 mg/kg per day, not exceeding a total dose of 100 mg/d. For the ABC-H, the primary outcome measure, improvement significantly favored atomoxetine. Adverse events were described as tolerable, with no tendency to increase stereotypy. Atomoxetine had an effect size similar to that shown in the MPH trial by the RUPP,[46] with effects mainly seen on hyperactive-impulsive behaviors. However, this study was small and allowed concomitant administration of other psychotropics, placing further limitations on generalizability.

Atypical antipsychotics

Secondary analyses of the ABC-H scale from large RCTs demonstrated that risperidone[16] and aripiprazole[20] are associated with large reductions of hyperactivity in children with ASD.

Other agents

Clonidine, an α2-agonist, was associated with a superior reduction in disruptive behaviors over placebo in a small, controlled trial.[49] Guanfacine, an α2A-adrenergic agonist, has been reported to demonstrate modest improvement in a retrospective study, in particular in irritability and explosive behavior. An additional open-label study of 25 children with ASD and high levels of ADHD symptoms suggested moderate benefit over 8 weeks.[50] However, no RCTs have been conducted for this class of agent.

Clinical implications

Hyperactivity is a frequent symptom that, when severe, interferes with educational and social interventions. As such, it is often the subject of requests for pharmacologic treatment. Unfortunately, none of the highly effective treatments for typically developing children have the same robust response in ASD, and the rate of side effects even at low doses is remarkably high. MPH is the best studied agent and although its use is off-label, it has the strongest evidence for modest effectiveness. MPH requires starting at doses roughly half that of usual doses in typically developing patients with ADHD and close monitoring of side effects, particularly irritability. α-Agonists deserve more research exploration, and often form a solid second-line treatment choice. While antipsychotics have also shown effectiveness for marked hyperactivity, their off-label use for this indication and potential significant toxicity make them a less favored choice.

Depression and Anxiety

The literature on effects of psychotropics for the treatment of depression and anxiety is sorely limited, despite the frequent description of dysphoria and apparent anxious behaviors in individuals with ASD. Although there is strong empirical support for the SSRIs as treatment for children with anxiety disorders, it is uncertain if benefits seen in typical children translate to children with ASD. It is interesting that some positive support exists for use of these medicines in adults with ASD,[51,52] but the high rate of significant adverse reactions to SSRIs in children, such as disinhibition, hyperactivity, and somatic complaints, greatly temper any enthusiasm for their common usage in youth with ASD.

Sleep Disorders

ASD patients experience sleep disorders at a much higher rate than typically developing children.[53] Various types of sleep problems have been described in this population, and may occur as a result of complex interactions between biological, psychological, social/environmental, and family factors, including child-rearing practices that are not conducive to good sleep.[54] Insomnia is the predominant sleep concern, and while its nature is also most likely multifactorial, abnormalities in the melatonin system have received the greatest level of consideration.[55] As per the ASD treatment principles discussed earlier and childhood insomnia treatment guidelines, pharmacology is recommended only when psychosocial treatments fail. A comprehensive review of such first-line approaches is described elsewhere.[56] Sleep disorders tend to be considered more benign than other associated problems such as aggression and repetitive behaviors; however, ongoing abnormal sleep patterns are very disruptive to the overall quality of family life and interfere with patient daytime functioning. Physicians receiving requests for medication are confronted with the lack of FDA-approved treatments for this problem. Although melatonin has been used off-label for many years, studies were sparse until several recent RCTs were conducted that, though of small sample size, have yielded encouraging results.[55] These studies found that melatonin in doses of up to 6 mg/d was effective and caused no significant side effects. However, long-term treatment has not been thoroughly examined.

SUMMARY

As reviewed in this article, clear progress has been made in defining approaches to evaluate the use of psychopharmacologic agents in ASD. While core features of ASD have shown limited improvement from treatment with well-known psychotropics, several high-quality studies have shown success using various drug classes for the management of commonly associated behaviors. Although effective, these medicines also carry a high risk of untoward effects that limit their widespread use. Therefore, psychopharmacologic approaches should always be viewed as one component of a broader, comprehensive treatment that addresses educational, behavioral, and social functioning with multimodal interventions. Within this framework, pediatricians can play an important role in the oversight of ASD treatment benefit and safety.

At present, evidence-based support exists for the role of psychotropics, particularly atypical antipsychotics, in the treatment of the following targeted symptom domains: (1) aggression and severe irritability; (2) hyperactivity; and (3) repetitive behaviors. The broad benefits in behavior observed in antipsychotic studies make these agents a common treatment choice, especially in the face of severe symptoms and failure of other agents with lesser side-effect burdens. Substantial unmet need exists for interventions targeting mood and anxiety symptoms and severe, persistent insomnia. Therefore, polypharmacy, as well as the use of complementary medicine agents, are commonplace in community treatment of individuals with ASD, even though these practices have not been thoroughly tested. Reducing medication exposure by lowering dosing and evaluating appropriateness for discontinuation should be considered when treatment goals are achieved. Given the increased psychotropic use in ASD, primary care pediatricians can benefit from greater familiarity with recommended dosing, types of side effects, and suggested monitoring in order to render the safest care possible. It is hoped that in the near future, emerging knowledge of underlying molecular pathophysiology in ASD will point to new and more effective medical interventions.

ACKNOWLEDGMENTS

The authors wish to thank Aaron Kaplan for his helpful comments during the preparation of this article.

REFERENCES

1. American Psychiatric Association. Diagnostic and statistical manual of mental disorders. text revision. 4th edition. Washington, DC: APA; 2000.
2. Levy SE, Mandell DS, Schultz RT. Autism. Lancet 2009;374:1627–38.
3. Rutter M. A selective scientific history of Autism. In: Hollander E, Kolevzon A, Coyle J, editors. Textbook of ASD. Washington, DC: APPI; 2011. p. 5–21.
4. Myers SM, Johnson CP. Management of children with ASD. Pediatrics 2007; 120(5):1162–82.
5. Krishnaswami S, McPheeters ML, Veenstra-Vanderweele J. A systematic review of secretin for children with autism spectrum disorders. Pediatrics 2011;127(5): e1322–5.
6. Guy W. ECDEU assessment manual for psychopharmacology—revised (DHEW Publ No ADM 76-338). Rockville (MD): U.S. Department of Health, Education, and Welfare, Public Health Service, Alcohol, Drug Abuse, and Mental Health Administration, NIMH Psychopharmacology Research Branch, Division of Extramural Research Programs; 1976. p. 218–22.
7. Aman MG, Singh NN, Stewart AW, et al. The Aberrant Behavior Checklist: a behavior rating scale for the assessment of treatment effects. Am J Ment Defic 1985;89:485–91.
8. Rating scales and assessment instruments for use in pediatric psychopharmacology research. Psychopharmacol Bull 1985;21(4):714–1124.

9. Scahill L, McDougle CJ, Williams SK, et al. Children's Yale-Brown Obsessive Compulsive Scale modified for pervasive developmental disorders. J Am Acad Child Adolesc Psychiatry 2006;45(9):1114–23.

10. Kanne SM, Mazurek MO. Aggression in children and adolescents with ASD: prevalence and risk factors. J Autism Dev Disord 2011;41(7):926–37.

11. Campbell M, Anderson LT, Meier M, et al. A comparison of haloperidol and behavior therapy and their interaction in autistic children. J Am Acad Child Psychiatry 1978;17:640–55.

12. Mandell D, Morales K, Marcus SC, et al. Psychotropic medication use among Medicaid-enrolled children with autism spectrum disorders. Pediatrics 2008; 121:e441–8.

13. Anderson LT, Campbell M, Grega DM, et al. Haloperidol in the treatment of infantile autism: effects on learning and behavioral symptoms. Am J Psychiatry 1984; 141(10):1195–202.

14. Campbell M, Armenteros J, Malone RP, et al. Neuroleptic-related dyskinesias in autistic children: a prospective, longitudinal study. J Am Acad Child Adolesc Psychiatry 1997;36(6):835–43.

15. Posey DJ, Stigler KA, Erickson CA, et al. Antipsychotics in the treatment of autism. J Clin Invest 2008;118:6–14.

16. RUPP. Risperidone in children with autism and serious behavioral problems. Research Units on Pediatric Psychopharmacology (RUPP) Autism Network. N Engl J Med 2002;347:314–21.

17. RUPP. Risperidone treatment of autistic disorder: longer term benefits and blinded discontinuation after six months. Research Units on Pediatric Psychopharmacology (RUPP) Autism Network. Am J Psychiatry 2005;162:1361–9.

18. Sharma A, Shaw S. Efficacy of risperidone in managing maladaptive behaviors for children with autistic spectrum disorder: a meta-analysis. J Ped Health Care 2011. [Epub ahead of print]. DOI:10.1016/j.pedhc.2011.02.008.

19. Marcus RN, Owen R, Kamen L, et al. A placebo-controlled, fixed-dose study of aripiprazole in children and adolescents with irritability associated with autistic disorder. J Am Acad Child Adolesc Psychiatry 2009;48(11):1110–9.

20. Owen R, Sikich L, Marcus RN, et al. Aripiprazole in the treatment of irritability in children and adolescents with autistic disorder. Pediatrics 2009;124:1533–40.

21. Potenza MN, Holmes JP, Kanes SJ, et al. Olanzapine treatment of children, adolescents, and adults with pervasive developmental disorders: an open-label pilot study. J Clin Psychopharmacol 1999;19(1):37–44.

22. Malone RP, Delaney MA, Hyman SB, et al. Ziprasidone in adolescents with autism: an open-label pilot study. J Child Adolesc Psychopharmacol 2007; 17(6):779–90.

23. Martin A, Koenig K, Scahill L, et al. Open-label quetiapine in the treatment of children and adolescents with autistic disorder. J Child Adolesc Psychopharmacol 1999;9(2):99–107.

24. Correll CU, Kane JM. One-year incidence rates of tardive dyskinesia in children and adolescents treated with second-generation antipsychotics: a systematic review. J Child Adolesc Psychopharmacol 2007;17(5):647–56.

25. Correll CU. Antipsychotic use in children and adolescents: minimizing adverse effects to maximize outcomes. J Am Acad Child Adolesc Psychiatry 2008;27: 9–20.

26. Guy W, editor. ECDEU assessment manual for psychopharmacology: Publication ABM 76-338. Washington, DC: US Department of Health, Education, and Welfare; 1976. p. 534–7.

27. Kaplan G, Newcorn JH. Pharmacotherapy for child and adolescent attention-deficit hyperactivity disorder. Pediatr Clin North Am 2011;58(1):99–120.

28. Handen BL, Johnson CR, Lubetsky M. Efficacy of methylphenidate among children with autism and symptoms of attention-deficit hyperactivity disorder. J Autism Dev Disord 2000;30:245–55.

29. Quintana H, Birmaher B, Stedge D, et al. Use of methylphenidate in the treatment of children with autistic disorder. J Autism Dev Disord 1995;25:283–94.

30. Hollander E, Chaplin W, Soorya L, et al. Divalproex sodium vs placebo for the treatment of irritability in children and adolescents with autism spectrum disorders. Neuropsychopharmacology 2010;35:990–8.

31. Parikh MS, Kolevzon A, Hollander E. Psychopharmacology of aggression in children and adolescents with autism: a critical review of efficacy and tolerability. J Child Adolesc Psychopharmacol 2008;18(2):157–78.

32. Mandell DS. Psychiatric hospitalization among children with autism spectrum disorders. J Autism Dev Disord 2008;38(6):1059–65.

33. Kanner L. Autistic disturbances of affective contact. Nerv Child 1943;2:217–50.

34. Leekam SR, Prior MR, Uljarevic M. Restricted and repetitive behaviors in autism spectrum disorders: a review of research in the last decade. Psychol Bull 2011; 137(4):562–93.

35. McCarthy M, Kolevzon A. Serotonin reuptake inhibitors and other serotonergic medications. In: Hollander A, Kolevzon A, Coyle JT, editors. Textbook of autism spectrum disorders. Washington, DC: American Pyschiatric Publishing; 2011. p. 439–55.

36. Hollander E, Phillips A, Chaplin W, et al. A placebo controlled crossover trial of liquid fluoxetine on repetitive behaviors in childhood and adolescent autism. Neuropsychopharmacology 2005;30:582–9.

37. SOFIA. Available at: http://www.autismspeaks.org/about-us/press-releases/autism-speaks-announces-results-reported-study-fluoxetine-autism-sofia. Accessed July 28, 2011.

38. King BH, Hollander E, Sikich L, et al. Lack of efficacy of citalopram in children with autism spectrum disorders and high levels of repetitive behavior: citalopram ineffective in children with autism. Arch Gen Psychiatry 2009;66(6):583–90.

39. Owley T, Walton L, Salt J, et al. An open-label trial of escitalopram in pervasive developmental disorders. J Am Acad Child Adolesc Psychiatry 2005;44(4): 343–8.

40. McDougle CJ, Scahill L, Aman MG, et al. Risperidone for the core symptom domains of autism: results from the RUPP Autism Network study. Am J Psychiatry 2005;162:1142–8.

41. Hollander E, Soorya L, Wasserman S, et al. Divalproex sodium vs. placebo in the treatment of repetitive behaviours in autism spectrum disorder. Int J Neuropsychopharmacol 2006;9(2):209–13.

42. McCracken JT. Disruptive behaviors. In: Hollander E, Kolevzon A, Coyle JT, editors. Autism spectrum disorders. Washington, DC: American Psychiatric Publishing; 2010. p. 159–67.

43. Murray MJ. Attention-deficit/hyperactivity disorder in the context of autism spectrum disorders. Curr Psychiatry Rep 2010;12(5):382–8.

44. Gadow KD, DeVincent CJ, Pomeroy J. ADHD symptom subtypes in children with pervasive developmental disorder. J Autism Dev Disord 2006;36(2):271–83.

45. APA DSM-5 Development. Available at: http://www.dsm5.org/ProposedRevision/Pages/proposedrevision.aspx?rid=383. Accessed July 28, 2011.

46. RUPP. Randomized, controlled, crossover trial of methylphenidate in pervasive developmental disorders with hyperactivity. Research Units on Pediatric Psychopharmacology (RUPP) Autism Network. Arch Gen Psychiatry 2005;62(11): 1266–74.

47. Paykina N, Greenhill L. Attention deficit hyperactivity disorder. In: Findling RL, editor. Clinical manual of child and adolescent psychopharmacology. Washington, DC: American Pyschiatric Publishing; 2008. p. 33–87.

48. Arnold LE, Aman MG, Cook AM, et al. Atomoxetine for hyperactivity in autism spectrum disorders: placebo-controlled crossover pilot trial. J Am Acad Child Adolesc Psychiatry 2006;45(10):1196–205.

49. Jaselskis CA, Cook EH Jr, Fletcher KE, et al. Clonidine treatment of hyperactive and impulsive children with autistic disorder. J Clin Psychopharmacol 1992; 12(5):322–7.

50. Scahill L, Aman MG, McDougle CJ, et al. A prospective open trial of guanfacine in children with pervasive developmental disorders. J Child Adolesc Psychopharmacol 2006;16(5):589–98.

51. Fatemi SH, Realmuto GM, Khan L, et al. Fluoxetine in treatment of adolescent patients with autism: a longitudinal open trial. J Autism Dev Disord 1998;28(4): 303–7.

52. McDougle CJ, Naylor ST, Cohen DJ, et al. A double-blind, placebo-controlled study of fluvoxamine in adults with autistic disorder. Arch Gen Psychiatry 1996; 53(11):1001–8.

53. Richdale A. Sleep problems in autism: prevalence, cause, and intervention. Dev Med Child Neurol 1999;41:60–6.

54. Cortesi F, Giannotti F, Ivanenko A, et al. Sleep in children with autistic spectrum disorder. Sleep Med 2010;11(7):659–64.

55. Sánchez-Barceló EJ, Mediavilla MD, Reiter RJ. Clinical uses of melatonin in pediatrics. Int J Pediatr 2011;2011:892624.

56. Vriend JL, Corkum PV, Moon EC, et al. Behavioral interventions for sleep problems in children with autism spectrum disorders: current findings and future directions. J Pediatr Psychol 2011;36(9):1017–29.

Transition from School to Work for Students with Autism Spectrum Disorders: Understanding the Process and Achieving Better Outcomes

Carol Schall, PhD[a,b,*], Paul Wehman, PhD[a,c], Jennifer L. McDonough, MS, C.R.C[a]

KEYWORDS

- Autism spectrum disorders • Early adulthood
- Social competence • Employment models

Darius was diagnosed with autism when he was 6 years old. He displayed all of the classic characteristics of the disorder around the age of 3, but his physician was uncomfortable with the disorder and reluctant to "label" Darius at such a young age. Specifically, Darius spoke his first word at 2 years old. By 3, he was using one-word phrases. He did not like playing with others and did not play pretend ever. Instead, he stacked blocks while watching the same part of a children's movie repeatedly. He was a difficult child as well. His parents struggled to get everyday community activities done because he screamed and cried whenever his daily routine changed. As a young child with a communication delay, he received 1 hour of speech therapy per week from an early-intervention provider. The early-intervention provider met with the family and child care providers, and taught them to withhold items he wanted

[a] Rehabilitation Research and Training Center, Virginia Commonwealth University, Richmond, VA 23284, USA
[b] Special Education and Disability Policy, Virginia Autism Resource Center, VCU Autism Center for Excellence, Virginia Commonwealth University, Richmond, VA 23284, USA
[c] Physical Medicine and Rehabilitation, Virginia Commonwealth University, Richmond, VA, USA
* Corresponding author. Special Education and Disability Policy, Virginia Autism Resource Center, VCU Autism Center for Excellence, Virginia Commonwealth University, Richmond, VA 23284.
E-mail address: cmschall@vcu.edu

Pediatr Clin N Am 59 (2012) 189–202
doi:10.1016/j.pcl.2011.10.009
0031-3955/12/$ – see front matter © 2012 Published by Elsevier Inc.

until he named the item he wanted. By the time Darius entered school; he used two-word phrases to request items and repeated verbatim sections of dialogue from his favorite children's movie.

Once he entered school, Darius' school team prepared an Individualized Education Program (IEP) and served him as a child with autism. At that point, Darius' physician also diagnosed him with autism. When meeting with the doctor, Darius' parents had many questions for the medical professionals about his future. The parents wondered whether Darius would be able to get a job, live independently, have a girlfriend, and partake in all the other activities that most other individuals without disabilities experience; they asked their family physician about Darius' future and asked what they should do to plan for his life. The physician did not have many answers for them. In fact, she was not even sure what to tell them about planning for Darius' schooling. Instead, she suggested that they talk to the school psychologist in his special education program. After turning to the school psychologist and the other medical and psychological professionals, the parents still did not have many answers about how to plan for Darius' future, so decided to take his educational and behavioral treatment year by year and leave their worries about his future for later.

Throughout his schooling, Darius did make progress. For example, he acquired more language, albeit with a loud, pedantic voice tone. He learned to read and complete simple mathematical problems to a third-grade level. Because of a new practice called inclusion, Darius also had the opportunity to attend some classes with his peers without disabilities. During these classes, he displayed somewhat more flexibility in respect of his daily routines. At home, he continued to spend his free time watching sections of the same movie repeatedly. As he entered high school, he continued to work on academic skills and activities designed for elementary school children. Because of the progress he made through his school career, as a 20-year-old young adult he did not display the classic signs of autism that were present at the age of 3; nevertheless, he continued to display many characteristics typical of adolescents and adults with autism spectrum disorders (ASD).[1]

Darius desires to live a full and connected life in his adulthood. He represents the beginning of a wave of students with ASD who are entering adolescence. As the measured incidence of ASD has increased, most of the research available to describe evidence-based practices has focused on young children between the ages of 3 and 6 years.[2,3] At the same time, many more individuals will enter adolescence and young adulthood in the coming years.[4–6] It is essential to increase understanding of the essential elements of support necessary to assist Darius and his peers with ASD in successfully transitioning from school to adulthood. In other words, while Darius is still in school it is important to redesign his school program to prepare him for adult life. Thus, the purpose of this article is to: (a) describe the characteristics of autism in adolescence and young adulthood, (b) identify the needs of individuals with ASD as they transition from school services to adulthood, (c) describe the employment supports and models for adults with ASD, and (d) discuss implications of these supports for medical professionals.

THE CHARACTERISTICS OF ASD IN ADOLESCENCE AND EARLY ADULTHOOD

ASD is a behavioral disorder that includes deficits in communication and social interaction, and a series of behaviors described as "repetitive, restricted, and stereotyped patters of behaviors, activities, and interests."[7] Darius displays many of these characteristics, as described above. Specifically, he continues to display challenges related to communication and social interaction. He also continues to rely on routines to guide his behavior, even with some increased flexibility.

As individuals with ASD move into adolescence, the characteristics associated with ASD change somewhat.[1] Specifically, individuals with ASD, like Darius, who have had the opportunity to interact with their peers without disabilities, demonstrate improved communication and social interaction. In addition, there may be a lessening of the impact of the restricted behaviors associated with the disorder.[1,8–10] Thus, by adolescence many of the original symptoms that lead to initial concerns abate somewhat. Nevertheless, Seltzer and colleagues[10] suggest that, while there is an abatement of symptoms, the developmental trajectory for individuals with ASD is splintered, with improvement in some behaviors that define autism. These investigators also note that some individuals with ASD experience periods of regression in the areas of behavioral challenges and insistence of sameness. Finally, they note that some individuals experience a worsening of symptoms. Thus, the developmental trajectory for individuals with ASD through adolescence is neither uniform nor linearly ascending. Seltzer and colleagues report findings indicating improvement in communication; however, continued impairment, particularly in social communication, persists into adulthood.

Gilchrist and colleagues[8] found that by adolescence, individuals with Asperger syndrome show similar behavioral characteristics to individuals with high-functioning autism in adolescence. These investigators found that delays in language development for individuals with high-functioning autism were ameliorated by adolescence, leading to the finding that individuals with Asperger disorder were similar to individuals with high-functioning autism. This final point adds support to the proposed changes in the *Diagnostic and Statistical Manual of Mental Disorders*, Fifth Edition (DSM-V). In fact, proposed changes to DSM-V include the elimination of Asperger disorder as a separate diagnosis (Proposed Revision, APA DSM-5, unpublished data, 2011). Though controversial, it appears that this change will not result in significant changes related to diagnosis in adolescence. In addition, the American Psychological Association proposes a change from 4 symptom categories to 3. **Table 1** shows the proposed changes to the diagnosis of ASD between the *Diagnostic and Statistical Manual of Mental Disorders*, Fourth Edition, Text Revised (DSM-IV-TR) and DSM-V.

These changes in diagnostic requirement are likely to have little impact on adolescents, with a few exceptions. First, it is possible that some adolescents did not present the full characteristics of ASD under the old criteria, but will present as such under the new diagnostic criteria. Second, the loosening of the age of onset of symptoms is likely to assist diagnosticians in identifying individuals with symptoms after early childhood. Finally, the merging of deficits in social and communication abilities into one symptom category may decrease the emphasis placed on symptoms, such as nonverbal communication, that are both social and communicative in nature.

In addition to these primary diagnostic symptoms, there are secondary symptoms that can be as impactful and debilitating as the primary characteristics. Such indications include mental health diagnoses and behavioral challenges. In fact, there is evidence that adolescents with ASD are at greater risk of experiencing depression and anxiety disorders.[11–13] Finally, the combination of primary and secondary characteristics affects individuals' abilities to adapt and be successful at work, at home, and in relationships with others. Consequently, individuals with ASD have experienced lower rates of success in adulthood than those with other types of disabilities. Research indicates that adults with ASD are chronically unemployed and underemployed at relatively high rates.[14–18] Nevertheless, individuals with ASD can achieve employment and independence in life when provided with a personal goal-focused

Table 1
Proposed changes to the new diagnostic characteristics from DSM-IV-TR to DSM-V

Characteristic	Current Characteristics in DSM-IV-TR	Proposed Changes in DSM-V	Description of Proposed Changes
Title of disorders	Pervasive Developmental Disorders	Autism Spectrum Disorder	Placing Autism in name of category and including the word "spectrum" in title
Disorders included in category	Autism, Pervasive Developmental Disorder Not Otherwise Specified, Asperger Disorder, Rett Disorder, Childhood Disintegrative Disorder	Autism Spectrum Disorder with notation of severity across symptoms, Level 1 "requiring support," Level 2 "requiring substantial support," Level 3 "requiring very substantial support"	Rett Disorder will be categorized as a medical disorder and therefore removed from the DSM altogether. All other disorders will be considered "autism spectrum disorder." Levels of intensity of support noted across symptoms
Deficits in communication	Qualitative Impairment in Communication: Four different symptom descriptions, diagnosis required at least 1 of the 4 noted symptoms	This category is combined with deficits in social interaction to become "Persistent deficits in social communication" There are 3 symptom areas. Must meet criteria for all 3 of the descriptions	The notation of communication deficits becomes a part of the behaviors described under "Persistent deficits in social communication"
Deficits in social interaction	Qualitative Impairment in Social Interaction: Four different symptom descriptions, diagnosis required at least 2 of the 4	This category is combined with deficits in communication to become "Persistent deficits in social communication" There are 3 symptom areas. Must meet criteria for all 3 of the descriptions	The notation of social interaction deficits becomes a part of the behaviors described under "Persistent deficits in social communication"
Excessive repetitive behaviors, routines, activities, and interests	Restricted, Repetitive, and Stereotyped Patterns of Behavior, Activities and Interests: Four different descriptions of behaviors, Diagnosis required 1 of the 4 descriptions	Restricted, Repetitive Patterns of Behavior, Interests and Activities. Four different descriptions of behaviors. List now includes "Hypo or Hyper reactivity to sensory input." Must meet criteria for at least 2 of the 4 descriptions	The only major change in this category is the inclusion of different responses to sensory input
Age of onset	Onset prior to age 3 y	Onset in early childhood while noting that symptoms may not be fully manifested until demands exceed capacity	Slight loosening of the age of onset with the notation that symptoms may not be salient until social demands exceed individual's ability to respond

From Proposed revision, APA DSM-V. Available at: http://www.dsm5.org/ProposedRevision/Pages/proposedrevision.aspx?rid=94. Accessed June 15, 2011.

curriculum and intensive structured instruction.[1,19–22] The next section of describes the elements of quality transition programs for adolescents and young adults with ASD.

TRANSITION NEEDS FOR YOUTH WITH ASD

Much of the early research on children with ASD has focused on the younger ages, with less attention to the transition issues and challenges they face.[23] According to the US Department of Education there are 6,608,446 youths in special education, with 10% between 14 and 21 years of age.[24] It is known that more than 90% are unemployed on exiting school[17] and that relatively few go to college and complete a degree. In addition, it is known that as these children become adolescents they are among the most expensive to rehabilitate through the federal state vocational rehabilitation program, as well as having among the poorest outcomes.[25] The vocational rehabilitation system in the United States has not considered young people with ASD as good candidates for employment.

Transition has been defined in the Individuals with Disabilities Education Act (IDEA) 2004 as follows.

Transition services mean a coordinated set of activities for a student with a disability that:

A. is designed to be within a results-oriented process, that is focused on improving the academic and functional achievement of the student with a disability to facilitate the student's movement from school to postschool activities, including:
- postsecondary education,
- vocational education,
- integrated employment (including supported employment),
- continuing and adult education,
- adult services,
- independent living, or community participation;
B. is based on the individual student's needs, taking into account the student's strengths, preferences and interests; and
C. includes instruction, related services, community experiences, the development of employment and other postschool adult living objectives, and, if appropriate, acquisition of daily living skills and functional vocational evaluation (IDEA; 2004 [34 CFR 300.43(a)] [20 U.S.C. 1401(34)].

IEPs for students aged 16 years and older must reflect specific transition planning. Some states (Virginia, Delaware, Rhode Island) have moved this to age 14. According to IDEA, the IEP must include a statement of

- appropriate measurable postsecondary goals based on age-appropriate transition assessments related to training, education, employment and where appropriate, independent living skills;
- the transition services (including courses of study) needed to assist the (student) in reaching those goals [34 CFR 300.320(b) and (c)] [20 U.S.C. 1414 (d)(1)(A)(i)(VIII)].

TRANSITION OUTCOMES

Public education has not been very effective in meeting the needs of adolescents and young adults with ASD, as the aforementioned data demonstrate. A primary source of information about postsecondary outcomes for students with ASD is the National

Longitudinal Transition Study 2 (NLTS2). The NLTS2 followed a large representative sample of youth enrolled in special education as they transitioned into young adulthood from 2001 to 2009, with a cumulative age range of 13 to 26 years. From the overall sample (N = 11,000), 922 youths were from the autism category. Newman and colleagues[17] reported that students with ASD only participated in general education about 33% of the time, with most coursework provided in special education (62%). Even though the majority of time modifications to the curriculum were in place in general education settings, students with ASD were substantially less engaged than their typical peers in general education settings. In a recent study, Shattuck and colleagues[26] examined patterns of service use among youth with ASD from the NLTS2 sample. Data analysis on youth who exited high school revealed that 32% attended postsecondary education schools, 6% had competitive jobs, and 21% had no employment or education experiences at all. Further, 80% of these individuals were living with their parents, 40% reported having no friends, and only 36% had a driver's license. Unfortunately, youth from families with lower socioeconomic levels had worse outcomes on all measures.[26]

Hence, the question becomes what can help influence these outcomes in a more positive manner? Some educational practices are favorably associated with better outcomes. The next section describes such practices.

FACTORS ASSOCIATED WITH FAVORABLE TRANSITION OUTCOMES
Vocational Competence and Employment Perspective

Vocational capacity, employment, and the opportunity to advance in a career is a major underpinning of success in American society.[27] Adults frequently describe their success by their earning ability, the type of work that they do, the regularity with which they are employed, the type of environment in which they work, and their long-term work potential. It is known that those youths with ASD who work in school are more likely to be employed as adults.[28,29] Thus, the first practice associated with favorable transition outcomes is the design of high school internships that result in employment before the individual graduates from high school. It is critical that educators and community support programs emphasize employment as a desired and measured outcome prior to graduation from high school.

Implementing Evidenced-Based Practices that Increase Independence

The use of the Internet, automation, greater efficiency in the workplace, and technology enhance the success of all workers. Youth with ASD can be empowered in the workplace with the use of equipment such as smart phones and personal digital assistants.[30] In addition, educators and community support staff must increase access to programs implementing scientifically based practice for this age group.[31] At the same time, there is a need for more research toward defining program practices and design that result in employment outcomes for students with ASD. While this literature is growing, it is not currently meeting the needs of the educational community to provide guidance for those students currently in school. The discovery and implementation of evidence-based practices are essential in improving student learning so that individuals with ASD can maximize their work capacity in American society.[2,3]

Increasing Social Competence

Many believe that demonstrating interpersonal skills and social competence in a variety of environments are the most important features of success in life. Unfortunately, many young people with ASD are ultimately unable to achieve this level of competence.[20] Using effective social skills and knowing how to behave in a variety of social situations can make the difference in successful outcomes in the workplace as well as at home and in the community. Youth with ASD who are verbally inappropriate most likely will not develop effective social relationships. Many of the precipitating factors that lead to problem behaviors in the classroom are predicated on poor social skills. On the other hand, using practices such as role playing, counseling, behavior rehearsal, and targeted instruction on social skills frequently results in overcoming the problems associated with poor social skills. Social competence and the demonstration of positive social skills are critical to successful transition.

Self-Determination and Self-Advocacy

Self-determination is the capacity to choose and to act based on those choices. In addition, individuals who are self-determined can make plans and adjust those plans based on circumstances beyond their control. For individuals with ASD, self-determination results in individuals being able to identify their strengths, preferences, and interests, and to identify potential careers that match their strengths and interests.[32] The emphasis on self-determination for people with ASD and other disabilities can be traced to the independent living and self-advocacy movements that emerged in the 1970s. Most people develop self-determination in childhood and adolescence as they receive greater responsibilities and freedom from their parents and teachers.[33] Individuals cannot self-advocate if they have not developed self-determination skills. Self-advocacy ultimately will be the way for young people with ASD to navigate the challenges they face as they enter adulthood.[32]

Self-determination requires that the teenager with ASD learn the knowledge, demonstrate the competency, and identify the opportunities necessary to exercise freedom and choice in ways that are valuable to him or her. Little doubt remains that those people who are self-directed, and have the initiative and ambition to be successful while also practicing a reasonable degree of work ethic do better in life than those who do not.[34] There is, of course, room for debate regarding how much the schools are able to instill these important skills.[35] Self-determination is related to personal attributes that result in better outcomes for students with ASD.[36] Therefore, curriculums that result in increased self-determination are an important aspect of transition programs.

Parental Involvement

In a word, good parents are awesome. Good parents do make a difference, with their values and their contacts in the community and workplace. For a student with ASD seeking employment on graduation, the family and extended family play a very important role. The transition to adulthood is both an exciting and challenging time for youth with ASD and their families. Although this period is critical for all individuals, for people with autism the development of appropriate supports during the transition process is crucial. Indeed, individuals with ASD may be described by the supports they need in relation to the demands in specific environments. For example, these individuals may have support needs in areas of intellectual functioning, adaptive skills, motor development, sensory functioning, health care, or communication. These areas necessitate identifying strategies and supports that will assist these individuals in being successful and achieving desired outcomes. The family frequently acts as case manger and the conduit through which many of these needs are identified and skills practiced. Transition programs that result in excellent outcomes for youth with ASD involve families in the process throughout the youth's school years.

School and Community Inclusion

The inclusion of students with disabilities into general education classrooms is a substantiated transition best practice.[31] Young people with disabilities cannot feel part of a high school if they do not have access to the general curriculum, interact with students in the school, participate in extracurricular activities, and abide by the school rules. Working in real jobs, shopping, and volunteering in the community cannot be preformed competently without the foundation of being in a regular school. Perhaps one of the most useful applications of the original school "mainstreaming" concept has been collaborative teaching.[37] In this approach a special education teacher or paraprofessional works collaboratively in the general education classroom with the regular education teacher. This collaboration can take place in a tutoring mode, a team teaching mode, or any collaboration model that benefits the students with ASD who are in the classroom.

According to Snell and Janney[37]:

> The nature of high schools present greater obstacles for co-teachers because of the emphasis on content area knowledge, the need for independent study skills, the faster pacing of instruction, high-stakes testing, high school competency exams, less positive attitudes of teachers, and the inconsistent success of strategies that were effective at the elementary level. (p. 36)

Despite these points, the fact remains that collaborative teaching opens up the doors for students to have many more opportunities to interact with nondisabled students and general education teachers. This forward step results in higher expectations of students with ASD, higher aspirations by parents, greater access to activities with their nondisabled peers, and a much richer set of opportunities for enhanced self-esteem and adjustment.[38]

Postsecondary Education

A final theme that continually emerges in successful transition outcomes is the need for postsecondary education.[39] Many individuals with disabilities have difficulty in the workplace throughout their lives, and also have difficulty with social skills and personal self-esteem. One way to overcome such drawbacks is education. Earning an associate's degree or a bachelor's degree from a 4-year college course will be an outstanding asset to add to one's résumé. Even so, being able to take courses and assimilate new information into life and work can also make a significant difference.[40] Adding new skills to one's knowledge base, identifying new interests, hobbies, and avocations, and making new friends are all mediated in a very effective way through postsecondary education and life-long learning experiences. For those students with ASD for whom postsecondary education is an option, inclusion of such experiences for the purposes of a diploma or for personal growth and development is a final important ingredient in an exemplary transition program.

The authors propose that these elements are essential to ensuring a successful transition from school to work for individuals with ASD. The next section reviews the employment supports that further the success of young adults with ASD in their quest for a full and connected life.

EMPLOYMENT MODELS FOR INDIVIDUALS WITH ASD

As noted earlier, individuals with ASD can work with proper supports. In fact there is a growing literature suggesting that individuals with ASD achieve many desirable outcomes when they are able to work independently in a community-based environment.[21] Even so, individuals with ASD may require support to achieve these outcomes. This section describes supported employment for individuals with ASD and reviews some specialized vocational models that are reporting preliminary success.

Supported employment is an approach that helps individuals with ASD acquire, learn, and maintain competitive employment in a regular job for a competitive wage. Wehman and colleagues[29] described such a program whereby individuals with ASD achieved and maintained employment in a suburban hospital in a variety of paraprofessional positions at a competitive wage. The Federal Register defines supported employment as "competitive employment in an integrated setting with ongoing support services for individuals with the most severe disabilities" (Federal Regulations Register, 2002). **Table 2** displays the 4 major components required for implementing a supported employment program.

Supported employment is arguably the single most influential practice that results in employment for youth with ASD. Incorporating this support, there are other emerging models of employment that are resulting in employment in "real jobs" for individuals with ASD: business partnerships, customized employment, and self-employment. Each is described here.

Business Partnerships

Individuals with ASD have tremendous personal strengths that make them excellent employees. For example, the insistence on a consistent routine, attention to details, and general preference for visual order make adults with ASD successful employees at particular kinds of tasks. Although individual differences may exist, many adults with ASD display some or all of the characteristics listed in **Box 1**.

Because of these strengths, many businesses are collaborating with disability-specific employment organizations to increase the employment of individuals with disabilities. Examples of these employment partnerships result in "real jobs for real pay" for individuals with ASD and other disabilities. The partnerships are successful

Table 2
Four components for implementation of a supported employment program

Component	Description for Individual with ASD
Job-Seeker Profile and Assessment	Collect information about the person's strengths, interests, needs, and previous experiences. Develop a clear picture of the job seeker's skills and needs
Job Development and Career Search	Finding and matching job requirements, employment, social, and communication environment, and job seeker. This step is critical to the success of the person's work life. Persons with ASD are particularly affected by subtle aspects of an employment environment that can lead to success or cause the person to leave the job early
Job-Site Training and Support	Once on the job, a job coach will teach the person every aspect of the job from the necessary social "soft" skills to the job requirements. This step frequently requires the implementation of visual supports, applied behavior analytical teaching strategies, and the use of adaptive aids such as the iPod Touch to increase independence at work
Long-Term Support and Job Retention	Continuing to follow individual with ASD through changes in work and job assignments and to provide additional training as needed

---

Box 1
Strengths observed in workers with ASD

- Attends regularly due to resistance to changes in routine
- Demonstrates high rate of accuracy once task is learned
- Attends to small details and can become adept at self-correction
- Prefers visually organized environments and will bring order to disorganized environments
- Displays excellent memory for details
- Enjoys completing tasks
- Prefers work over socialization
- May have detailed information in area of special interest

---

in Walgreens, Bank of America, Marriot Bridges and, most notably, Cincinnati Children's Hospital Project SEARCH, which has been replicated internationally at numerous sites.[1,41,42] In this model, supported employment is used to support workers in these specialized businesses until the employee is independent. One specialized demonstration of this model for individuals with ASD has resulted in graduating adults with ASD acquiring employment at a suburban hospital.[43]

Customized Employment

Customized employment is a model that allows a person with ASD to negotiate a personalized job independently or through a job negotiator. The job coach frequently acts as the job negotiator.[44] In one example of this model, a job coach met with the owner of a small coffee and sandwich shop in a college town to negotiate a job for a person with ASD. In this example, the job coach arranged for the individual to prepare vegetables for sandwiches, stock the drink cooler, and deliver orders within a 4-block radius of the store. These tasks did not comprise the typical job in this establishment, but did serve the needs of the business and the employment needs of this individual with ASD.

Self-Employment

In this model of supported employment, individuals with ASD have the opportunity to develop a community-based or home-based business that capitalizes on their personal strengths.[45] Due to personal circumstances such as challenging behavior or intensity of support needs, individuals with ASD can develop their own business whereby they can define their job and the time they will devote to that job. Perhaps one of the most notable examples of this model is Poppin Joe's Kettle Korn in Louisburg, Kansas (see: http://www.poppinjoes.com/home).[46,47] Joe is a young man with ASD. With support from his family members, Joe now owns and operates a very successful kettle popcorn business. He specializes in popping and selling a variety of different-flavored popcorn.

As noted earlier, Darius' family asked the family physician what Darius' future held. Would he be able to work, live independently, have friends, and even have a girlfriend? If he is provided with an excellent transition program that results in employment and other desired outcomes, the answer is a resounding yes. In fact, when provided with the proper educational and work supports, adults with ASD are living full and connected lives and are working in their communities.

IMPLICATIONS FOR HEALTH PROFESSIONALS

The transition issues faced by youth with ASD have serious implications in communication with and planning by health professionals. Like Darius and his family, most of these students and their families will have the following questions:

- Can I go to college?
- Will I be able to work?
- Should I plan on my child living with me forever?
- How does our family manage behavioral and psychiatric problems that are presented by my child?
- How do we manage issues related to sleeping, restlessness, and other somatic issues?

For health professionals such as physicians and school psychologists to answer these questions, it is important to be knowledgable about the vocational, social, and postsecondary capacity that many of these students may demonstrate. More importantly, however, health professionals should recognize the tremendous capacity that students with ASD have to become fully contributing members of their communities.

It is a fact that many of these students will participate in school programs that do not enhance these positive outcomes, because of curriculum and instruction that does not reflect best practices. Nevertheless, as the authors have suggested, the potential of these students is quite substantive when given the proper training and support.

Physicians, especially pediatricians and experts in adolescent medicine, must be aware of the impact that excellent transition programs, evidence-based strategies, supported employment, and specialized employment models can have for students with ASD. Likewise, school psychologists must be highly sensitive to what teachers and families are doing to help these students. Finally, all health professionals who serve individuals with ASD must communicate the tremendous outcomes that can be achieved for individuals with ASD when they receive meaningful educational interventions across their entire school careers. With new advances in providing support and teaching, individuals with ASD are achieving successful outcomes and increasing their quality of life.

REFERENCES

1. Schall CM, McDonough JT. Autism spectrum disorders in adolescence and early adulthood: characteristics and issues. Journal of Vocational Rehabilitation 2010; 32:81–8.
2. National Autism Center. National Standards Report; 2009. Available at: http://www.koegelautism.com/Report_NACStandardsReport.pdf. Accessed June 15, 2011.
3. National Professional Development Center on ASD. Evidence Based Practice Briefs; 2010. Available at: http://autismpdc.fpg.unc.edu/content/briefs. Accessed June 15, 2011.
4. Centers for Disease Control. Prevalence of autism spectrum disorders (ASD's) in multiple areas in the United States, 2004 and 2006. Washington, DC: Department of Health and Human Services; 2009.
5. Table 1-3. Number of students ages 6 through 21 served under IDEA, Part B, by disability category and state: Fall 2009. (2010, July 15). Data Tables for OSEP: State Reported Data. Available at: https://www.ideadata.org/arc_toc11. Accessed June 15, 2011.

6. Rice C. Prevalence of autism spectrum disorders. Autism and Developmental Disabilities Monitoring Network, United States, 2005. Atlanta (GA): Dept. of Health and Human Services, Centers for Disease Control and Prevention; 2009.

7. Diagnostic and statistical manual of mental disorders (text revision). 4th edition. Washington, DC: American Psychiatric Association; 2000. Author.

8. Gilchrist A, Cox A, Rutter M, et al. Development and current functioning in adolescents with Asperger syndrome: a comparative study. Journal of Child Psychology and Psychiatry 2001;42:227–40.

9. McGovern CW, Sigman M. Continuity and change from early childhood to adolescence in autism. Journal of Child Psychology and Psychiatry 2005;46:401–8.

10. Seltzer MM, Shattuck PT, Abbeduto L, et al. Trajectory of development in adolescents and adults with autism. Mental Retardation and Developmental Disabilities Research Reviews 2004;10:234–47.

11. Bradley EA, Summers JA, Wood HA, et al. Comparing rates of psychiatric and behavior disorders in adolescents and young adults with severe intellectual disability with and without autism. Journal of Autism and Developmental Disabilities 2004;34:151–61.

12. Schall CM. Positive behavior support: Supporting adults with autism spectrum disorders in the workplace. Journal of Vocational Rehabilitation 2010;32:109–15.

13. White SW, Oswald D, Ollendick T, et al. Anxiety in children and adolescents with autism spectrum disorder. Clinical Psychology Review 2009;29:216–29.

14. Howlin P, Goode S, Hutton J, et al. Adult outcome for children with autism. Journal of Child Psychology and Psychiatry 2004;45:212–29.

15. Hurlbutt K, Chalmers L. Employment and adults with Asperger's syndrome. Focus on Autism. 2004;19(4):215–22.

16. Mawhood L, Howlin P, Rutter M. Autism and developmental receptive language disorder—a comparative follow-up in early adult life. Journal of Child Psychology and Psychiatry 2000;41(5):547–59.

17. Newman L, Wagner M, Cameto R, et al. Comparisons across time of the outcomes of youth with disabilities up to 4 years after high school. A report of findings from the National Longitudinal Transition Study-2 (NLTS2). Menlo Park (CA): SRI International; 2010.

18. Wagner M, Newman L, Cameto R. Changes over time in the secondary school experiences of youth with disabilities. In: A report from the National Longitudinal Transition Study-2 (NLTS2). Menlo Park (CA): SRI International; 2004.

19. Beard R. For some with autism, jobs to match their talents. Opinion - Opinionator - NYTimes.com. Available at: http://opinionator.blogs.nytimes.com/2011/06/30/putting-the-gifts-of-the-autistic-to-work/?src=tptw. NYTimes.com; 2011. Accessed July 7, 2011.

20. Carter EW, Sisco LG, Chung Y, et al. Peer interactions of students with intellectual disabilities and/or autism: a map of the intervention literature. Research & Practice for Persons with Severe Disabilities 2010;3(4):63–9.

21. Cimera RE, Cowan RJ. The costs of services and employment outcomes achieved by adults with autism in the US. Autism 2009;13(3):285–302.

22. Garcia-Villamisar D, Wehman P, Navarro MD. Changes in the quality of autistic people's life that work in supported and sheltered employment. A 5-year follow-up study. Journal of Vocational Rehabilitation 2002;17:309–12.

23. Kluth P, Shouse J. The autism checklist: a practical reference for parents and teachers. San Francisco (CA): Jossey-Bass; 2009.

24. Statement by Assistant Secretary Alexa Posny on the Fourth Annual World Autism Awareness Day on Saturday, April 2. US Department of Education; 2011. Available at: www.ed.gov/news/press-releases/statement-assistant-secretary-alexa-posny-fourth-annual-world-autism-awareness-d. Accessed June 15, 2011.
25. Cimera RE, Wehman P, West M, et al. Do sheltered workshops enhance employment outcomes for adults with autism spectrum disorder? Accepted: Autism. The International Journal of Research and Practice, in press.
26. Shattuck PT, Grosse S, Parish S, et al. Utilization of Medicaid-funded intervention for children with autism. Psychiatric Services 2009;60:549–52.
27. Wehman P, Inge KJ, Revell G, et al. Real work for real pay: inclusive employment for people with disabilities. Baltimore (MD): Paul H. Brookes; 2007.
28. Wehman P, Lau S, Moore C, et al. Supported employment for young adults with autism spectrum disorder: Preliminary data. Submitted to: Research and Practices for Persons with Severe Disabilities, in press.
29. Wehman P, McDonough J, Molinelli A, et al. Project SEARCH for youth with autism spectrum disorders: Increasing competitive employment upon graduation from high school, in press.
30. Gentry T, Wallace J, Kvarfordt C, et al. Personal digital assistants as cognitive aids for high school students with autism: results of a community-based trial. Journal of Vocational Rehabilitation 2010;32:101–7.
31. Wehman P, Smith M, Schall C. Autism and the transition to adulthood: success beyond the classroom. Baltimore (MD): Paul H. Brookes; 2009.
32. Schall C, Wehman P. Understanding the transition from school to adulthood for students with autism. In: Wehman P, Smith MD, Schall C, editors. Autism and the transition to adulthood: success beyond the classroom. Baltimore (MD): Brookes; 2009. p. 39–94.
33. Wehmeyer ML. Self determined assessment: critical components for transition planning. In: Sax CL, Thoma CA, editors. Transition assessment: wise practices for quality lives. Baltimore (MD): Paul H. Brookes Publishing Co; 2002. p. 25–38.
34. Cobb B, Lehman J, Newman-Conchar R, et al. Self-determination for students with disabilities: a narrative metasynthesis. Career Development for Exceptional Individuals 2009;32:108–14.
35. Lee S, Wehmeyer ML, Palmer SB, et al. Self-determination and access to the general education curriculum. The Journal of Special Education 2008;42:91–107.
36. Carter EW, Owens L, Trainor AA, et al. Self-determination skills and opportunities of adolescents with severe intellectual and developmental disabilities. The American Journal on Intellectual and Developmental Disabilities 2009;114:179–92.
37. Snell ME, Janney R. Collaborative teaming. 2nd edition. Baltimore (MD): Paul H. Brookes; 2005.
38. Murawski WW, Dieker LA. Tips and strategies for co-teaching at the secondary level. Little Rock (AR): The Arkansas Special Educator Unit; 2005.
39. Getzel EE, Wehman P. Pursuing postsecondary education opportunities for students with disabilities. In: Wehman P, editor. Life beyond the classroom: transition strategies for young people with disabilities. 3rd edition. Baltimore (MD): Brookes; 2006. p. 355–68.
40. Eskow KG, Fisher S. Getting together in college: an inclusion program for young adults with disabilities. Teaching Exceptional Children 2011;36:26–32 Federal Register, (2002 June 26). 67(123), 43154–9.
41. Luecking R. The way to work: how to facilitate work experiences for youth in transition. Baltimore (MD): Paul H. Brookes; 2009.

42. Rutkowski S, Daston M, Van Kuiken D, et al. Project SEARCH: A demand-side model of high school transition. Journal of Vocational Rehabilitation 2006;25:85–96.
43. Bell N. NBC 12 News, Weather, Sports, Traffic [Television broadcast]. Richmond (VA): NBC; 2011.
44. Targett P, Inge K, editors. Q & A on customized employment: employment negotiations. Boston: Virginia Commonwealth University and the Institute for Community Inclusion, University of Massachusetts; 2005.
45. Griffin, Hammis. 2003.
46. Kettle Korn Retail, Wholesale, Fundraisers Greater Kansas City, Missouri, Kansas. Available at: http://www.poppinjoes.com/hom. Accessed August 3, 2011.
47. Schall C, Wehman P, Doval-Cortijo E, et al. Application for youth with autism spectrum disorder. In: Wehman P, editor. Life beyond the classroom: transition strategies for young people with disabilities. 3rd edition. Baltimore (MD): Brookes; 2006. p. 535–76.

Sensory Processing in Children with Autism Spectrum Disorders and Impact on Functioning

Michelle A. Suarez, MOT, OTR/L

KEYWORDS

- Autism • Sensory processing disorder • Children

Children who have autism spectrum disorders (ASDs) exhibit impairments in communication and social skills and have restrictive or repetitive interests that limit functioning.[1] In this population, dysfunctional or unusual processing of sensory information has been noted since the earliest descriptions of autism.[2] Rates of unusual response to sensory information for children with autism may be as high as 90%,[3–6] and sensory processing disorder (SPD) is correlated with many diagnostic symptoms of autism and levels of everyday functioning. Better understanding by medical professionals of the impact of SPD and the resources available for identification and treatment may lead to increased functioning and participation for children with autism and their families.

SPD DEFINED

Sensory processing is defined as the brain's ability to register, organize, and make sense of information received from one's senses.[7] Although most children with autism exhibit symptoms of SPD, this condition is also common in children who have other developmental disabilities and may occur in typically developing children.[6] When sensory processing is dysfunctional, the individual may struggle with behaving in line with the demands of the environment, contributing to broader functional difficulties.[3–6] A variety of terms have been used to describe SPDs. **Box 1** provides a glossary for commonly used terminology.[7]

To increase diagnostic precision for research and treatment purposes, a unified nosology has been proposed for the discussion of sensory processing dysfunction.[7] In this nosology, several categories of SPD have been suggested to describe different

---

The author has nothing to disclose.
Occupational Therapy Department, College of Health and Human Services, 1903 West Michigan Avenue, Kalamazoo, MI 49008-5333, USA
E-mail address: michelle.a.suarez@wmich.edu

Box 1
Glossary of terms related to SPDs

Sensory integration dysfunction: this term was used previously to describe the dysfunctional motor, behavioral, emotional, and attentional responses to sensation that were caused, theoretically, by the brain's inability to process tactile, visual, olfactory, gustatory, proprioceptive, and/or visual information. The recommended term used to describe this dysfunction is SPD.

SPD: this condition includes sensory-based processing challenges that result in behavioral dysfunction. The condition encompasses impaired processing that affects the ability to modulate (sensory modulation disorders), motor plan (sensory-based motor disorders), and discriminate between the qualities of sensation (sensory discrimination disorders).

Sensory defensiveness: also called sensory overresponsivity. Individuals with this condition have a low threshold for sensation that causes them to avoid or overreact to sensory information. This condition includes tactile defensiveness, gravitational insecurity (extreme sensitivity to vestibular information), and auditory defensiveness.

Occupational therapy–sensory integration: this therapy uses a sensory integration approach to remediate dysfunction associated with SPDs.

---

patterns of behavioral dysfunction: sensory-based motor disorder, sensory discrimination disorder (SDD), and sensory modulation disorder.[7] Their hierarchical relationships are illustrated in **Fig. 1**. Sensory-based motor disorder is described as poor motor planning and/or postural instability resulting from ineffectual processing of information from the senses and can present as discoordinated or immature movement patterns. SDD is described as the inability to interpret differences and similarities between information received from the senses. For example, difficulty discriminating visual information may present with inability to distinguish between letters, making acquisition of reading skills a challenge. Sensory modulation disorders are described later and are of particular relevance to a discussion on children with autism.[8]

Sensory modulation disorder constitutes a cluster of disorders characterized by impairment in the intensity and nature of behavior in response to sensory input.[7] As a result, the response to sensation is out of synchrony with the demands of the environment, and attentional and emotional regulation is affected. Three subcategories of sensory modulation disorder have been hypothesized: sensory overresponsivity, sensory

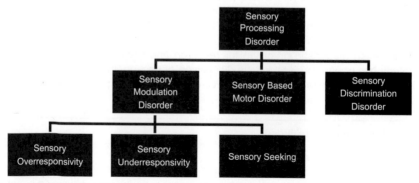

Fig. 1. SPD hierarchy. (*From* Miller LJ, Anzalone ME, Lane SJ, et al. Concept evolution in sensory integration: a proposed nosology of diagnosis. Am J Occup Ther 2007;61(2):137; with permission.)

PHYSIOLOGIC EVIDENCE FOR DISTINCTION OF SENSORY MODULATION DISORDERS

In the 1970s, Jean Ayres was one of the first to describe what seemed to be a sympathetic nervous system fight-or-flight reaction to sensation for children demonstrating difficulty modulating their arousal level.[19] Physiologic measurement tools are now available that make it possible to explore the neurologic correlates of sensory modulation disorder. Using tools such as electrodermal sensors, research is beginning to capture the physiologic response of individuals with behavioral abnormalities to sensory information, implicating the autonomic nervous system in this dysfunction. Two key studies point to differences in sympathetic and parasympathetic response to sensation for children with clinically identified sensory modulation disorder compared with children developing typically.

In a study of the physiologic responses to sensation in children clinically identified with sensory modulation disorder, McIntosh and colleagues[9] demonstrated connections between different patterns of sensory processing, electrodermal responses (EDR), and functional behavior. The researchers chose EDR as the objective physiologic measure of sympathetic nervous system activity based on prior research that had shown associations of EDR activation with startling or threatening stimuli and during positive and negative emotional events. EDR changes were measured for the study in the context of an innovative space ship–themed protocol, dubbed the Sensory Challenge Protocol, which was designed to present sensory stimulus in a nonthreatening manner. Each of the sensory modalities was stimulated during the protocol (eg, tactile stimulus, feather touched to the skin; vestibular stimulus, child tipped back in the chair; olfactory, smell of wintergreen under nose; auditory and visual, series of bright lights and sounds). The physiologic responses of children who had been identified clinically as having sensory modulation disorder were compared with those of children without such a diagnosis.

The study revealed that there were significantly more children in the sensory modulation disorder group who failed to exhibit EDR response to stimuli than in the typically developing group. This finding tentatively points to a decrease in sympathetic nervous system response in children with sensory underresponsivity. The children who did not respond to the stimulus were then removed from the next analysis. Physiologic evidence for the overresponsivity pattern of dysfunction was provided with the greater response and higher number of responses to sensation in the remaining sensory modulation disorder group. These findings provided physiologic support for the distinction between sensory underresponsivity and sensory overresponsivity. Specifically, as expected, there was both a decrease and an increase in EDR response to sensory stimuli in children with sensory modulation disorder consistent with the clinical presentation of sensory underresponsivity and overresponsivity compared with typically developing children.[9] These data provided support for the unique physiologic pattern of processing sensory information in children clinically diagnosed with sensory modulation disorder and served as the basis for additional research into the nature and causes of sensory modulation disorder.

A subsequent study provided evidence for indirect implication of the sympathetic nervous system and involvement of the parasympathetic system. Schaaf and colleagues[10] conducted a pilot study of differences in parasympathetic functioning of children with clinical symptoms of sensory modulation disorder that were age matched to children functioning typically. They used the cardiac vagal tone index as the primary measure of parasympathetic activity based on its demonstrated validity in a variety of clinical populations and age groups for this purpose. Data on cardiac vagal tone were collected during the Sensory Challenge Protocol described earlier.

underresponsivity, and sensory seeking. Although these subcategories are cur
hypothetical, physiologic research is emerging to support these distinctions.[9,10]

Sensory overresponsivity is the subtype of sensory modulation disorder that is
acterized by fast, intense, sustained reaction to sensory stimuli that is out of pro
tion with the situation.[7] People with sensory overresponsivity are hypothesized to
an unusually low threshold for sensation in any or all of the sensory systems (ta
vestibular, proprioceptive, visual, olfactory, gustatory, and/or auditory).[11] As a re
people with sensory overresponsivity may overreact to sensations that are typi
not perceived as threatening or even noticed by most people. Symptoms may inc
inappropriate behavioral outbursts that may be triggered by the feeling of texture
skin (clothing, socks, food on fingertips), movement activities (swinging, riding in
car), and loud or unexpected noises (bell ringing at school, toilet flushing). Often,
dren with sensory overresponsivity seem to be excessively cautious, become up
with changes in routine, and have difficulty with transitions between activities. Th
automatic and inappropriate responses prevent effective functioning in daily life tas
Sensory overresponsivity is often most evident when the person is faced with un
pected or novel situations or during transitions from one activity to another. Insister
on sameness and difficulty in discontinuing or initiating an activity are common behavi
in children with autism that may be related to dysfunctional sensory processing.[12–16]

Sensory underresponsivity is a subtype of sensory modulation disorder that
believed to result from an unusually high threshold for sensation.[7,11,17] Sustaine
loud, bright, fast, or otherwise intense input is required to get the attention of someo
with sensory underresponsivity.[17] Symptoms might include not responding wh
name is called, extreme preference for sedentary activities, and failing to respond
pain. The lack of ability to register sensation may lead to a child being described a
unresponsive or unaware of their surroundings, both common concerns in childre
with autism.[3]

The sensory seeker subtype of sensory modulation disorder is characterized by th
appearance of an excessive insatiable drive for sensory experiences.[7] Children wit
this subtype may climb to unsafe heights, mouth nonfood items, or touch peopl
and/or food objects to the point of annoying others.[17] Children with sensory seeking
may also engage in dangerous movement activities not in line with their motor skil
level or demonstrate disruptive behavior that limits their ability to integrate into classroom or group situations. Sensory-seeking behavior has the potential to cause injury
and disrupt the development of meaningful routines and relationships. This could be
particularly problematic in children with autism who already have difficulty with relationship formation.[18]

Sensory modulation disorders of any type can be disruptive to a child's development. Children with ASD demonstrate high levels of sensory modulation disorders
across ages and severity of autism.[3] The presentation of these symptoms is
heterogeneous, with highest incidence of sensory underresponsivity followed by
overresponsivity and sensory seeking. Links between sensory modulation disorders
and psychological dysfunction may contribute to autism symptom severity and
deficits in everyday functioning, in effect, compounding the severity of autism
symptoms.

Investigation into the underlying neurologic causes of sensory modulation disorders are ongoing, with significant discoveries emerging. Technological advances
have made it possible to measure physiologic functioning related to the behavior
observed in response to sensory input. The research into the physiologic correlates of sensory modulation disorders can provide insight into this comorbid
condition.

The results indicated that children with sensory modulation disorder had significantly lower cardiac vagal tone measurements, suggesting that these children have less effective parasympathetic functioning compared with typical controls.[10] The investigators discussed the implications of sensory modulation disorder on functioning, suggesting that a compromised parasympathetic system may disrupt the child's ability to maintain a calm focused state in the face of sensations encountered in everyday life.

IMPACT OF SENSORY MODULATION DISORDERS ON FUNCTIONING FOR CHILDREN WITH ASD

The functional difficulties associated with the diagnostic symptoms of autism pose daily obstacles for many children. The presence of sensory modulation disorders in these individuals is correlated with and may compound the symptoms of autism. If the child's sympathetic and parasympathetic systems are not working to allow the maintenance of a calm alert state, this may make participation in meaningful daily activities an even greater challenge.[17]

Participation in meaningful activities is key to achieving a high quality of life.[20] Symptoms of autism have a debilitating effect on participation in daily activities.[21] Sensory modulation disorders, which are associated with many of the symptoms of autism, may compound dysfunction and further decrease life engagement. This includes the relationship between sensory modulation disorders and diagnostic features of autism, such as restrictive/repetitive behaviors and social skill deficits as well as comorbid feeding dysfunction.

Restrictive and Repetitive Behavior

Restricted repetitive behaviors (RRBs) are included as one component of the diagnostic criteria for autism[1] that has been linked to SPDs in the literature.[3] It has been suggested that these dysfunctional, repetitive, and inappropriate behaviors may represent an effort to relieve stress produced by difficulty in processing sensory information.[16] RRBs can range from lower to higher order.[12] Lower-order RRBs include stereotypy, such as hand flapping or self-injurious behavior (eg, head banging, scratching, or biting). These behaviors can be found in children with severe developmental disabilities as well as autism.[22] Higher-order RRBs are more exclusively found in children with autism.[22,23] These behaviors encompass compulsions, insistence on sameness, and restricted interests. Children with autism sometimes have odd attachments to and/or unusual preoccupation with objects (eg, fascination with spinning the wheels on a toy truck or gazing at ceiling fans). They also can have a narrow range of interests and compulsively try to steer conversation to discussion of these interests. These behaviors can restrict participation in functional activities.[23]

Several studies have provided growing evidence that sensory modulation disorders are highly correlated with and may contribute to the frequency and severity of RRBs.[12–16] For example, Gal and colleagues[15] examined the relationships between SPD and stereotyped movement in 221 children with and without developmental disorders (including autism). The researchers used the Short Sensory Profile (SSP) to measure SPD, Stereotyped and Self-Injurious Movement Interview, and Repetitive Behavior Interview to measure potentially related behaviors. They found that the within-group and between-group differences in stereotyped movement could be accounted for by differences in SSP scores.

This relationship between sensory modulation disorders and RRBs may be especially strong for sensory overresponsivity. Chen and colleagues[13] looked at the relationship between the SSP and the Childhood Routines Inventory (measuring compulsivelike behaviors) in 29 children diagnosed with high functioning autism or Asperger syndrome. The investigators found a significant relationship between the frequency and intensity of behaviors in the Childhood Routines Inventory and tactile, visual, and auditory sensitivity (all constructs included in sensory overresponsivity).[13] Similarly, Joosten and Bundy[16] found that children with autism and intellectual disability were significantly more sensitive to sensation and went to greater means to avoid sensation than children with intellectual disability alone. The investigators combined these results with a previous study of the same participants that revealed that stereotyped repetitive behaviors of children with autism are commonly associated with anxiety. The combined results suggested that the use of RRBs might be a result of the child's effort to relieve anxiety produced by sensory input.[16,24] Using repetitive motor movement or demonstrating the need to control the conversation may be an effort to reduce feelings of anxiety resulting from discomfort with sensory stimulation. RRBs can lead to a lack of flexibility and isolation that limits the play repertoire and opportunity to engage with others.[25] This has significant implications for participation in meaningful and purposeful activities for children with autism.

Social Functioning

Social competence is gained through interactions with others during social activities.[21] Difficulty with the development of social relationships is another diagnostic characteristic of ASD,[1] and, here too, the presence of sensory modulation disorders may further amplify these deficits. Several studies have described links between deficits in social competence and/or decreased social participation and sensory modulation disorders. Hilton and colleagues,[26] for example, found a strong relationship between sensory responsivity and social responsiveness, irrespective of the child's intelligence quotient score. This relationship was particularly true for the proximal (ie, tactile, oral, and olfactory sense items) and multisense items. The investigators suggested that this made sense given the multisensory and proximal nature of communication and socialization. Similarly, Lane and colleagues[27] found a clear association between sensory processing dysfunction and impairments in communicative skills. Children with autism and sensory modulation disorders participate less frequently in activities outside the school and home settings and report enjoying those activities less than children with autism who have less prominent sensory modulation deficits.[18] Meaningful social engagement is one hallmark of satisfaction with life. Sensory modulation disorders may exacerbate the social deficits found in autism and present increased challenges for the development of meaningful socialization.

Feeding and Eating

Children with ASD frequently demonstrate dysfunction in feeding and eating (ie, food selectivity), and it has been suggested in the literature that this may be related to sensory modulation disorders as well, specifically sensory overresponsivity. In the population of children with autism, 40% to 60% of children have food selectivity, meaning they have a restricted range of foods that they will eat.[28–30] This food selectivity poses a significant concern for parents because it has been associated with inadequate nutrition[29] and is often accompanied by disruptive mealtime behavior.[31]

Clinicians and parents describe children with autism who choose foods based on their presentation and texture. For example, some children with autism only eat foods of a particular texture, color, or flavor; off a particular plate; and/or with certain utensils.[28–30] Cermak and colleagues[32] suggested that food selectivity might be partially a result of sensory modulation disorders. This is in keeping with the fact that children with sensory overresponsivity but who were otherwise developing typically were found in one study[33] to eat fewer fresh fruits and vegetables and gagged more when eating than those without sensory modulation disorders. Also, children with autism often are very particular about the texture of foods,[32] which may implicate a lower threshold for sensation in the tactile system. Further investigation is needed to establish the factors associated with food selectivity in the autistic population, including close examination of the link to sensory modulation disorder.

Summary

Sensory modulation disorders have been associated with key diagnostic features of autism and comorbid feeding dysfunction. Researchers and clinicians are just beginning to understand the role of the autonomic nervous system in the behavioral manifestation of sensory modulation disorders in the autistic population. In addition to the functional deficits caused by the symptoms of autism, if the child is unable to maintain physiologic homeostasis due to sensory modulation disorders, little energy may be available for participation in meaningful functional activities that are the cornerstone of quality of life.

WHEN TO REFER

From time to time, all children experience some difficulty modulating their arousal level in response to sensation from the environment.[17] When typically developing children are stressed, tired, or overwhelmed, they may tune out or act out when faced with sensory experiences that they usually handle in their stride. However, when a child consistently has a behavioral response to stimuli that is extreme and inconsistent with the demands of the environment, a referral for treatment may be indicated. Children on the autism spectrum, in particular, should be referred as soon as possible so that intervention can begin early. Attending to warning signs (**Table 1**) can allow for the provision of treatment for possible increases in functioning.[17] Beyond informal observation, the SSP is a quick and easy screening tool that can help to confirm clinical observations that point to a sensory modulation disorder.[34] This caregiver questionnaire has 38 items and takes approximately 10 minutes to administer. Using a Likert scale, parents report the frequency of the occurrence of behaviors related to sensory dysfunction. The measure yields results that quantify no, probable, or definite differences in the behavioral output in response to sensory stimulus compared with typically developing children. Knowing the warning signs and investigating further with screening tools can facilitate appropriate referrals to clinicians, such as occupational therapists (OTs), who have training to treat sensory modulation disorders.[17] Treatment can ease the burden of this disorder for children and their families.[17]

TREATMENT AND OUTCOMES

The goal of OT treatment of children with sensory modulation disorder is to decrease the functional limitations caused by the SPD.[17] The treatment includes several overlapping and integrated elements. Components of treatment include remediation for underlying sensory processing dysfunction, environmental modifications to reduce sensory stressors in the environment, and task practice to increase competence in specific skill areas.[35] Each of these components is addressed briefly in the sections that follow.

Table 1
Examples of behaviors associated with sensory modulation disorders

Sensory Overresponsivity	Sensory Underresponsivity	Sensory Seeking
Is upset by tags in clothing and the seam in socks and/or only wears clothing with particular textures	Does not respond when name is called repeatedly	Is in motion from the moment of waking until falling into bed to sleep at night
Struggles excessively to avoid grooming tasks such as brushing teeth or having nails clipped	Does not react to injuries and seems to have a very high pain tolerance	Takes risks during play such as climbing too high, jumping off high surfaces, and moving too quickly for safety
Hates messy play (eg, finger painting). Becomes very concerned when hands get dirty	Often appears disheveled and does not notice food left on face or clothing twisted on body	Appears driven to touch everything in the environment
Covers ears and/or becomes very distressed with loud or unexpected noises	Difficulty with toilet training and has frequent accidents	Frequently crashes and bumps into people and objects
Avoids movement activities such as swinging or climbing	Extreme preference for sedentary activities	Mouths nonfood objects
Is picky about food textures and frequently gags on food or the smell of nonpreferred food	Does not notice things going on around the room	Makes nonfunctional noises
Has extreme difficulty with changes in routine, novel activities, and anything unexpected	Overstuffs food in mouth	Likes spicy or flavorful foods

Remediation

To remediate the underlying deficits related to sensory modulation disorders, the OT seeks to integrate the client's sensory system through response to multisensory activities that get increasingly more difficult as the child gains skill. This approach, often called Occupational Therapy–Sensory Integration (OT-SI) has a specific set of elements that must be present for fidelity to be maintained.[36] The treatment should be designed to involve active client participation in activities that provide enhanced sensation and require the client's adaptive response. Activities should be client driven and support optimal arousal, leading to the client's ability to self-regulate during the experience of sensation. Motivation for participation is encouraged through the therapeutic relationship, collaboration on activity choice, and a play context. The child is set up for success and assisted to learn through experiences with sensory stimuli. Through these activities, the goal is for the child to learn to respond appropriately to a variety of sensory stimuli.

Environmental Modification and Tools for Adaptation

In addition to remediation of underlying sensory dysfunction, several other treatment elements may be aimed at increasing functioning of individuals with autism and sensory modulation disorder. OTs, speech and language pathologists, physical therapists, special education teachers, parents, and others may be involved in aspects of treatment of sensory modulation disorders beyond the remedial sensory integration approach.[17,35] Consideration of the context is important for facilitating functional gains in children with autism and sensory modulation disorders.[37] Different environments (eg, home, school) hold different challenges. In collaboration with parents, the clinician or teacher can provide recommendations for environmental modifications to minimize sensory challenges and capitalize on the child's strengths.[17] For example, a child with sensory overresponsivity often has extreme difficulty with changes in routine, making a class field trip very difficult. To decrease the stress associated with this experience, the therapist may write a story describing what the child should expect during the trip,[38] offer calming music to listen to on the bus ride, and allow the child to take a break in a quiet space with a trusted adult when the experience becomes over-whelming. Environment modifications and support may allow for greater participation in meaningful activities for the child with autism and sensory modulation disorders.

Specific Task Practice

After providing remediation to minimize underlying deficits and modifying the environment to increase the child's comfort and success, task practice may be necessary for specific skill development.[39] For example, a child with sensory modulation disorder and autism may have been uncomfortable with sensations associated with self-care tasks and lacked the attention required to practice these skills. As a result, they may experience lack of development in this area. Treatment of sensory modulation disorders requires specific task practice (eg, zipping coat, tying shoes, brushing teeth) using a multisensory approach to increase skill in specific areas.

Sensory Integration Treatment Research

Sensory integration treatment is one of the most frequently used therapies for autism and sensory modulation disorders.[40] Despite the frequency of use, however, little evidence is available, and there are no adequate-sized high-quality randomized controlled trials to confirm the effectiveness of this approach. Research on OT-SI and associated components described previously for sensory modulation disorders has suffered from lack of uniform terminology, lack of fidelity to sensory integration theory, lack of homogeneity of treatment groups, and lack of sample sizes large enough to detect changes.[41]

Efforts are underway to address these issues. Studies are emerging that use man-ualized treatment approaches administered by adequately trained providers to ensure that important elements of treatment are upheld.[40] Better inclusion and exclusion criteria are being developed to ensure that samples include subjects who experience similar dysfunction. For example, Miller and colleagues[40] completed a pilot random-ized control design with the treatment group participating in OT-SI and controls including an activities placebo group and wait-list group. Homogeneous samples were obtained using several clinical measures and physiologic data (ie, EDR to stimuli) to verify sensory modulation dysfunction. Despite the small sample size, the OT-SI group was shown to achieve statistically significant improvement on a measure of goal attainment and on a parental report measure of attention and social skills. High-quality research on the sensory integration treatment approach is emerging, but much work is still needed to determine conclusively the efficacy of this approach.

SUMMARY

Children with autism experience many challenges that affect their ability to function. SPD and, specifically, sensory modulation disorder can compound dysfunction and further inhibit participation in productive activities. Through detection of and referral for sensory modulation disorders, treatment can be accessed. Emerging treatment evidence points to functional gains for autism and sensory modulation disorder that can ease the burden that this combination of symptoms has on the everyday life of children with autism.

REFERENCES

1. American Psychiatric Association. Diagnostic and statistical manual of mental disorders. Text Revision. 4th edition. Washington, DC: American Psychiatric Association; 2000.
2. Kanner L. Early infantile autism. J Pediatr 1944;3:211–7.
3. Ben-Sasson A, Hen L, Fluss R, et al. A meta-analysis of sensory modulation symptoms in individuals with autism spectrum disorders. J Autism Dev Disord 2009;39:1–11.
4. Baranek GT, David FJ, Poe MD, et al. Sensory experiences questionnaire: discriminating sensory features in young children with autism, developmental delays, and typical development. J Child Psychol Psychiatry 2006;47:591–601.
5. Leekam SR, Libby SJ, Wing L, et al. Describing the sensory abnormalities of children and adults with autism. J Autism Dev Disord 2007;37:894–910.
6. Tomchek SD, Dunn W. Sensory processing in children with and without autism: a comparative study using the short sensory profile. Am J Occup Ther 2007; 61:190–200.
7. Miller LJ, Anzalone ME, Lane SJ, et al. Concept evolution in sensory integration: a proposed nosology of diagnosis. Am J Occup Ther 2007;61(2):135–40.
8. Baker AE, Lane A, Angley MT, et al. The relationship between sensory processing patterns and behavioural responsiveness in autistic disorder: a pilot study. J Autism Dev Disord 2008;38:867–75.
9. McIntosh DN, Miller LJ, Hagerman RJ. Sensory-modulation disruption, electrodermal responses, and functional behaviors. Dev Med Child Neurol 1999;41: 608–15.
10. Schaaf RC, Miller LJ, Seawell D, et al. Children with disturbances in sensory processing: a pilot study examining the role of the parasympathetic nervous system. Am J Occup Ther 2003;57(4):442–9.
11. Dunn W. Performance of typical children on the sensory profile: an item analysis. Am J Occup Ther 2002;57:967–74.
12. Boyd BA, McBee M, Holtzclaw T, et al. Relationships among repetitive behaviors, sensory features, and executive functions in high functioning autism. Res Autism Spectr Disord 2009;3:959–66.
13. Chen Y, Rodgers J, McConachie H. Restricted and repetitive behaviours, sensory processing and cognitive style in children with autism spectrum disorder. J Autism Dev Disord 2009;39:635–42. DOI:10.1007/s10803-008-0663-6.
14. Gabriels RL, Agnew JA, Miller LJ, et al. Is there a relationship between restricted, repetitive, stereotyped behaviors and interests and abnormal sensory response in children with autism spectrum disorders? Res Autism Spectr Disord 2008;2(4):660–70.
15. Gal E, Dyck MJ, Passmore A. Relationships between stereotyped movements and sensory processing disorders in children with and without developmental or sensory disorders. Am J Occup Ther 2010;64:453–61.
16. Joosten A, Bundy AC. Sensory processing and stereotypical and repetitive behavior in children with autism and intellectual disability. Aust Occup Ther J 2010;57:366–72.

17. Miller LJ. Sensational kids: hope and help for children with sensory processing disorder. New York: G.P Putnam and Sons; 2006.

18. Hochhauser M, Engel-Yeger B. Sensory processing abilities and their relation to participation in leisure activities among children with high-functioning autism spectrum disorder (HFASD). Res Autism Spectr Disord 2010;4:746–54.

19. Ayres J. Sensory integration and the child. 11th edition. Los Angeles: Western Psychological Services; 1994.

20. Simeonsson RJ, Leonardi M, Lollar D, et al. Applying the International Classification of Functioning, Disability and Health to measure childhood disability. Disabil Rehabil 2003;25:602–10.

21. Reynolds S, Bendixen R, Lawrence T, et al. A pilot study examining activity participation, sensory responsiveness and competence in children with high functioning autism spectrum disorder. J Autism Dev Disord 2011;41(11):1496–506.

22. Carcani-Rathwell I, Rabe-Hasketh S, Santosh PJ. Repetitive and stereotyped behaviours in pervasive developmental disorders. J Child Psychol Psychiatry 2006;47(6):573–81.

23. Lam KS, Bodfish JW, Piven J. Evidence for three subtypes of repetitive behavior in autism that differ in familiality and association with other symptoms. J Child Psychol Psychiatry 2008;49(11):1193–200.

24. Joosten AV, Bundy AC, Einfeld SL. Intrinsic and extrinsic motivation of stereotypic and repetitive behaviors. J Autism Dev Disord 2009;39:521–31.

25. Prelock PA. Autism Spectrum Disorders: Issues and Assessment Intervention. Pro-Ed; 2006. p. 230.

26. Hilton CL, Harper JD, Holmes KR, et al. Sensory responsiveness as a predictor of social severity in children with high functioning autism spectrum disorders. J Autism Dev Disord 2010;40:937–45.

27. Lane AE, Young RL, Baker AE, et al. Sensory processing subtypes in autism: association with adaptive behavior. J Autism Dev Disord 2010;40:112–22.

28. Schreck KA, Williams K. Food preferences and factors influencing food selectivity for children with autism spectrum disorders. Res Dev Disabil 2006;27:353–63.

29. Cornish E. A balanced approach towards healthy eating in autism. J Hum Nutr Diet 1998;11:501–9.

30. Williams KE, Gibbons BG, Schreck KA. Comparing selective eaters with and without developmental disabilities. J Dev Phys Disabil 2005;17:299–309.

31. Ahearn WH, Castine T, Nault K, et al. An assessment of food acceptance in children with autism or pervasive developmental disorder-not otherwise specified. J Autism Dev Disord 2001;31:505–11.

32. Cermak SA, Curtin C, Bandini LG. Food selectivity and sensory sensitivity in children with autism spectrum disorders. J Am Diet Assoc 2010;110(2):238–46.

33. Smith A, Roux S, Naidoo NT, et al. Food choices of tactile defensive children. Nutrition 2005;21:14–9.

34. Dunn W. Sensory profile. San Antonio (TX): The Psychological Corporation; 1999.

35. Bundy AC, Murray AE. Sensory integration: a. Jean Ayres theory revisited. In: Bundy AC, Lane SJ, Murray EA, editors. Sensory integration: theory and practice. 2nd edition. Philadelphia: FA Davis; 2002. p. 3–33.

36. Parham LD, Cohn ES, Spitzer S, et al. Fidelity in sensory integration intervention research. Am J Occup Ther 2007;61(2):216–27.

37. Case-Smith J, Arbesman M. Evidence-based review of interventions for autism used in or of relevance to occupational therapy. Am J Occup Ther 2008;62(4):416–29.

38. Howley M, Arnold E. Revealing the hidden social code: social stories for people with autism spectrum disorders. London: Jessica Kingsley; 2005.

39. Bundy AC. The process of planning and implementing intervention. In: Bundy AC, Land SJ, Murray EA, editors. Sensory integration theory and practice. 2nd edition. Philadelphia: FA Davis; 2002. p. 211–25.
40. Miller LJ, Coll JR, Schoen SA. A randomized controlled pilot study of the effectiveness of occupational therapy for children with sensory modulation disorder. Am J Occup Ther 2007;61(2):228–38.
41. Miller LJ, Schoen SA, James K, et al. Lessons learned: a pilot study on occupational therapy effectiveness for children with sensory modulation disorder. Am J Occup Ther 2007;61(2):161–9.

Index

Note: Page numbers of article titles are in **boldface** type.

A

Aberrant Behavior Checklist, 177
Abnormal Involuntary Movement Scale, 179
N-Acetylaspartate studies, 68–69
Adaptation, for sensory modulation disorders, 210–211
Adenosine deaminase deficiency, 116–117
Adenylosuccinate lyase deficiency, 116
Adolescents
    language and communication in, 132–133
    transition to work for, **189–202**
Ages & Stages Questionnaires, 95, 134
Aggression, treatment of, 177–180
American Academy of Pediatrics, Autism Expert Panel, 31
Americans with Disabilities Act, 3
Amphetamines, 182
Anatomic traits, of autism, 35
Androgen receptors, 81–82
Angelman syndrome, 49
Antidepressants, 181
Antidiuretic hormone, 78–79
Antipsychotics, 178–179
Antivaccination movement, 3, 5–7
Anxiety, 153, 183
Apelin, 79
Arginine vasopressin, 78–79
Arginine:glycine amidinotransferase deficiency, 117
Aripiprazole, 178–181
ASDs. *See* Autism spectrum disorders.
Asperger, Hans, 4–5, 19
Asperger Support Network, 171
Asperger syndrome
    diagnostic criteria for, 20–21
    language and communication in, 131–132
    serotonergic transmission in, 67
Atomoxetine, 182
Attention-deficit/hyperactivity disorder, with autism, 31
Atypical antipsychotics, 181, 182
Auditory processing, 52–54
Autism A.L.A.R.M., 31, 91
Autism and Developmental Disabilities Monitoring network, 27–28
Autism Diagnostic Interview, 24, 107–108

Pediatr Clin N Am 59 (2012) 215–224
doi:10.1016/S0031-3955(11)00180-5
0031-3955/12/$ – see front matter © 2012 Elsevier Inc. All rights reserved.

pediatric.theclinics.com

Autism Diagnostic Observation Schedule, 24, 107
Autism Research Institute, 5
Autism Society of America, 5
Autism Speaks, 89–90, 95–97, 171
Autism spectrum disorders
  anatomic traits with, 35
  assessment of, 133–134, 176–177
  behavioral interventions for, **147–164**
  best practices in, 105–108
  clinical features of, **19–25,** 45–46
  diagnosis of, **19–25,** 45–46, **103–111**
    challenges in, 104–105
    recent changes in, 191–192
  differential diagnosis of, 24
  endocrine factors in, **75–88**
  epidemiology of, **27–43**
    incidence, 27–28
    prevalence, 21, 28–31
  first use of term, 3
  genetic evaluation of, **113–128**
  genetic syndromes associated with, 35
  historical perspectives on, **1–10**
  importance of, 108
  instruments for, 23–24, 91–96, 107–108, 134
  language and communication in. *See* Communication; Integrated view of language
    and communication.
  morbidities with, 36–37
  mortality in, 37–38
  neurobiological basis of, **45–61**
  neuroimaging and neurochemistry of, **63–73**
  parent perspective of. *See* Parents.
  prognosis for, 35–36
  psychopharmacology of, **175–187**
  regressive, 3
  risk factors for, 32–35
  screening for, **89–102**
  sensory processing in, **201–214**
  social skills training for, **165–174**
  symptoms of, 21–22
  terminology of, 7
  transition from school to work with, **189–202**
  treatment of. *See* Interventions.
Autism Spectrum Screening Questionnaire, 92
Autism Tissue Program, 47–48
Autoimmune disorders, 83
Ayres, Jean, 206

B

Babbling, 94
Bedlam (hospital), 2

Behavior Analyst Certification Board, 151
Behavioral interventions, **147–164**
    collaboration in, 155
    early intensive behavioral intervention program, 149–152
    problem-focused outpatient and consultative services, 152–155
    resources for, 164
    terminology of, 148, 162
Bettelheim, Brun, 5
Birth weight, autism risk and, 34
Blair, Hugh, 2
Bleuler, Paul Eugen, 3
Books, for social skills training, 167, 170–171
Brain, dysfunction of, 46–48
Business partnerships, employment opportunities in, 197–198

C

Celiac disease, 83
Cerebral folate deficiency, 118
Chambliss Criteria, 150
Checklist for Autism in Toddlers, 91–93
Child Development Inventory, 95
Childhood autism Spectrum Test, 92
Childhood Routines Inventory, 208
Children's Psychiatric Rating Scale, 177
Children's Yale-Brown Obsessive Compulsive Scale Modified for Pervasive
    Development Disorder, 177
Cholesterol metabolism, disorders of, 118
Chromosome anomalies, 119–120
    16p11.2 duplication or deletion, 119–120
    17q12 deletion, 120
    22q13 deletion, 120
    15q13 deletion or duplication, 120
    7q11.23 duplication, 119
Circadian system, abnormalities of, 51–52
Citalopram, 181
Clinical Global Impression Scale, 176–177
Clonidine, 182
Clumsiness, 54–56
Cognitive behavioral therapy, 153
Collaboration, in behavioral interventions, 151
College education, 196
Communication. *See also* Integrated view of language and communication.
    gesture, 94
    impairment of, 21–22
    parent perspective of, **13–18**
Communication and Symbolic Behavior Scales, 93, 107
Community agencies, 95–97, 196
Comorbid conditions, 22, 24, 31–32, 36–37
Competence
    social, 194–195, 208
    vocational, 194

Consultation, for behavioral interventions, 152–155
Core symptoms, of ASD, 21–22, 130–131
Cortisone, 80–81
Creatine transport and metabolism, disorders of, 117
Creatinine transporter 1 deficiency, 117
Customized employment, 198

D

Depression, 31, 183
Developmental delay, with autism, 31–32
Developmental Profile Infant-Toddler Checklist, 93
Developmental regression, 50–51
Diabetes mellitus, 83
Diagnostic and Statistical Manual of Mental Disorders, 19–21
Diagnostic Interview for Social and Communication Disorders, 24
Disabilities Education Act, 97, 193
Discrete trial training, 148
Disintegrative disorders, 50–51
Divalproex, 180, 181
Dopamine precursor and transporter studies, 65–66
Drugs, for ASD, **175–187**
Dysmorphic features, 35
Dyspraxia, 54–56

E

Early intensive behavioral intervention program, 149–152
Eating, dysfunctional, 208–209
Education
    parental, as autism risk, 33
    postsecondary, 196
Education for All Handicapped Act, 2–3
Eisenberg, Leon, 4
Electroencephalography, 49–51
Electronic health records, 98–99
Employment
    models for, 196–198
    transition to, **189–202**
Endocrine disrupters, 84
Endocrine factors, **75–88**
Environmental factors, 34–35, 210–211
Epilepsy, ASD association with, 22–23, 37, 48–51
Escitalopram, 181
Estrogen, 82
Ethnic factors, in autism, 35
Extreme male brain theory, 81–82

F

Feeding, dysfunctional, 208–209
First Signs, 89–90
Fluorodopa studies, 65–66

Fluoxetine, 181
Folate deficiency, 118
Food selectivity, 54
Fragile-X syndrome, 49, 122
Freud, Sigmund, 3

G

Gait disorders, 54–56
Gamma-aminobutyric acid studies, 67–68
Gaze avoidance, 54
Gender differences, in autism, 33
Genetic factors, in autism, 33–34
Genetic syndromes, 31–32, 35, **113–128**
    chromosomal anomalies, 119–120
    evaluation of, 113–116, 122–124
    metabolic disorders, 116–118
    mitochondrial disorders, 119
    monogenic disorders, 120–124
Gestational age, autism risk and, 34
Gesture communication, 94
Global Assessment of Functioning Scale, 36
Glutamate-glutamine studies, 69–70
Grandin, Temple, 53
Groups, for social skills training, 167–169
Growth factors, 77
Growth hormone, 77
Guanidinoacetate methyltransferase deficiency, 117

H

Haloperidol, 178
Head circumference, 35, 46, 77
Hippocrates, 2
Hyperactivity, treatment of, 181–183
Hyperacusis, 54
Hypothalamo-pituitary-adrenal axis, 80–81
Hypotonia, 56

I

Independence, promotion of, 194
Individualized education programs, 171, 193
Individuals with Disabilities Act, 3
Infants, communication observations in, 132
Insomnia, 51–52, 183
Insulinlike growth factor-1, 77
Integrated view of language and communication, **129–145**
    assessment in, 133–134
    description of, 130–133
    events in infancy and, 132
    family support in, 134–135
    in subthreshold diagnoses, 131–132

Integrated (*continued*)
    intervention approaches in, 135–139
    later academic and social learning and, 132–133
Intellectual disability, 22, 31–32
Interventions, **147–164**
    behavioral, **147–164**
    collaboration in, 155
    early intensive behavioral intervention program, 149–152
    for sensory modulation disorders, 209–211
    for social skills, 166–171
    in integrated view of language and communication, 135–139
    pharmacologic, **175–176**
    problem-focused outpatient and consultative services, 152–155
    resources for, 164
Irritability, treatment of, 177–180
Itard, Jean, 2

J

Joint attention, 94
Joint laxity, 54–56

K

Kanner, Leo, 4, 19
Kennedy, Rosemary, 2
Kinesthetic processing, 52–54

L

Landau-Kleffner syndrome, 50
Language. *See also* Communication; Integrated view of language and communication.
    regression of, 50–51
Learn the Signs, Act Early campaign, 31, 89–90
Legislation, on disabilities, 2–3
Literacy, 135–139
Løvaas, Ole Iva, 6
Luther, Martin, 2

M

Magnetic resonance spectroscopy, 68–70
Magnetoencephalography, 49
Medical Home, 97
Melatonin, 52, 79–80, 183
Mental retardation, 37
Mental status examination, 23
α [^{11}C]Methyl-L-tryptophan, in PET, 66
Methylphenidate, 179, 182
5-Methyltetrahydrofolate deficiency, 118
Mindfulness training, 169
Mirror neuron system, 46–47
Mitochondrial disorders, 119
Modified Checklist for Autism in Toddlers, 91–95, 99, 134

Monogenic disorders, 120–124
Morbidities. *See* Comorbid conditions.
More Than Words–The Hanen Program, 135
Mortalities, 37–38
Motor issues, 54–56
Multidisciplinary approach, 105–106
Multimodal Anxiety and Social Skills Intervention, 153
Muscle tone abnormalities, 54–56
Myotonic dystrophy, 121–122

N

Naltrexone, 180
National Autism Center, 136, 139
National Longitudinal Transition Study, 193–194
National Research Council Committee on Educational Interventions for Children
    with Autism, 105, 107
National Survey of Children's Health, autism incidence in, 28
Navigating the Social World, 168
Neurofibromatosis type 1, 121
Neuroimaging, **63–73**
    magnetic resonance spectroscopy, 68–70
    positron emission tomography, 64–67
    single photon emission computed tomography, 64–67
Neurologic issues, 37, **45–61**
    brain function and dysfunction, 46–48
    developmental regression, 50–51
    epilepsy, 22–23, 37, 48–51
    in diagnosis, 45–46
    motor, 54–56
    sensory, 52–54
    sleep problems, 51–52
Neurotensin, 82–83
"Nick's Story" (video), 15–17
Nutritional deficiencies, 54

O

Observation Scale for Infants, 93
Obsessive-compulsive disorder, 31
Occupational therapy-sensory integration, 204, 210
Offit, Paul, 6
Olanzapine, 179
Olfactory processing, 52–54
Outpatient services, for behavioral interventions, 152–155
Oversensitivy, to touch, 53–54
Oxytocin, 77–78

P

Parents
    antivaccine movement among, 5–7
    characteristics of, as autism risks, 32–34
    experiences of, **13–18**

Parents (*continued*)
    in transition from school to work, 195
    support of, 134–135
Patient Protection & Affordable Care Act, 98–99
Pediatric Evaluation of Developmental Status, 95
Peer mentoring, for social skills training, 166–168, 170
Pervasive developmental disorder, autism as, 130
Pervasive Developmental Disorders Screening Test, 92–93
Phenylketonuria, 116
Physical examination, 23
Physical traits, of autism, 35
Picture books, for social skills training, 167, 170–171
Pivotal Response training, 168
Plato, 2
Polysomnography, 51–52
Positron emission tomography, 64–67
Preterm infants, autism risk in, 34
Proprioceptive processing, 52–54
Psychiatric disorders, with autism, 31–32
Psychopharmacology, **175–187**
    for aggression, 177–180
    for anxiety, 183
    for depression, 183
    for hyperactivity, 181–183
    for repetitive behaviors, 180–181
    for sleep disorders, 183
    outcome measurement tools for, 176–177
Purine metabolism, disorders of, 116–117
Purkinje cell abnormalities, 46

R

Reciprocal social deficits, 21–22
Red flags, for ASK, 133–134
Referral, in sensory modulation disorders, 209
Regression, 50–51
Regressive autism, 3
Relaxation training, 169
Remediation, for sensory modulation disorders, 210
Repetitive movement and behavior, 54–56, 180–181, 207–208
Response to name, 94
Restrictive behavior, 207–208
Rett disorder, language and communication in, 131–132
Rheumatoid arthritis, 83
Rigid ritualistic interests, 21–22
Rimland, Bernard, 5–6
Risperidone, 178, 181
Rutter, M., 19

S

Screening, 23–24, **89–102**
    early, 93–94

electronic health records and, 98–99
information for, 89–92
integrated view of, 133–134
pediatrician role in, 91, 93
positive results in, 96–97
reimbursement for, 97–98
statistics on, 90–91
suggestions for, 93–94
Screening Tool for Autism in Toddlers and Young Children, 91–93, 107
Secretin, 82
Seizures, ASD association with, 22–23, 37, 48–51
Selective serotonin reuptake inhibitors, 181, 183
Self-advocacy, 195
Self-determination, 195
Self-employment, 198
Self-injury, treatment of, 177–180
Sensory Challenge Protocol, 206–207
Sensory defensiveness, definition of, 204
Sensory integration dysfunction, definition of, 204
Sensory integration treatment, research on, 211
Sensory issues, 52–54
Sensory modulation disorders
    definition of, 204–205
    physiology of, 206–207
    referral in, 209
    treatment of, 209–211
Sensory overresponsivity, 205, 210
Sensory processing, **203–214**
    definition of, 203–204
    disorders of. *See also* Sensory modulation disorders.
        nosology of, 201–205
Sensory seeker, 205, 210
Sensory underresponsibity, 205, 210
Serotonin precursor, transporter, and receptor studies, 66–67
Services, access to, 171
[^{18}F]Setoperone, in PET, 67
Shakespeare, William, 2
Single photon emission computed tomography, 64–67
Sleep problems, 51–52, 154, 183
Smith-Lemli-Opitz syndrome, 118
Smoking, maternal, as autism risk, 34–35
Social Communication Questionnaire, 92–93, 108
Social competence, 194–195, 208
Social functioning, 208
Social interaction, with doctors, 15–16
Social skills, **165–174**
    deficits of, 165–166
    interventions for, 166–171
Social Skills Picture Book, 171
Social smiles, 94
Social STAR, 168

Social Stories intervention, 16–17, 167, 170–171
Somatosensory processing, 52–54
Specific task practice, for sensory modulation disorders, 211
Stereotypies, 54–56
Stimulants, 182
Succinic semialdehyde dehydrogenase deficiency, 117
Support
    for employment, 196–198
    groups for, 171
    resources for, 134–135

T

Taste processing, 52–54
Testosterone, 81–82
Think Social! 168
Thyroid hormone, 80
Toe walking, 54–56
Touch response, 52–54
Transition, from school to work, **189–202**
    ASD characteristics and, 190–193
    case report of, 189–190
    employment models for, 196–198
    factors promoting, 194–196
    heath professionals involvement in, 199
    needs in, 193
    outcomes of, 193–196
Tuberous sclerosis, 22–23, 49, 121
Twins studies, 33–34

V

Valproate, 180, 181
Vasopressin, 78–79
Vestibular processing, 52–54
Video modeling, for social skills training, 167, 169
Visual processing, 52–54
Vitamin D, 83
Vocational competence, 194

W

Wakefield, Andrew, 6
Wallace, Alfred Russel, 3
Williams syndrome, 119
Wing, Lorna, 5, 19
Work, transition to, **189–202**

Y

Yale-Brown Obsessive Compulsive Scale Modified for Pervasive Development
    Disorder, 177

Z

Ziprasidone, 179

Moving?

Make sure your subscription moves with you!

To notify us of your new address, find your **Clinics Account Number** (located on your mailing label above your name), and contact customer service at:

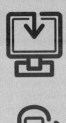

Email: journalscustomerservice-usa@elsevier.com

800-654-2452 (subscribers in the U.S. & Canada)
314-447-8871 (subscribers outside of the U.S. & Canada)

Fax number: 314-447-8029

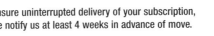

Elsevier Health Sciences Division
Subscription Customer Service
3251 Riverport Lane
Maryland Heights, MO 63043

*To ensure uninterrupted delivery of your subscription, please notify us at least 4 weeks in advance of move.

ELSEVIER